Praise

"Illness *is* a metaphor for our anguishe   harrowing and haunting, but also joyfu.   Malpede's memoir of a life lived in the c   book that forces us to sit with death and   teaches us new ways to be alive. We've becc   as we have to *war*. Malpede's honest, limpid   us to feel again, not merely to assign meaning to sickness—our own and that of our loved ones—but to see sickness in its social totality. A bracing and true book."
GREG GRANDIN, PULITZER PRIZE WINNING AUTHOR OF
The End of the Myth

"A wonderful, important book about the theater and about love."
KATHLEEN CHALFANT, AWARD WINNING STAGE AND SCREEN ACTOR

"Karen Malpede's *Last Radiance* is a stunning work—a book that somehow manages to be a coming of age story, a memoir of deep love and searing loss, and a sweeping cultural history of New York City avant-garde theater and activism spanning from the 1960s to the present. Malpede's voice is strong and her eyes are clear; she examines her own history through a well-earned, unafraid lens, looking at everything, knowing fully what is important. If only we were all this devoted—to love, to art, to writing, to seeing the world so clearly. A deep, moving work; Malpede's story will stay with me."
NELLIE HERMAN, AUTHOR OF *The Cure for Grief*
AND *Season of Migration*

"Lucky you to have found this book by playwright Karen Malpede! Herein lies a deeply human secret history; a poetic memoir of the American avant-garde. This is a world of magic and passion that only someone who lived it can transmit. No dry academic theories here! This is a jewel box of lived politics, lived aesthetics, lived poetry and lived art that is disappearing. Savor it! Carry the history."
PENNY ARCADE, PERFORMANCE ARTIST

"George Bartenieff lived an exemplary life in the theater, using his great gifts as an actor not just for his own fulfilment, but always, practically and imaginatively, for the fulfilment of others."
DAVID HARE, PLAYWRIGHT

"Karen Malpede achieves the writer's dream—a simultaneity of unheard past, screaming present, and cresting future where 'language could hurt' but 'absolute kindness, fierceness of vision, and commitment to act … bring grace into a world through luminous gaze and deep attention.' Only Malpede's own words from this astonishing book match the intensity of its bravery and truth. Although cancer and grief are its alleged subjects, its subterranean magma erupts to command us to 'wonder at life every moment' and to be equal to it."
RITA CHARON, FOUNDING CHAIR, NARRATIVE MEDICINE, COLUMBIA UNIVERSITY

"What an important book it is in several different ways—as a memoir of cancer (and indictment of cancer treatment and healthcare in general), a biographical portrait of George Bartenieff and others, a memoir of a marriage, and a history of poetic theater."
JOAN WICKERSHAM, NATIONAL BOOK AWARD FINALIST AND AUTHOR OF *THE SUICIDE INDEX*

"Truly eloquent and very, very moving. The writing is a form of poetry, only much less abstract and the metaphors are all tangible. The description of being alive while dying made me cry. It's such a brave testament to what all of us are terrified of and it's full of love and softness, too."
AVRA SIDIROPOULOU, DIRECTOR, PERSONA THEATER, GREECE

"Fascinating and moving. Karen Malpede takes us on a searlingly personal tour of her life in art at the beating heart of the avant-garde political theater movement based in New York City. She bears passionate witnes to the roots of today's experiemental theater and makes us feel we've lived through it ourselves while navigating through a perilous dance of cancer treatments, poised on the edge of life and death."
JAY O. SANDERS & MARYANN PLUNKETT, NEW YORK CITY-BASED ACTORS

"Across decades, Karen Malpede has safeguarded embers of unpopular feminisms with fierce humility. She chose not to compromise in her commitment to seeing accurately, and to remembering. She models a life lived in conscious proximity to disconcerting and existential truth. And she showed me how to uphold motherhood in the face of annihilation, amnesia, and erasure."
ANOHNI

About the Author

Karen Malpede is the author/director of twenty-two plays produced in the United States and Europe. Her plays have been translated into Albanian, Arabic, French and German. She co-founded New Cycle Theater in 1978 and co-founded Theater Three Collaborative in 1995 with George Bartenieff and Lee Nagrin. Play anthologies: *4 by Malpede plus an Intervention*, *Plays in Time: The Beekeeper's Daughter, Prophecy, Another Life, Extreme Whether, A Monster Has Stolen the Sun and Other Plays*. Editor/contributor: *Acts of War: Iraq and Afghanistan in Seven Plays, Women in Theater: Compassion and Hope, Three Works by the Open Theater, People's Theater in Amerika*. Her short fiction, nonfiction and drama are published in many periodicals, including: *The Kenyon Review, TriQuarterly, Theater Quarterly, American Theater, Theater Topics, Confrontations, Torture Magazine, The Typescript, Kairos, Courtship of Winds*, and *The New York Times*. OBIE award *I Will Bear Witness*. McKnight National Playwrights fellow. CAPS, New York State, playwriting fellowship. She has taught theater, playwriting, ecofeminism, and environmental justice at Smith College, New York University, and John Jay College-CUNY. MFA Columbia University.

www.theaterthreecollaborative.org

Last Radiance

Radical Lives, Bright Deaths

KAREN MALPEDE

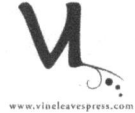

www.vineleavespress.com

Last Radiance
Copyright © 2025 Karen Malpede

All rights reserved.
Print Edition
ISBN: 978-3-98832-176-3
Published by Vine Leaves Press 2025

No parts of this publication may be reproduced, stored in a retrieval system, or transmitted in any form or by any means, electronic, mechanical, photocopying, recording, or otherwise, without the prior written permission of the copyright owner.

This book is sold subject to the condition that it shall not, by way of trade or otherwise, be lent, resold, hired out, or otherwise circulated without the publisher's prior consent in any form of binding or cover other than that in which it is published and without a similar condition including this condition being imposed on the subsequent purchaser. Under no circumstances may any part of this book be photocopied for resale.

Cover design by Jessica Bell
Interior design by Amie McCracken

For: Carrie Sophia
who lived it
and
For our grandchildren: Abel, Eben & Briana
who might wish to know what we were about

Author's Note

LAST RADIANCE. I had meant the title to pay homage to my protagonists—the artists, thinkers and nonviolent activists who grace its pages. Only now, I see, since the book will be published in October 2025, that the title takes on added resonance. Beginning in the sixties, ending in 2024, its pages become a record of a time gone by, of an avant-garde that expanded boundaries, envisioned a world free from violence, created, lived and loved wildly. If we failed to bring into being this world of harmony with nature and ourselves we envisioned, it is worth remembering the art we made and the ideas of justice for which we lived. The current times appear dark, yet around the world a chorus of the young has taken up the work and amplifies the call.

No one remembers events in exactly the same way. I have tried to be faithful to my own memories, and as truthful as I could be about personal and charged situations. Others who experienced the same events from a different angle might retain different memories and might have different interpretations of the same events. I use real names throughout. When I have not wished to identify by name, I use initials, or I identify by title, as in "doctor." So many of the people I write about are now dead and cannot, therefore, rise to their own defense. I have tried to tell their remarkable stories as well as I am able. In one way or another, I have loved everyone I recall in these pages.

Prologue:
Father, A Terminal Case

If I had not loved my father fiercely, loved him fiercely to this day, and remember him as a fine, if hurt, person, these scenes would not bear such resonance for me, nor would they be, as they became, predictors of my fate. If I had not been fiercely loved and wounded by this man who was my father I would not have become as I am—nothing would have followed as it did had it not been predetermined by a fate before my own, his fate, which I know only in part, a fate I carry and cannot forget.

His skin shriveled and yellowed from disease, his dark red uncircumcised penis flapping helplessly between his bony legs, he ran, kitchen knife in hand, yelling expletives like these, "whore, dirty fucking whore," and worse, after her, my naked mother, her breasts flapping against her chest, chasing her through the living room, dining room, kitchen, the hall by the den, the marble-tiled front entrance way, waving the knife, not yet close enough to strike, again into the living room, with its purple carpet and its pale purple drapes; round and round they went until exhaustion took them upstairs, where, perhaps, if they could, though he was very sick by then, they made love, while my boyfriend and I sat in a corner on the purple carpet, against the purplish white walls and watched. He with amusement, I almost thought. I, numb, as I'd learned to become over years. My twin brother recalls a similar scene (there were others), when with a baseball bat, he was chasing her, naked again both of them. She took refuge in her son's room, begging for rescue. My brother wrested the bat away. He was weak, after all, with not long to live.

Earlier, quite soon after his terminal cancer diagnosis, before, that is, he'd made it up, in this torturous fashion, with his once unfaithful wife, he'd taken me into his car: a bronze and white Oldsmobile with fins, the kind executives drove, and he was one of those. He gestured me into the front seat. He called me darling, baby, those sorts of words, as he wrapped his arms around me. He told me he was dying, that he had cancer, as if I hadn't heard. And he needed me, now, to care for him, like a wife, he said, and he put his wet tongue deep inside my throat and kissed me hard. Then, he stopped as abruptly as he'd begun. He escorted me out of the car. I'd been willing against my will, the way one is, catapulted into illicit sex as if shot from a cannon. I'd been willing to become his because he had no other. Who else but I ought to nurture my dying father. "I'm dying," he wept. "Yes, yes," I promised him, in my head. I was silent, I think. I don't think I said, "yes." I froze. My stiffness brought him back to his senses. Must have. He decided to make it up with my mother after the kiss. We are repairing our marriage, they said. He was forgiving her affair with a television producer, with whom she'd been caught crawling out the window of an empty house. A thoughtful neighbor turned them in, that is, told my father. Who was not yet sick. From that moment on, every dinner was interrupted with my father's rage. His swearing in his astonishingly scatological tongue, like none other I've heard, an amazing litany of sexual, semi-rhyming words, like a chant or a song, like a spewing out of hurt and hate, nearly beautiful in its alliterative sounds, its cadence, its force, the glory of the English language turned inside out. Whore, filthy whore, no good cunt, slut, but far more imaginative than that. Or he'd stand and whip off his leather belt and threaten us, his no-good twin progeny sitting right there eating his food, undercooked. She, a reluctant housewife, had come home late, turned the oil up high and thrown the frozen chicken piece by piece from across the room into the sputtering pan so it looked crusty and cooked on the outside, at least, ready the minute he walked in the door, done with his sixty-mile drive from Chicago's South Side where the chemical factory was to the North Shore and his suburban home. Belt in his hand, he'd threaten to beat us to a pulp as we deserved. Then, abruptly, he'd sit. It was a threat, that was all. Everyone kept eating the chicken, raw at the bone. No one but he said a word. Sometimes, though, my brother would start to laugh uncontrollably, and my father's rage would recur. Sometimes, my mother would murmur "Joe," in that little voice of hers. I do not remember ever speaking up; certainly, I did not laugh.

He'd had his tongue in my mouth. He'd wept. He was afraid. He was dying by then. Eaten from the insides. His stomach cancer, I thought, had grown from this. His rage was his disease. For a while before his diagnosis, though he was already ill, being treated for an ulcer, and the discomfort from the illness made him rage even more, I thought we wouldn't all live. He'd kill at least one. Her, or my brother, or all of us in a car crash as he drove drunkenly home from Sunday visits to his parents. He was always drunk when he left his Italian-Catholic parents' home with us, his Jewish wife and his unbaptized children. We'd eaten lasagna, roast, cannoli, from the bakery our aunt and uncle owned, over which they lived. He'd be drunk and swerving. We would pretend to be asleep in the back seat, but I'd be squinting at the street signs. Once we reached "Taylor Street," roughly halfway home, I'd breathe a sigh of relief. But then, the cancer was discovered, too late, and I realized we were saved. He was going to sacrifice himself.

I loved him madly because when he wasn't in the grip of his rage, he was kind, smart, considerate, principled, funny. I'd always been called "his" child. "Little Joe." My fair-skinned, freckled twin brother was my mother's son. I was dark like him in looks and temperament. Dark, fiery. I thought he was made of finer stuff than it often seemed. That his rages were not him but something terrible inside put there by someone else. His mother, perhaps. Horrible things must have been done. He'd been burned by his mother on the penis with a fireplace poker, so I'd heard from my mother, to toilet train. There must have been other abuse as terrible. I could not imagine. I saw him as a good man in the control of a beast, an eruption inside, his astonishing perversion of the English language, his dirty mouth, so terribly sexual, numbing but also exciting, rolling, rhythmic, alliterative. Language could do that. Make one quake. Language could wake one up. Language could hurt. But words also brought the insides out. Language revealed what was hidden. Listening to him taught me to write. I would have done as he asked, had he persisted. Nursed him through his illness, been his little wife.

I'm very grateful that he did not. It was a mark of his goodness that he held himself back. I did not have to take care of him while he died. My mother and he made it up, in a manner of speaking. I had only to watch. I could go on with my life. Buried deep inside, for years and years, the muddled feelings I had that I ought somehow to be punished—for having seen, for having been "his child," for having been kissed by him. It was almost as if I had been betrothed to him, almost, and my twin brother given to my mother to be cherished and to love.

Later, closer to death, more emaciated even than he'd been when he brandished the knife, chasing our mother around the house, he came outside one night, where I was with my actual boy lover, whose last name was Taylor—like the street that signaled safety to me, once we reached it we were halfway home from his parents' house and his rage began to ebb. We had just made love in the same car, in the Oldsmobile's back seat parked in the garage that smelled like oil. We'd emerged and straightened our clothes. We were saying goodnight, standing together on the dark asphalt driveway that sloped up to our faux French Provincial house on a small hill at one end of the subdivision. He came outside, without warning, threatening to kill the boy who'd deflowered his daughter. How had he known, I wondered? He started screaming at him, the boy who had just made love to the daughter he had French kissed in the car he owned, who had been exchanged for the beautiful wife, who trailed after, in her tiny voice, whispering, "Joe, Joe."

"I'm sorry you feel that way, Mr. Malpede," said the boy who had just had his dick inside me in the back seat.

"You fucking bastard. I should wring your fucking neck, you miserable son-of-a-bitch ..." he went on for a while inventing, in his scatological, melodious way—like the Italian father in some village, defending his "ruined" property.

"Joe, Joe," she quietly insisted.

"Fucking bastard."

"I'm sorry, Mr. Malpede."

I was silent. The boy went home; he lived around the cul-de-sac. Then my cancerous father knocked me down, took me by the leg and dragged me up the driveway into the house. "Joe, Joe," she murmured, following after. I do not remember saying a word. But my fate was sealed. Later, at my mother's urging, I would marry that same boy my father threatened to murder on our suburban street in Wilmette, Illinois, and live unhappily, and unfaithfully, for a year or more.

On the low table next to my father's side of their bed stood a collection of small plastic saints painted in purples, dark blues, and gold. "Little people," my mother called them. "Oh, Joe, I knocked over your little people," she said. Educated by the Jesuits, he had gone back to the Church in his illness, while nearing his death. He, a religious Catholic. She, a secular Jew. We were unbaptized, the twins, and were despised, "those no-good kids," his mother, our devout Catholic grandmother called us. She died three weeks before he did. "I see her and she's beautiful," she said, about the Virgin Mary who appeared at her side. Her last words. We were not asked to go to her funeral, nor was our father told of her death. He was nearing his own, lying in his hospital bed, tethered to machines; he never knew why his mother stopped coming to visit him—a final abuse. He must have thought himself unworthy, if he could still compose thoughts in his head. But, perhaps, he knew little by then. The cancer was in his brain. The last time I saw him alone, he was sitting up, bound with a wound sheet to a chair, a hospital table in front of him. On the table was a child's wooden puzzle of a duck. He held a yellow wing in his hand. He was trying to fit it where it belonged, in the gaping space between the other pieces, yellow, black, and green, concentrating as hard as he could. He did not seem to know who I was.

My father was diagnosed with terminal cancer after being treated for six-or-so months for ulcers by the family doctor. Finally, the doctor performed an exploratory operation one sunny June day, at Evanston Hospital where the Amish worked, their buggies parked outside, their chestnuts and bays waiting in harness—patiently. After surgery was complete, the doctor and a nurse took us into a private room—my mother, young and beautiful, my twin and I, seventeen—and gave us little paper cups of warm water with little white pills to swallow. As the sedation kicked in, I was sitting on a windowsill, the sun hot at my back, feeling nothing, as I had trained myself to do at the dinner table without medication; one of them, perhaps the family doctor himself, told us our father and husband would be dead in three months, the cancer, inoperable, was inevitably fatal. They had put a feeding tube into his stomach. He would never eat again. When he woke up, he would be told to put his affairs in order and get himself ready to depart this world. There was nothing to be done. My mother woke up. "He ate yesterday," she said. "Take the feeding tube out." And, not in a tiny voice at all, she said: "No, you cannot tell him he is going to die." She was going to get other opinions. I was impressed.

A friend of my brother's mother had recently died of breast cancer. Cancer was shameful then, kept secret as long as one could. Whispered about, if that, as if its victims were at fault. The new widower spoke with my mother about the cancer research hospital at the University of Chicago called Billings, where the latest treatments were available, and he introduced my mother to the cancer specialist who had treated his wife. Dr. John Van Prohaska took on my father's case. A few years after my father's death, my mother married the widower who recommended the cancer doctor, and they lived happily ever after, more or less.

My father ate lots of meat—Italian sausage grilled or fried for a long time, bacon, pork, beef, lamb—there was meat at every meal. He had grown up on relief in the Depression, eating prunes from cans. Meat was proof of well-being, proof of financial success. He was the Vice President–Comptroller of a chemical company just outside of the city. The executive offices were located in the same building where the chemicals, pesticides, and Pam Dry Fry were manufactured. One of their best sellers was the pesticide my father sprayed weekly on the roses he grew. He sprayed large amounts—it was free, after all—bending down low. My mother, in her little voice, would whisper, "Joe, please wear a mask." He'd swear at her in response. She had begged him to get a second opinion, too, about that pesky ulcer. He refused, and just kept getting sicker, belching more, always in pain, and more easily enraged. He smoked. He gave me my first cigarette in our living room before we moved into the bigger house the next suburb over. He had seen me through the window, pretending to smoke. Cavalierly, he shook the pack, so the cigarette stuck out. He walked across the room. He let me pull the Pall Mall out and put it to my lips. He flicked his lighter. I must have been fifteen. We inhaled. Immediately, I began to buy packs of cigarettes from the machine at the hamburger joint where I worked part-time. The slight tobacco high made waiting tables easier to endure.

My father ate himself up, I thought when I learned he was dying. He turned his rage inward. We were only collateral damage, a phrase I did not know then. Cancer was not yet a ubiquitous disease, a disease of chemicals and discord. Cancer was still coming into its own as the second killer, after heart attacks, of Americans. Its treatments were primitive, too. The untargeted chemo and radiation Dr. Prohaska offered a terminally ill man were by today's standards brutal. My father had fantastic insurance. He lived another year and a half—with enormous suffering, with the cancer invading ever more organs. Was he a research object, someone upon whom new drugs could be tried? A hopeless case, kept alive with draconian treatments, which he never refused, for the purpose of medical science? Did his suffering benefit others? It certainly did not help him. His suffering intensified during the year-and-a-half that he lived until he had lost his mind and weighed ninety-eight pounds. Then he died.

There was, in the midst of this terrible trajectory an unforgettable moment of grace, when it became clear for an instant who the man really was, if he could have become himself amid the terrors of whatever abuse he suffered, the pressures of working himself up from unlettered poverty to the middle class and of leaving his church to elope with my mother, against the wishes of his family and hers. Immediately, he enlisted in the air force, intending to become a fighter-bomber pilot in World War II, but he was not found stable enough to fly planes in combat and was given a desk job as an accountant at Sheppard Air force Base in Wichita Falls, Texas, a severe humiliation, which only intensified his rages. My mother worked as a secretary on the base until her ninth month of pregnancy. She was huge, but no one knew she was carrying twins. She was so heavily drugged she remembered nothing of our birth. I was born first, supposedly the doctor walked away when the nurse called him back, "there's another baby in here." My brother was born with a collapsed lung and nearly died. He was in an incubator for six weeks. My mother, prone to anxiety, was a wreck. My father, prone to anger, was no help; the weak boy-child reminded him of himself. I sat on my brother in the womb was the family myth; a fratricide, averted by chance. A soldier on the base donated blood to my brother, and told my mother not to worry, everyone to whom he gave his blood survived.

Both our parents hated racism and antisemitism and raised us on cautionary tales of the terrible things they heard rural Texans say about Black people and Jews. Now, our father was dying at forty-four years old. He had been lying nearly comatose, curled up like a babe, naked under his hospital gown, and we, my mother, brother, and I were standing around his crib-like bed with the bars raised. All of a sudden, he awoke and pulled himself up straight; he was very close to death, and this might have been his last coherent speech. He looked hard at us and he declared his love to each one in turn—the wife he had beaten, the son he had denigrated with words, the daughter he had almost incested, if "almost" is an apt concept here. He told us to look after one another. He said he had done the best that he could. He loved us, he said. He blessed us, each in turn. And we saw, then, the man he was, or might have been, gracious and brave, freed from demonic rage and free, for the moment, of his physical pain and decay. He summoned all he had left in order to speak. It was a scene that seemed to be happening out of time, an epiphany, a vision. Improbable, impossible, in fact, yet it did happen. And it taught me that another way might always be possible, that lurking underneath there is always grace. We are not destined forever to remain as we are. We are more than we seem. We can transform in an instant. And who is to say what is real.

I learned many things from my father—the power of language was one, I learned how to write from the cadence and verse of his scatological tongue. I learned to be diligent, hardworking, persistent. I learned, also, that the good can be subsumed by trauma, by rage, but nevertheless good exists and might, at any time, become present as a force.

Not long after the magical scene when he sat up in the bed to bless us each in turn, I stood next to my mother at his deathbed. He was tethered to monitors, unresponsive. He would be dead at any moment. Suddenly the nurse turned to my mother and told her that I should leave the room. "You don't want her to see this," the nurse said. My mother told me to leave.

And I went, against my will. I was wrong to obey, I knew, as I mechanically walked out the door, and left him to breathe his last without me there.

When he died, I was lost. I had not the ability to grieve. There was a tangle of feelings inside, one of which was relief.

His funeral was a nightmare, in fact. Held on Yom Kippur, and as he'd worked for a Jewish firm, he had mainly Jewish pallbearers, in the large Catholic cathedral where I'd gone to midnight mass with him. This was a high mass, nearly unheard of at a funeral, done at his bereaved father's request, whose wife, our Italian grandmother, had died of a heart attack three weeks before his only son. The priest who ministered to our father while he was in hospital called our mother "a woman of valor" though he knew she was Jewish, not Catholic. She stayed by her husband's side through all his suffering. Often, she read him Twenty-third Psalm, "Yea, though I walk through the valley of the shadow of death, I shall fear no evil, for thou art with me …" The priest promised my mother he would speak of her valor at her husband's funeral; he would praise her, the Jewish wife, also in front of her husband's family, for her devotion. But he was abruptly transferred to a new parish. A new priest officiated. "Joseph Malpede died for his sins: marrying out of his religion and having two unbaptized children," he said. The words fell like blows. Even if we, my mother, brother, and I, did not believe them, we felt their blunt force. Then he was buried in consecrated ground. If my mother wished to be buried next to him, she would have to be encased in lead so that her heathen, Jewish flesh would not pollute blessed earth. I have never since visited his grave. I wrote a poem as an undergraduate, its refrain, "Where are you buried, here, here in my heart." I never saw my Italian family again. They threw us out. "Don't come back." We upset the grandfather and aunts who had just lost wife and son, mother and brother. In our unbaptized state, we were responsible for having killed Christ. Years later, in Italy, a philologist of the Italian language told me the surname Malpede (bad foot) is a Sicilian nickname actually meaning "hard way to walk." Like Oedipus (swollen foot) in fact. Years later, too, Italians to whom I told this story were shocked. I'd written a version for an anthology of Italian-American women writers. Educated Italians did not behave as my peasant family had. Italians do not disown children, these Northern Italians said, though we had been disowned.

I will never know what happened to my father in his early life, what abuse ignited his rages since out of nowhere they came, inexplicable and terrible, also, for him. Often he would weep and apologize once the explosion was done, as if he had been snatched and was shocked himself. I came to wonder if my father was being medically tortured with treatments and drugs for the sake of cancer research, if he had become a body on which to experiment, as there was never the slightest hope of curing him. I thought that the family doctor who had wrongly mistreated him for an ulcer for six months might have been right once the cancer was diagnosed, too late. My father ought to have been helped to die, without radiation or chemotherapy, without so much suffering. Indeed, the doctor's prognosis was correct. He enjoyed three months of "normal" life in which he returned to work, then he was kept alive as he died by radiation and chemotherapies. But, of course, the family doctor had been harsh, "tell him to get his affairs in order," and there was no palliative care, then. I knew my mother wanted him alive. He was paid his full executive salary as long as he lived, surely that played a part; she was frightened of becoming a widow, at age forty-two. She would have to get a job. Although she strove for a life of her own—she acted, modeled and had her own radio show, "Something for the Girls," it was called, and on it she'd interviewed Eleanor Roosevelt—none of this paid the bills. But her compassion also played a part and he, a slipped, now repentant Catholic, only forty-four, was terrified of death. They wished to repair their marriage, they both said. They were both willing for him to endure any amount of terrible treatment to forestall the inevitable end. He retched, he shook, he lay on a mattress of ice. He lost weight and strength. I gave him an art book for Christmas. He wept when he could not lift it. They did what the doctor wanted, what he deemed best, if, indeed, they were ever asked by the oncologist to consent, and not just given whatever treatment Dr. Prohaska, whom we were taught to regard with awe, like a demigod, deemed to be next. I had not been asked my opinion, of course. I would not have given it even if asked. I'd been demoted after one brief night in a car from designated caretaker-wife back to daughter without voice. I watched.

I left home for college. I hardly returned to the comfortable suburb for more than a weekend. I never looked back. Instead, I dragged the whole tangle of events along with me, a ball and chain that retarded every yearning to be free and would take decades to unlock. Being unable to grieve, furiously going on, leaving the family home, I threw myself into studies, work, and the antiwar movement. Stopping cruelty to others seemed paramount after the violence we'd endured in our home and the medical violence that was called cancer treatment. If our father's near-nightly rages made our home a war zone, the cancer made my father's body a battleground.

Nor was cancer done with me. Twice more in my life I would be flailed by the disease, not in my body, but in the bodies of those I loved. In this way, I am like everyone because no one is spared confrontation with cancer. There is no such thing as being "cancer free." Cancer is everywhere, in our friends, in our family, ourselves, in the plastic particulates in our food, in the air we breathe. Twice more, I'd be asked to attend to cancer as best I could. This, then, is the story of that—cancer treatment from the point of view of a woman who has cared for its sufferers and, in this way only, suffered it.

What helped me were the lessons I was able to take away from the father who died when I was nineteen: he worked himself from poverty through Loyola University (as a bill collector, one of the least pleasant of jobs); he married up, and become a well-paid comptroller of a chemical firm. That dogged work ethic was something I learned. He was honest, too, and without prejudice (when in his right mind). But, more than that, my sorrow at his sorrow, my pain at his pain became the deep well from which I drew. I could not have become a writer without him, not just his rhythmic, scatological tongue, the boundaries he broke, and the ways in which he suffered and lived, but without his love. He was a fine person overcome by traumas he had not the wisdom to understand. Few people did, then. The cancer that struck him seemed like fate, and what matters with fate is how we become who we are when confronted with the impossible choice. Do we rise to a compassionate height or fall into numbness or rage, self-blame, or do it all, in a tangle, a mess. How we writhe in the grip of fate, how we must make choices, make decisions of how now to be, is the essence of drama, and the choices we make in crisis reveal our character. My father had shown me the essence of my craft: that night in the car—a desperate, misguided need, he renounced; then, its opposite, by sitting up straight in his hospital bed to bless us in turn with his dying breath—the purity of that love. The drama of the thing and its opposite. Increasing our tolerance for ambiguity may be the true purpose of art—so we can hold opposites within ourselves without anger or fear, and we become larger by doing that. True to the poem I wrote: "where are you buried, here, here in my heart," he lived inside—in memory but also in deed, in things that I chose to do, and things I had no choice but to do. In the ways I rebelled, and could, with him dead. I took him with me where I went, to this day. Memorializing him in my work, and, yes, in my heart.

Through writing first theater history, and, then, twenty-two plays, my life took on a trajectory. I became part of the culture of the New York downtown avant-garde, and it was there, among those extraordinary people, that I found my elective family. And through them, I would meet cancer twice more, but both times everything would be different. Each cancer story prepared me for the next. My father's sent me to Julian Beck's bed, and what I learned from Julian's grace allowed me to introduce Julian to Barbara Deming, another extraordinary pacifist artist, also with terminal cancer, and, then, to minister to my partner, another artist-activist, George Bartenieff, when the time came. They were alike, these three, in their absolute kindness, the fierceness of their individual visions, their commitment to making art and to encouraging others to create. They were alike in that they nurtured many. Their eyes lit with wonder as they gazed upon whoever it was. They shone as if from within. It was as if all of my father's latent goodness, which I imagined and loved, suddenly materialized in the flesh of these others, long after his death. And two of them, Julian and George, loved me with intensity, boundaries, and grace. "You need someone who will let you be," Julian, who was homosexual, said to me. The words reverberated as if through an underground cavern. I'd never thought of such a thing, *let me be*. George was that one who allowed me to become.

Just as my first play, *A Lament for Three Women*, a re-envisioning of my father's cancer death, solidified my place as a young artist in Julian's world, so the play I wrote after Julian died, *Us*, including yet another version of my father's cancer, his violence for the first time, and which was dedicated to Julian, led me to George, who starred in it. George became my partner in life and work for the next thirty-five years. I wrote and directed ten plays with him as a lead, knowing what shape shifting he could perform on stage. In this story, our colleagues and friends themselves artists and writers, make cameo appearances: Judith Malina, Allen Ginsberg, Andrea Dworkin, Grace Paley, Dorothy Dinnerstein, Barbara Deming, Noam Chomsky, Peter Schumann, Joseph Chaikin, Karl Bissinger, Erika Duncan, Kathleen and Henry Chalfant, Tony Giovannetti, Sally Ann Parsons, Lee Nagrin, Anohni, Basil Twist, Ynestra King, Jan Clausen, Christen Clifford, my twin John Malpede, and many others.

If we have been largely shaped before we are capable of self-knowledge, then the work of a lifetime is to reconstruct that making, to dig ourselves out of the rock of event and inchoate feeling and emerge as close as we can as to our true self formed by self-knowledge. Then, our life story might illuminate the way for others in their very same work of becoming. Then, we shine with luminosity, a word I use often in this book in reference to its heroes, Barbara Deming, Julian Beck, and George Bartenieff. These three understood language to be our best defense and only way to change a culture. Barbara and Julian wrote poetry, plays, and political theory. George was an unpublished diarist and he was an actor completely committed to language on the stage. He was also a producer with unerring taste who sought out language writers, acted in their plays and promoted them over years.

Pacifists, ecologists, artists, Barbara, Julian and George, such people reckon with grace; they bring grace into the world by their actions, by their attention to others, by the intensity of their listening, the penetration of their gaze, how they seem to hold you still enough so that you might look inward, driven inward by their deep attention. Brilliant artist-activists each, they shared a vision of a nonviolent world, a world in which just the sort of interactions they engaged in and their deep self-examination would become the established way. In the world they created around them, all creatures are held within a penetrating and luminous gaze that looks in and out, that comprehends self and the selves of others. How humans bring light into the world is their story. How they may bring light even as they die is the focus. How, dying, those with such grace bestow upon others light divine.

Chapter One:
Julian Beck
With Barbara Deming

Julian Beck "You need someone who will let you be."
Barbara Deming "We cannot live without our lives."

Prophetically, as if aware of my future life, the young man my father threatened to kill on our driveway wooed me with tales of the Living Theatre's work in New York. He had seen *The Connection* at their Fourteenth St. theater, a first play by twenty-seven year-old Jack Gelber about heroin addiction and jazz that made Jack; Judith Malina, its director; and Julian Beck, designer; the two founders of the Living Theatre, sudden celebrities, and rising stars. Although "the Becks" as they were often called were already well known in the downtown avant-garde world—they had been staging poetic plays, first in their living room, since the late forties, they were now international artists to be reckoned with—it was a British critic, Kenneth Tynan who first discovered them and his appreciation sent American critics to their Fourteenth St. theater for another look. Because the Becks believed in Jack's play and in their production, they kept it running for months until, yes, critical opinion reversed itself and word-of-mouth brought audiences eager to get in. In a dark corner next to my house, D. passed me a joint and described *The Connection* in detail while my heart beat faster: its jazz score by Freddie Redd, the acting so realistic that people struggling with their own drug problems vomited in the audience, its mix of fine actors like Warren Finnerty with nonactors off the street, some of them addicts. I was awed. D. was so cool. Fucking with D. in the back seat of my father's bronze and white Oldsmobile was an initiation having as much to do with aesthetics as sex.

At the University of Wisconsin, where I began sophomore year the fall of my father's death, I buried myself in classes and work. I wrote culture pieces for the *Daily Cardinal*. The student newspaper was under investigation by the state legislature for supposed Communist infiltration—Wisconsin was Joe McCarthy's home state, as well as home to a populist movement—and its staff was proud and on-edge. The paper was printed each night on a big letterpress. I set the headlines for my stories myself. Then the frames holding the lead type were locked in. We would ink them with a roller, press down a sheet of paper and give a final proofread. It was thrilling to hear the loud metallic clank of the big press and grab the first copies at 4 am. The Madison campus was home to a growing antiwar movement. I went to teach-ins by radical graduate assistants and junior faculty members, and learned the colonial history of Vietnam and the folly of the US invasion. At my first anti-war protest, I marched around the State Capitol building with about thirty others. We watched the FBI agents on the balconies snap our photos. I read Buchner's antiwar play, *Woyzeck*, and the German Expressionists from between the two World Wars, Toller and Kaiser, and learned how traumatic violence affects literary form. The fad in the English department was the Irish literary revival—Yeats, Synge, O'Casey, Shaw. I took every class and discovered how plays might revive a people's soul during a long occupation, and support their fight for independence and cultural pride while being extraordinary theater, too. I also encountered, though of her fifty plays none was mentioned, must less, taught, my first woman playwright, Yeats's co-founder, without whom the Abbey Theatre would not exist, Lady Augusta Gregory.

In my senior year, D. flunked out of his Florida college and, no longer protected by being a student, was immediately drafted. He visited me in Madison for a final fling before the Army. I was dating a graduate student. D. did not write, and I forgot all about him. I forgot about the graduate student, too, after my period was weeks late and I feared I was pregnant. "You will go to a home for unwed mothers," he counseled, "I'll write to you." A few days later, overcome by sudden cramps in class, I began to hemorrhage through my clothes onto the wooden seat, a first-term miscarriage, perhaps; I rejoiced, despite the humiliation. I graduated and moved to New York. In 1967, my first year out of college, I marched on the Pentagon with many thousands. I half expected to find my drafted driveway ex-lover standing there in the long line of soldiers my age aiming their rifles at our heads. We didn't know their guns were not loaded when we broke through their line—and, Hibiscus, one of the Harris family who founded the avant-garde theater Angels of Light, a company George produced, stuck a flower down the barrel of a rifle, creating the iconic photo. I was in the same phalanx as Norman Mailer, who memorialized the march in his book *Armies of the Night*, and I spent the night on the same Pentagon steps. Unable to pee for over thirty-six hours, afraid to squat down in public even in a skirt, a red, faux-leather mini, though the men were gleefully spraying the stone walls, I became very ill and had to stay out of work, a terrible editing job at an electronics magazine, for several weeks.

On weekends and nights, I was researching and writing an article on assignment about off-off Broadway for a Wisconsin arts journal. I worked on my story for nearly a year and the editor liked it when I sent it in. He came to New York and took me to dinner, got me very drunk, took me back to his hotel room and then into bed, but I froze under his touch. I got dressed and left. When the "article" came out, he had cut all the words I had written, leaving only the many photos I'd collected and my captions. I was ashamed of myself. I thought it was my fault that he ruined my work, that I deserved retribution for not fulfilling his sexual desire. But I'd been accepted at the new Columbia School of the Arts. And so, as I'd done with the cataclysm of my father's death, I moved on without excavating my woundedness. I buried my rage and my grief deeper still, and lived with self-blame. I'd found an apartment uptown on 108th and Broadway with a friend when D. reappeared, done with his two years in the infantry. By manipulating his file, he'd avoided Vietnam and been sent to Germany where he designed sets for an army theater. D. moved in with me and my friend left.

It was 1970. I was studying at Columbia. D. was designing a set for the Long Warf Theater in New Haven and I went up for the weekend, not so much to visit him as to take part in the mass protest in support of the Black Panthers planned for that Saturday, May 1, one of the more extraordinary political events in which I have ever taken part. It was the start of two Panther trials. Bobby Seale and Ericka Huggins had not killed their fellow Black Panther, Eric Rackley, who, suspected of being an FBI informant, had been tortured and murdered, but the two stood accused. Seale was the National Chairman of the Panthers and Huggins was head of the New Haven chapter. I went on foot from the Warf, walking under the highway toward the city. It was like entering a war zone. Trucks full of armed National Guard filled the access road. I slipped between two trucks and continued toward town. It was eerily quiet. All the stores on the main streets were closed with their windows boarded up. The town was deserted. Robert Brustein, then Dean, had closed the Drama School, shuttered the Yale Theater, and removed himself to his country home, which struck me as wrong. There was enormous fear of a Black riot—or so the University and the shopkeepers explained themselves.

No one but armed police and protestors were on the streets, moving quietly toward the town green in front of the courthouse where the demonstration would take place, a hundred yards from the gates of the Yale campus. Anti-Vietnam war fervor was at its height on campuses all over the country. We stood shoulder-to-shoulder on the courthouse green, so many of us we could not move. Were there 25,000 people, as later reported? Might have been. On every roof stood National Guard and police snipers with rifles pointing down at us. They could pick us off one by one. We were defenseless and in clear view. The word had just gone out from the Nixon White House to shoot antiwar students. But this was Yale. Our protest was peaceful; we were committed to nonviolence, all of us. There were not even insults hurled at the soldiers or the police, who after all were the same age as most of us—only not as privileged as the Yale students. We were very well behaved, smashed together, looking at the raised stage in front of the courthouse steps. The Reverend William Sloan Coffin spoke. Then Chaplain of Yale, Coffin had been arrested many times as a civil rights and anti-war activist. There were other speakers I do not remember. Then came Jean Genet, in his black leather jacket. I was thrilled; he was one of my playwright heroes. In high school, our English teacher took us to see Genet's *The Blacks* on tour, the first avant-garde play I had ever seen. I was blown away, as I also was when the same teacher showed us Ingmar Bergman's *The Seventh Seal* and had us read James Joyce' *Portrait of the Artist as a Young Man*. Genet spoke to the crowd in French. Someone must have translated, but I have no memory of what he said—a version of what everyone was saying of course, Seale and Huggins were innocent. They had not committed the murder, we all knew; they had been set up. After they spent two years in prison, the judge would declare a mistrial and dismiss the charges against both of them.

Years later, I learned from one of the Yale student organizers, that they had negotiated with the New Haven police and National Guard to make certain there would be no live ammunition in the rifles; in return, they promised a nonviolent protest. But, of course, most of us did not know then that the guns pointing down at our heads were not loaded. Days later, on May 4, the Ohio National Guard opened fire indiscriminately and killed four students on the Kent State campus. On May 14, two students were killed and others wounded at Jackson State, Mississippi, a Black college. The nation had turned from assassinations of prominent leaders JFK in 1963, Malcolm X, 1965, and in 1968-'69, Martin Luther King, Jr, Bobby Kennedy, and leader of the Panthers Fred Hampton, killed while he slept by the Chicago police, each one of them shot at the moment they put things together, saw oppressions as interlinked, war, poverty, race. Now, in 1970, we were seeing the murders of young antiwar protesters on college campuses, but Yale—white, wealthy, savvy—was spared.

I never saw Genet again, although he was a good friend of my soon-to-be close friend Julian Beck; they were both homosexual. Julian toured Europe playing Solange in the Living Theatre's version of Genet's *The Maids*, directed by Judith Malina, who followed the playwright's request, usually ignored, that the two women servants be acted by teenage boys—men in this case. Nearly twenty years later, I dedicated my play *Us*, also directed by Judith, and in which George Bartenieff starred, to the memories of Julian Beck and Jean Genet as both had recently died. Judith told me Genet had clear disdain for women and she did not like to be around him, nevertheless, the women characters in his plays are marvelously astute. The two servants in *The Maids*, locked in a jealous rage at the mistress they emulate and detest or in *The Screens*, Leila, the ugliest woman in Algeria, she must wear a cloth to cover her face. She is the only woman Said, the poorest man, can afford to buy for his wife; loyal and brave, she is forever embarrassed by herself.

    Born to a prostitute, raised on the streets, in and out of jail for petty theft, and due to Sartre's praise, a hero of the intelligentsia, Genet had been a young French soldier in the French-Algerian war, fighting on the aggressor's side, but his allegiance lay elsewhere. Along with his brilliant plays on the subject of colonial domination, his support of the Black Panthers and of the Palestinians once he became a famous author was another way of making amends for having fought as a conscript in the colonizer's army. In all his work and his later life, he aligned himself with his people—the wretched of the earth, as Franz Fanon called them. Years later, when I knew Julian Beck well, he often told and retold a favorite story. At a border crossing, the French customs officer reached into his sling bag, and pulled out his silken costume for *The Maids*, holding up slip and thong underwear, looking them over, putting them gingerly on the counter. "That is my costume for Jean Genet's play," Julian explained. The customs officer nodded. Reaching back in, the customs official pulled out a large piece of hashish. "And what is *this?*" he demanded. Julian, replied in his haughtiest voice he saved for moments like this, "*That* is a piece of *bark* from a *tree* in *Voltaire's* garden." Sniffing it, handing it back, "And some very good shit, too," the custom's officer said, letting Julian pass. Genet was revered in France. So was the Living Theatre of Judith Malina and Julian Beck.

    I didn't want a long-term relationship with D, but I had been handed to him by my father that night on the driveway as surely as if we still lived in a Calabrian village, and my mother's admiration of D. for not getting into a physical fight with a dying man reinforced our primitive betrothal. "If you are living together …" She called every week. My mother's insistence wore me down. D. agreed to marry if we used the wedding money to buy a BMW motorcycle, on which, predictably, we were almost killed. With me seated in back, holding tight to his waist, D. lost control on the George Washington Bridge and the BMW, he and I skidded across the highway in front of oncoming cars. Miraculously unhurt, we scrambled back on the dented bike. D. designed my wedding dress, an off-white, high-necked, lace Victorian gown. My marriage to D. could not have been more arranged had livestock been exchanged, had a dowry been given. Driving back to Chicago from the wedding in the Columbia University chapel and the fancy family dinner at the Algonquin hotel, my mother suddenly wondered, "Why did I make her marry him?" And once home in our Wilmette subdivision, a neighbor asked the same, how could she have allowed her daughter to "marry that kid?" But I, also, had an ulterior motive in mind—being married, myself, would make me a safer choice for the married playwright, Jack Gelber, who was teaching at the Columbia School of the Arts. D. and I had never been faithful.

My MFA thesis on the thirties workers' theaters was expanding into a book that would become a history of people's theater in America from 1929 to 1972. I was under contract to Drama Book Specialists whose publisher, Ralph Pine took me to long, drunken lunches at the Russian Tea Room, next door to his office. We returned to speak about my manuscript while I squirmed away from his touch. I determined to interview Jack Gelber about his fourth play *The Cuban Thing*. I thought it his finest work since *The Connection*. So did he, but the play had been a trauma for Jack. "I still have nightmares about it," he told me. Jack was enamored of Castro. He loved his revolutionary machismo. He smoked Cuban cigars in homage. He had been to Cuba twice, once as a tourist, the second time as a reporter. His play mixed documentary footage of the Cuban revolution with domestic scenes of a middle-class family adjusting to their new lives in Castro's Cuba. It was pro-revolution; in fact, the middle-aged central character regains his sexual potency as he embraces the revolutionary program. But Jack's play also critiqued Castro's oppression of homosexuals. Jack directed the Broadway production, which opened on September 24, 1968. The theater was surrounded by New York City police protecting the first night audience and the critics from about a hundred anti-Castro Cuban exiles marching outside protesting the production. Inside the theater were even more militant protesters who had bought tickets and who with catcalls, stink bombs and jeers disrupted the performance. The producers closed Jack's play after one night. The reviews were hostile and the Cuban exiles had issued bomb threats should the play continue. Jack taught playwriting at Columbia along with Arthur Kopit, his good friend. I was not a playwright, yet, and something told me I should not take a playwriting class with either of them. Instead, I was studying dramatic literature. I was not Jack's student.

Jack and I stood next to each other during a fire drill, outside in the courtyard behind the theater building, located then on 110th St. Like two animals in heat, their smells irresistible, we could barely restrain ourselves from coupling there on the asphalt, in full view. We lunched at a Cuban restaurant on Broadway and began the interview about his play. When I next visited him in his office, wearing the one sweater I owned, a pink turtleneck, he smiled and said, "You have beautiful breasts." He had those breasts in his hands in an instant. Soon after, the chair of the theater department, a Shakespearian scholar, whose PhD seminar I attended at his invitation, gave Jack and me offices next to each other in an abandoned building under the 125th St. elevated subway tracks. The chair of the theater department acted as my mentor and pimp, so to speak. We made love on his desk or mine, or in borrowed apartments, for several years. "I love the sound of dick in cunt," Jack said in a prayerful voice. He was kind and communicative in all the ways my husband D. was not. He was an attentive, tireless lover, a listener, an altogether kind and giving man, married, for life, to a woman, Carol, but helpless before his sexual urges—she, of course, knew about his affairs, but I prided myself on being a good mistress who never made a single demand.

"Of course, he doesn't love me," I'd said to Jack one afternoon as we lay together on a friend's fold-out couch. "That's not good. You ought to be loved," Jack said, who did love his wife. But I had no sense I deserved more. I would be, forever, the other woman: the one French kissed in a car, his tongue down my throat, then dropped for her mother, or as I was, naked in a borrowed bed with someone else's husband. I was still sleepwalking through my life. Married unhappily to D., a narcissist, my book was published. It was well reviewed and admired. Everything was about to change.

One night I'd had enough. I left the marriage with an apple in my hand. "If you are going, take the dog," were D.'s final words. I did. My Sheltie, Malcolm, and I were alone in the world. My twin brother stopped speaking to me. He and D. had a carpentry business and together they also made street theater, using large wooden constructions they built. For the first few weeks, I slept on the couch of an Upper West Side communal house. Then, I was lent a small apartment in the West Village. I broke up with Jack. "I don't want to do this anymore." His last words, "I knew you would leave me when you moved down here." (Jack died of blood cancer in 2003. I dressed in a long skirt and stood at the back of his crowded memorial.) But if I had been wooed, first by tales of Jack's play *The Connection* in its Living Theatre production, on the driveway at my parents' house, then by Jack, himself, or, rather, Jack and I wooed one another is a more accurate way to say it as I never once felt taken advantage of by Jack—he was too fine a spirit, if highly sexed, for that. My future beloved, George Bartenieff, also had a life-changing epiphany because of the Living Theatre's production of Jack's first play. It was as if we were all already an elective family of sorts—Jack, Judith, Julian, George, and I, the directors Joseph Chaikin, and Peter Schumann, I had written about, too, were going to enter my life. We were bound by aesthetic ties that made our hearts beat faster. Though their work was unique to each and my playwriting when it happened would also be, there was in common among us a drive toward a heightened reality, and a shared theme of transformation, the urgent belief that the world could be different. George told his part of the story to performance artist, Penny Arcade, in our home in 2016, with his omnipresent enthusiasm, as if it had happened yesterday:

> *1960 was the real turning point for me. What happened was I went to the Living Theatre to see this controversial production of* The Connection *which was about heroin addiction in the jazz world, okay, and there was a live jazz band on stage and the actor really shot up, or it was so totally realistic you believed he actu-*

ally shot up, the acting was just amazing, the whole production was really amazing. They had really destroyed the fourth wall. You really felt you were in the room, you're just sitting in the back of the room in which these people live, that's the feeling you got and it was totally electrifying and mind-blowing that you could really, really really really create that reality, and in the intermission one of the musicians comes up to you and says (whispering), "I really really need some money, the guy is coming and I've got to have money for him" and you absolutely could not tell if this is real, or is this part of the show. It was the Living Theatre and I said to myself I've got to get into a company that can do things like this. This was the first time that I really got electrified by a company of actors that had a style, that had a philosophy. For two years I tried to get into the company. I auditioned and I auditioned and I got nowhere. Right after that I got into Judson (Poet's Theater). While I was doing those things (Irene Fornes and Rosyln Drexler's first plays) I suddenly heard that Joe Chaikin was leaving the Living Theatre to form his own company and they were looking for an actor to play the lead in The Dog Beneath the Skin *by W.H. Auden, another play in verse; I read for it, I auditioned for it and I got the part. And I thought, "wow, finally.*

—

I stood among a crowd of women gathered in the lobby of the Quaker Meeting House on Gramercy Park at the end of a women's theater weekend in the spring of 1972; I had been told by a member of the Living Theatre not to leave, that Judith Malina was coming to find me, but I hardly believed it. Then, I saw a small, dark-haired woman pushing her way toward me. "Karen Malpede," she sang into my ear in her tremulous voice, "I finished your book at 4 am and I feel so close to you." She threw her arms around me and hugged me tight.

We had never before actually met. I'd seen the Living perform on their fabled '69 American tour. Their first time home in many years, fresh from their participation in the French uprisings of 1968, with four new, large works, including *Paradise Now*, in which audience members joined the actors on stage, stripping off their clothes, sometimes having sex, smoking weed, walking or being carried outside to bring the beautiful nonviolent revolution (as they called it) from the theater into the streets. Seminaked, actors and audience were immediately arrested at Yale, where the tour began, but not in Brooklyn. At the Brooklyn Academy of Music, I'd watched *Paradise Now*, but I did not participate. I'd been mesmerized by Judith's highly choreographed direction of the chorus in her adaptation of Brecht's version of Holderlin's translation of Sophocles' *Antigone*, and by her fierce performance as the rebellious girl. Julian Beck played Creon with a Texas accent mimicking Lyndon Johnson, who was still sending more troops to kill and die in Vietnam. I'd been thrilled by their take on Mary Shelley's *Frankenstein*, with the huge creature—seeking love—they made out of many bodies hanging from Julian Beck's three-story set, holding on to each other. I tried to interview them, then, but they hadn't time for a graduate student, so I wrote about their work from research I did, without ever having met.

Now I was in Judith's arms because of my book. She spirited me across the sparkling river on the Q train to the Living Theatre squat in then-derelict Fort Greene, a crumbling brownstone on St. Felix St. We entered the basement kitchen where Julian Beck was cooking dinner for the Living Theatre company.

There is an iconic film interview with Julian in *Signals Through the Flames*, a documentary about their work, that looks antiquated and quaint from the vantage point of this beleaguered twenty-first century he did not live to see but warned us against. Who is this tall, thin man with the long, stringy hair, finely chiseled face, an accent no one could place—aristocratic, authoritative, unique—and the booming voice of a prophet, who is frantically chopping a carrot in a small kitchen in Rome, while explaining the connection between the desire to kill and the eating of animal meat, a portrait of Gandhi on the wall. ("Is there anything I haven't talked about," Julian asked his lover, Ilion Troya, in front of the filmmakers. "Vegetarianism," Ilion said, and so, he improvised the scene. There was only one carrot and a stick of butter in their Rome refrigerator.)

I stood in a Brooklyn kitchen, Judith at my side, watching Julian cook. He was moving about as if in a dance, his long arms seasoning and stirring a large pot of vegetarian stew. He wore a gauzy, loose, light green Indian embroidered shirt that just covered his thong underpants. "I like your book," were his first words, smiling down from what always seemed like a great height. He was tall, but not unusually so; it was the place from which he seemed to speak, a mountaintop with a 360-degree view that added the illusion of height. There was about him a glow; it emanated from his smile and his eyes, but it was an inner light of fierce devotion to a nonviolent cause. "I like your book, too," I answered back. "You see," Judith said, smiling, proud of me, as if she'd brought home a lost relative. Both Judith and I were small with large, dark eyes and dark hair. We might have been cousins. Her Jewish family from Poland through Germany arrived in New York in 1929, already running from rising fascism. Her father, the Orthodox Rabbi Max Malina, knew what was coming. My Jewish grandmother's family came from the shtetls of Odessa, fleeing pogroms of the previous century; her father, our Papa Joe, worked for the Democratic Party with his schoolboy friend, an Irishman called Hinky Dink who ran Chicago's First Ward.. My Jewish grandfather's family were horse traders from Alsace-Lorraine. In Chicago, they had a prosperous meat packing business at the Stockyards. My grandmother and grandfather quickly divorced. He was a compulsive gambler. She had an affair for many years with a married lawyer we called Mr. Landis; even though he was long dead, his photograph was always next to her bed. Our grandmother held family dinners every Friday night, but the word Shabbos was never mentioned, candles were not lit, nor were prayers said; we came together to share family gossip and eat. Liberals, all, devotion to Roosevelt and the New Deal substituted for religion. I knew very little of Judaism, then. Judith, a rabbi's daughter, part rabbi herself, would tutor me over the years.

Judith was writing a review of my book for *Liberation*, the literary pacifist magazine published by the War Resisters' League, co-edited by her former mentor, gestalt therapist and writer, Paul Goodman, some of whose plays the Living Theatre had produced, and by the writer-Freedom Rider-lesbian activist, Barbara Deming. Judith told me as we watched Julian prepare dinner. Judith never cooked; she was almost afraid of food—a vegetarian who refused to eat green vegetables, she subsisted on white things, bread, eggs, pastries, potatoes prepared by others. They were living in Brooklyn temporarily with members of their company, guests of the Brooklyn Academy of Music's executive producer Harvey Lichtenstein who lent them the decrepit brownstone and rehearsal space across the street in the BAM building. They erected their *Money Tower* in the top-floor rehearsal studio. Two fat capitalists acted their craving for more on the top of a spiraling five-level set, the stratified social order labored on platforms below, bureaucrats, police, secretaries, while many proletarian, bent, endlessly circled around on the floor, miming backbreaking work. Soon I would join their rehearsals and move in Judith's tightly choreographed workers' agony among them. The play was to open outside a factory gate in Pittsburgh where the Living Theatre was preparing to live among the American working class and continue to create their *Legacy of Cain* cycle of plays begun in the favelas of Brazil and meant to be performed on the streets. (As they said in *Paradise Now*, they had taken the theater into the streets, and made it free for all.)

People's Theater in Amerika, my book, escorted me into the world I had written about. The Kafkaesque "k" in the title, was intentional if brazen and a mistake in judgment as it branded me the "radical" I actually was. The illegal carpet-bombing of Cambodia occurred while I was completing my manuscript, and in it, I wrote, "as I type these words, Cambodia is being bombed." Julian had recently published *The Life of the Theater: The Relation of the Artist to the Struggle of the People*, a comprehensive, poetic statement of his aesthetic. Julian was forty-eight and world-famous. I was twenty-seven. He seemed ageless, always, innocent and ancient at the same time, neither old nor young, but wise, as if he had wandered out of the desert after a long time lost, to voice his incantatory commandment, do no harm. He opens his book:

> *There is a misery of the body and a misery of the mind, and if the stars, whenever we looked at them, poured nectar into our mouths, and the grass became bread, men would still be sad. We live in a*

system that manufactures sorrow, spilling it out of its mill, the waters of sorrow, ocean, storm, and we drown down, dead, too soon.

Theater is like a boat, it is only so big, but uprising is the reversal of the system, and revolution is the turning of the tides.

I had written in my chapter about the Living Theatre:

Between the time their loft-theater closed and 1959 when they opened a new Living Theatre on Fourteenth St., in an old building renovated by themselves and their friends, the Becks spent thirty days in prison for refusing to take part in an air raid drill. They had also received M.C. Richard's translation of Antonin Artaud's The Theater and Its Double. *Artaud's inspired ravings appealed to them immediately, because just at the time they were beginning to be punished for their peace actions, they glimpsed a theater whose poetry was active and aggressive and which was the idea of a man who spent World War II locked up in an insane asylum.*

It is here where the life of the prisoner meets the life of the artist that the history of the Living Theatre as it will remain to us began to be determined.

Judith and Julian felt seen by this younger woman standing in their kitchen and I felt suddenly accepted into a storied artistic world I had, up to then, only written about. We were all of us a bit thrilled. Judith led me up the creaking stairs to her bedroom on the top floor where we would pledge our love. If our sexual affair was short-lived, our devotion lasted the rest of her life and in my heart, beyond. At Judith's last Seder, five days before she died on April 10, 2015, I stood next to her holding her hand.

After their '68-'69 tour made the Living Theatre famous (again) in Europe and the U.S., the company split up. Those who remained with Judith and Julian went to Brazil, then under the rule of a military dictatorship that tortured and killed dissidents and at the same time fostered an economic revival that increased the gap between the poor and the bourgeoisie who kept the military junta in power. Working in the favelas, making theater for the streets with the poorest of the poor, Judith was fulfilling a promise she had made in 1949, when on a trip to Mexico with Julian, she'd encountered a small boy and wrote this pledge in her diary:

> *I look into his face and I see his sightless eyes. They are two sores that bleed a pus like tears along his cheeks.*
>
> *I want to give him, not a few centavos, but all my care, all my devotion, to cure his eyes—to stay in Mexico and cure them all— the entire plan of my life lies open in his sore eyes ...*
>
> *I screamed because I was leaving him, and I had already promised myself to him, and to do the work that I had to do for him, because in that pain and blindness he made it clear.*

The "crime" for which they were imprisoned was a Mother's Day play they were creating with children of the favela—though the charge was possession of marijuana, also true. "You can always get the Living Theatre on marijuana," Judith, who smoked constantly, said. The young performers, directed by Judith, used images from their dreams to create a theatrical gift for their caretakers to be presented outside in the slums. The company was arrested one night at an art gallery opening. Brazilian prisons were notoriously cruel and prisoners could be disappeared for years. But Judith and Julian were world-renowned artists and their jailing with other members of their company sparked an international protest. I gave a benefit for the Living's defense fund in a café in Woodstock where we showed the Mekas brothers' film of the final US performance of *The Brig*, made secretly, in defiance, after the IRS closed and padlocked the Living's theater on Fourteenth St. George played prisoner #6. Before screening the film for the public, I projected it against the refrigerator door in the one-room log cabin with sleeping loft in which I was living with D., while I finished my book. Even in a small, jerky frame against scratched white metal, I was staggered by *The Brig's* intensity. I had worked in the Woodstock Playhouse box office the previous summer and watched while the man I had recently married carried on his affair with a pretty, blond intern and George, a resident actor that summer, married, I knew, to Crystal Field, carried on his affair with another. George and I did not speak, though one day, he wormed his way past me in the narrow box office to use the phone, and our bodies touched for the first time. (Jack Gelber and I were on summer hiatus.) I sent the modest check with a brief note to Karl Bissinger, former celebrity photographer for Vogue, now working full-time at the War Resisters League, who was heading the international artists' campaign to free the Living from prison in Brazil. Judith called Karl "our angel" and he looked the part: small, white-haired, lithe, lively and kind. Karl escorted Julian's mother, Mabel, to Brazil so that she could bring Isha Manna, Judith and Julian's daughter, back to safety in the United States.

Karl soon became a close friend. In 1979, we were arrested together, with our mutual friend, the writer, Grace Paley, and eight others on the White House lawn after we unfurled a banner, "No Nuclear Bombs, No Nuclear Power USA-USSR." The Washington Lawn Eleven, we came to be called. We had gone on the White House tour, exited down the driveway and stepped carefully over the low chain between driveway and lawn. We walked slowly to the fountain, where our photo was taken. We were arrested almost immediately and bound with plastic handcuffs. We were booked, photographed and strip-searched. We spent the night in jail. Grace and I used our single phone calls to contact the pimps of the prostitutes in jail with us, so they could bail them out. At our trial, officers testified we climbed a fence and ran across the lawn. We had not done that. There were snipers on the White House roof, of course, and we would have been shot. Our small antinuclear protest became significant when our two-week trial received major coverage in the Washington Post, and the publicity helped to spark a nationwide antinuclear movement, which would see one million people marching in the streets of New York by 1982, demanding an end to nuclear weapons. In 1987, The Intermediate Range Nuclear Forces Treaty was negotiated and signed by Ronald Reagan and Mikhail Gorbachev—making the world a safer place, until Donald Trump abrogated the treaty during his first term as president. Like opposition to the war in Vietnam,

I saw and participated in small actions that helped spur mass movements, and I learned ordinary people might make a difference.

Julian kept my note inside the cover of his copy of my book. (I received the book back after Julian's death—it had become rare. He had covered it in plastic wrap and kept it behind glass on a shelf in his mother's upper West Side apartment.) There was never to be a question of the bond between us; it began when we read one another's words. We were lost family, found.

Judith and Julian were like no people I had known. Being with them was to live in heightened reality, stoned, of course—they were always stoned—but it was more than that, they were witty, urbane, learned, kind. They believed in the power of the theater to change lives and they believed in the efficacy of nonviolence. They were endlessly creative. "There's Sheridan Square where everything that ever happened to me in my life happened to me," Judith quipped driving across the Village, the four of us, crammed into a cab, Julian in front, Hanon, their lover who would be Judith's second husband, Judith and me in back. Or walking in front of the White Horse Tavern, a sign in their window, No loud singing, radio playing, No drinking on the street. "And no poets," Julian added ruefully. That was the bar where Dylan Thomas nearly drank himself to death. One of the theater spaces they rented was closed on suspicion of being a whorehouse. They were about to do a play by Ezra Pound. "How else cd u support a surus teater in ny," Pound wrote on a post card they liked to show. Cocteau had designed their letterhead, a lute-playing pen-and-ink Orpheus in mid-dance. Young Bob Dylan sang at Monday-night open mic sessions at their Fourteenth St. theater. They had read widely, the Moderns, the Romantics, Martin Buber, Gaster on myth, Sartre, the anarchists Kropotkin and Emma Goldman, Brecht, Lorca, Gertrude Stein, Genet, whose plays they staged. When they first met, they spent a week typing on sticky labels, "Ban the Bomb." They dressed in evening clothes and moved through the city one night pasting the labels on every surface they could without being caught. They were arrested and each spent a month in jail for sitting outside in a park, refusing to take shelter in what was a citywide mandated air raid drill. Judith shared her cell with Dorothy Day, founder of the Catholic Worker.

"It is just the atrocity of the day," Julian would say, a sad smile on his face, whenever the world was engulfed in some new horrific violence. "The atrocity of the day;" he explained, "will be repeated every day until we bring about the Beautiful, Nonviolent, Anarchist Revolution." He would shake his head and go back to work. Their theater was their revolution. They were broke when I first met them and had no food for the company; I had some money saved, so I offered to lend them $3000. It was hot. Julian met me at the bank on Second Avenue, wearing red shorts, a white tank top, rubber thongs, his hair in a ponytail. The teller called the bank officer and the man in the suit took me into a corner. "Do you know *that person? Do not* lend *him* money." But I did. I believed Julian when he said they would pay me back and he did, five years later when I asked him to do so. They were in Europe on tour and he wired the cash. I wanted to go to Europe, too, to Ireland, and to Greenham Common where women had established a peace encampment and lived in small tents in a magical forest just outside a nuclear base.

I visited the Living for a few days in Milan. Judith had just finished her feminist version of the Passover Haggadah. I could not stay for the first of the Living's Seders held that year in Milan and every year after for decades, but I helped her paste together the pages and tie the mimeographed booklets together with braided twine. I had no idea what a Haggadah was, then, so secular I had never attended a Seder. A decade and a half later, George and I hosted six annual Living Theatre Seders for sixty people or more seated on the floor in front of low tables that filled in the front two parlors of the big Victorian house we rented. In Judith's Haggadah, Allen Ginsberg's poem "Holy" was chanted, and, for the Seders in our home, I wrote a feminist version we, also, chanted as a companion piece. Ginsberg's "Holy the cocks of the grandfathers in Kansas" was followed by my "Holy the cunts of the grandmothers …" Baba Ben Israel, son of long time Living Theatre actor, Steve Ben Israel, told me he learned feminism from my answering "Holy."

Julian dropped out of Yale as a freshman to devote himself to his abstract expressionist painting. Judith had never been to college, but she'd studied with Erwin Piscater in his Actor's Workshop at the New School, where George was a student in the children's program, directed by Piscator's wife, Maria Ley. Piscator and Brecht were the two creators of Epic Theater, and both had to flee Germany as soon as Hitler came to power. "For we went changing our country more often than our shoes," Brecht wrote. Judith was the only woman allowed in the director's track; Piscator did not believe a women could direct, but she insisted and she convinced him. Judith was raised in the New York community of German exiles. Her father, Max Malina, brought his wife and two-year old daughter to New York in 1929; already he sensed what was coming. Ilion Troya, who met the company in Brazil and came back to the U.S. with them and was an intimate partner of Julian Beck for many years, knows Judith's early history well:

> *Max Malina was the young rabbi of the German-speaking congregation at New York's Central Synagogue on Lexington Ave. and E. 55th St. Among the congregants was the mystic philosopher Eric Gutkind, and among his non-followers, was Albert Einstein (hence little Judith's photo sitting on his lap), all involved in the rescue of German and Polish Jews. Max Malina's congregation was a center of political activism and Judith's consciousness-raiser as she overheard at a very young age the stories of atrocities from the arriving Jews.*

Her mother had wanted to act, a compromise was reached; she would become the rabbi's wife, but their daughter would be allowed to go on the stage.

In an interview with Italian Journalist Cristina Valenti, Judith remembered:

> *My father conducted the German Jewish Congregation and published a paper called "Der Zeitgeist" (spirit of the time) with which he sought to awaken people regarding what was going on in Germany and Poland, and was beginning to happen throughout the world; my mother gave a new poetry recital on occasion, we sent clothes to Germany, we collected money and organized public events to denounce the Nazis' persecution of Jews.*

As a child, Judith performed poems at anti-Nazi gatherings. Coached by a family friend, she was thought successful by the number of people she moved to tears and the amount of money they donated to help fleeing refugees. She sat at a table with envelopes of dry shampoo to be shipped to Germany; each tenth one was carefully opened, a small piece of paper inserted inside, "do you know what has happened to your Jewish neighbors?" and sealed again. Rabbi Max Malina arranged marriages between young Jewish refugees and elderly widows so they could get into and remain in the US. Rabbi Malina died of a (broken) heart attack early in the war, leaving Judith and her mother bitterly poor. Julian was from the comfortable Jewish middle class living on the Upper West Side of New York. Judith was introduced to Julian by a mutual friend, who asked her for money to buy a sandwich at the Horn and Hardart automat on Fourteenth Street, and an additional quarter to call Julian Beck, "you are going to meet the most wonderful man in your life." It was "the best quarter I ever spent," Judith said. Her brilliance enchanted Julian. He was, and remained, homosexual, but here was an intense, visionary, talented, vibrant and beautiful woman who turned him on. They decided to start a theater for poets. They married because Judith's mother threatened to put her head into an oven if they did not. Judith was pregnant with Garrick, their son. They decided to live as if in a dream of the way things could be if one were on fire with creativity all of the time. Being with them was to step into a morally charged fairyland, where freedom, intellect and wit reigned. They were quite simply intoxicating.

With Judith and Julian, all was simple. We loved one another that was it. "They even look alike," Julian said about Hanon Reznikov and me, sitting across from them at Schrafft's late one night. I was surprised because we did not look alike. They wanted us to be their protégés, I suddenly understood, and, in fact, Julian wrote me a long letter in which he asked me to become a company member and to ("p.s. to do their publicity") but I would never join the Living Theatre. I thought that was obvious. I was going to be a writer. The Living Theatre was no longer producing plays. Everything was "collectively created," meaning Judith and Julian were the auteurs and had the final say. It didn't matter that I turned them down and went my own way; we were family.

I no longer wished to become a theater critic. "If I could do anything, I would write poetic plays," I'd said to my twin brother one day years before when we were home from college. "Why don't you do it?" he'd asked. "Because I'm a woman," I snapped, as if the reason were self-evident. I had never yet read a play written by a woman, not in college, not even in graduate school, though "well educated." Until I heard about Augusta Gregory, I did not think there were any good woman playwrights. Of course, I found many when I started to look, and in 1984, published a book of women's artistic theories, *Women in Theater: Compassion and Hope*.

"Well met, without resistance to friendship or love," Joe Chaikin wrote in my copy of his just published book, *The Presence of the Actor*, which he brought to me as a gift at a party I held in the West Village apartment in which I was temporarily staying. He, too, had read *People's Theater* and was impressed by my praise of his Open Theater. How could he not have been? I was, perhaps, most enamored of his work which I had seen many times live, on stage in New York. The Open Theater's heightened physical expression and sparse, poetic language—their sense of loss, of grief and of wonder—struck a chord deep inside me. Joe was very beautiful; he, too, had striking blue eyes. He, too, radiated a heightened—a theatrical—presence, an aliveness. Soon enough Joe and I were in bed in his Westbeth loft. For a moment, I fantasized having a child, either with Joe or Julian, knowing they were both homosexual, but why not form a nontraditional family? I was not the only woman in Joe Chaikin's crowded love life. Walking down the long, narrow halls of Westbeth, the artists' subsidized housing building in the West Village, toward Joe's loft apartment for a tryst, I brushed shoulders with the voice teacher, Kristen Linkletter, obviously just leaving Joe's bed. She would get pregnant with Joe and miscarry. He told me about it later. She phoned him to meet her in the emergency room.

He sat and waited. "I wondered why I was there." A nurse appeared, "She wants me to tell you not to worry." "That is when, Karen, I understood why she asked me to come. I ought to *be worried*," Joe told me in his breathless, childlike voice, as if human emotions were to him a great mystery. He used his sense of wonder to great effect in his work, and in his life to manipulate people. "Karen, I have something to tell you," Joe sat me down on a bench on a then-dilapidated pier by the Hudson River. "Yes, Joe?" Long, significant pause, then, in a low tone: "I am dying." "What, Joe, can I do?" "Whatever I need. Whatever I ask you to do." From a poor, immigrant Russian Jewish family, Joe had scarlet fever as a child and he'd been sent away to a sanatorium to recover. He had a weak heart from which he would die several decades later. Open-heart surgery was then in its infancy. Joe was fragile. He was not, any longer, particularly close to Judith and Julian, though he had been the lead actor in their Fourteenth Street Theater. "We are not like they are, Karen," he said breathlessly, "we are *real*." But Joe was unlike Judith and Julian in other ways. If Judith and Julian seemed doctrinaire about nonviolence, vegetarianism, or refusing to vote—I always voted, we argued back and forth, but they never expected compliance with their views—Joe expected absolute loyalty. Really, to whatever he thought. In 1973, Joe said in his breathless voice: "Karen, you must come to my apartment. We are going to demand the Government send more arms to Israel." It was the start of the Yom Kippur War, also known as the Ramadan War. "I can't, Joe, I am a pacifist. I am going to hear Noam Chomsky speak at Brooklyn College."

"You are an anti-Semite," Joe hissed, furious that I would not do as he asked and he told our mutual friend, Grace Paley, I was; in fact, he told many people we both knew. I was hurt. I didn't understand, then, the hysteria among Jewish people whose proximity to the Holocaust was closer than mine. Joe's family emigrated from Eastern Europe during the rise of Nazi Germany. I am a Jew. Joe was a Jew, Noam was a Jew, Grace was a Jew. Judith and Julian, obviously. George, too. Each of us had different stories. Some of the people who believed Joe's accusation against me were not Jewish but they thought everything Joe said was gospel, or, rather, Torah. Over the years, Joe learned and he changed. He did theater work in Tel Aviv with Jews and Arabs. He began to understand the terrors of the Nakba and Occupation. He realized there is a difference between Judaism and Zionism. I learned, too; I had not understood the depth of the fear of annihilation he carried.

Noam's linguistic theories fascinated me as much as his political insights instructed: because syntax is innate, each of us first speaks an invented sentence. Humans are inherently creative. I referenced Noam's work when I wrote about two new plays that dealt with the acquisition of language, the Open Theater's *Mutation Show* and Peter Handke's *Kaspar* for an article in *Performance* Magazine. Merrill Brockway, the producer of the CBS Sunday morning arts show Camera Three, handed me his business card at a party. He commissioned me to write and narrate a four-part series based on my article. The two plays were filmed for television in the CBS studios while I watched, entranced. Merrill, a small crew and I drove to Massachusetts to film an interview with Noam Chomsky at MIT, where the linguist and antiwar activist taught; we sat outside on the lawn, with Stanley Aronowitz, labor organizer, scholar and mutual friend. We three talked linguistics and politics; we were all against war and for what Noam called "libertarian socialism," an egalitarian, free and inventive social order. I introduced the two plays for the television audience but my interview with Stanley and Noam was never shown on CBS television. Merrill called to tell me, "My mother says I will be fired if I put on Noam Chomsky"—so controversial were Noam's pacifist political views that the producer who commissioned and filmed the interview pulled it at the last moment. I doubt Noam was surprised. He had been censored many times. The surprise would have been had the interview aired.

I was now living a Spartan life on $35 spending money a week, in a minuscule one-room apartment on East Fifth Street whose sloping wooden floor I painted bright red. The rent was $95 a month. I was intentionally celibate, at last, and determined to write. But what? Over my desk, I pasted a quote from *Gravity and Grace*, by the French mystic philosopher and Nazi resister Simone Weil. We were all reading Weil in those days: "Writing is like giving birth: we cannot help making the supreme effort. But we also act in like fashion. I need have no fear of not making the supreme effort—provided only that I am honest with myself and that I pay attention." I had a door across two battered, gray, metal filing cabinets for a desk, the same desk I write at now, the same filing cabinets beneath, only the door has been replaced. I had an electric typewriter. I found two rickety chairs and a small table. There was a mattress on the floor. My Sheltland sheepdog, Malcolm, followed me, off-leash, wherever I went. "Malcolm is not a dog but a person," Joe used to say, in his childlike, wondrous way. But all dogs are persons in the sense that each is an individual soul, and the better they are treated, the more personable they become. "And if the body were not the soul, what is the soul," Julian liked to quote from Walt Whitman's hymn to beauty, "I Sing the Body Electric."

Though I was intimate with Joe, I knew nothing about his private life. I'd had an affair, brief though it was, with Joe. Worse, perhaps, in Jean-Claude's mind, as he knew Joe was not faithful, Joe and I did a book together, *Three Works by the Open Theater* that documented the theater's final three plays, but left out the play before, *The Serpent* by Jean-Claude. It had already been published and I had not seen it performed. One day, I joined a group of theater people summoned to Joe's loft to help him think about what was the next logical step for experimental theater to take now that he had disbanded the Open Theater. We sat in a circle and talked. I said words to the effect that the Open Theater broke through the well-made play. Actors can now give shape to the inner life. It's time for the poetic play to replace American realism.

"Yes, yes," Joe was enthusiastic and he and I went back and forth for a bit.

"It's easier to talk about it than to do it," Jean-Claude spat at me from directly across the circle.

I shut up. He's right, I thought. I went home to my tiny room of one's own and shut the door.

Feminist firebrand, Andrea Dworkin, lived across the street. I don't remember how we met. Perhaps walking our dogs. Andrea had a big German Shepherd named Gringo. Andrea was writing her first book. We became friends. I introduced Andrea to Julian and Judith and to Joe Chaikin. (Andrea would soon secretly marry Joe's assistant, John Stoltenberg, with whom I had been in graduate school, "for his health insurance" and live with him for many years.) Joe was smitten—her seeming sweetness, her brains and her large size—he wanted to put her on stage. She refused. Julian was less impressed. Andrea was critical of his close relationship with Judith. She thought Julian kept Judith dependent on him. But nothing could have been less true. Judith could not boil an egg, much less cross the street by herself, or pay for anything. She was dependent upon Julian, and whomever else was around, for the very basics of life, including raising their daughter Isha Manna (whose biological father was Karl Einhorn, a lover who fled).

Judith was equally reliant upon Julian for realizing her ideas for the stage. During their European exile, they discovered the works of Sacher-Masoch, the writer about whom the Austrian psychiatrist Kraft-Ebbing wrote: "During recent years facts have been advanced which prove that Sacher-Masoch was not only the poet of Masochism, but that he himself was afflicted with the anomaly." The Living would take the title Sacher-Masoch used before them for his unfinished series of novellas and call the series of short plays they created to perform in the streets of Brazil, the United States, Italy and France, *The Legacy of Cain*. Originally, this was to be a cycle of 150 plays "on themes of enslavement to the State, to Money, to Property, to Violence, to Death and the Love of Sexes, that is, sadomasochism proper," says Ilion Troya, who was a journalist in Brazil before becoming a company member and moving with them to United States upon their release from prison. "We are a small theater. We can't send money. What can we do?" Judith and Julian asked their cellmates upon their release. "Speak about what happens here. Speak about the torture," the Brazilian prisoners asked. The screams of those being tortured echoed through the prison each night. They were returned to their cells, wounded and traumatized. The American artists were spared but they saw what torture did. The Living returned to New York and created a meditative masterwork. They performed *Seven Meditations on Political Sado-Masochism* for many years. I saw it first at the Washington Square Methodist Church, now a celebrity's private home, then a center for art, worship and peace, whose minister, Reverend Finley Schaef, ran a referral service to trusted doctors for abortions, before Roe v. Wade became for the next decades, law, and where the Greenwich Village Draft Counseling Center was located when counseling young men to avoid the draft was also illegal.

"The First Meditation is called a meditation on domination and submission with a text on the repression of sexual love … in which we meditate on what has corrupted love." *Seven Meditations* was performed in a circle: the audience sat around a larger circle just outside the actors who circled through each meditation, offering short, poetic texts, accompanied by striking physical poses. There were seven scenes that visualized, in slow motion, with spiritual chanting in counterpoint to their violent physicality, the vicious realities of sexual and political violence, its sadism. In the most memorable scene, the actors "speak" about the torture as their Brazilian cell mates asked them to do: Tom Walker, a longtime company member, is hung naked on a parrot perch (a pole that goes underneath the torture victims bent and tied legs, so that they dangle, head down), electrodes are attached to their genitals. The actor writhes as the electricity is turned on, shocking his anus and testicles. The victim is carried around the circle of performers and audience, so we bear witness to this agony. The slow motion of the movements in each of the meditations, the chants, interspersed with screams, make the work an experience in which time is suspended and the audience is transported into a realm beautiful (bodies in space, voices chanting) and terrifying (relationships of torture and domination) at the same time.

We were all then engaged in discovering how personal and political submission/domination are connected. From a feminist perspective, the question was, how have women been instrumental in our own oppression by supporting and nurturing patriarchy? When I emerged from my room several months later with my play in hand, I took it to Joe to read. He liked it enormously. I was so pleased. He said he would direct *A Lament for Three Women*. I told him no. I did not trust myself to be able to hold my own around Joe. I wanted a woman to direct my feminist play. He was graceful. He introduced me to Eleanor Johnson, a director he mentored at NYU's School of the Arts, who with her partner, an Israeli draft resister, Judah Kataloni, took on the work. I have no memory, none, of the writing of this cancer play, *A Lament for Three Women*. I must have been very afraid. Much later, I would tell my students that writing is a conversation between the conscious and unconscious mind. I had lived very little when I wrote my first play but I had, within, a depth of unexplored sorrow. I had never properly mourned my father's death, nor fully experienced the relief when his death set me free of his rages. Writing is about the forbidden. And playwriting is social and expiatory. A ritual cleansing performed in front of an audience. Theater, for me, as it was, also, for Judith and Julian, for Joe, and for George, with these roots in unexplored loss, has always also been about what hasn't happened yet but yet might. *Tikkun olam*, to heal the world. *A Lament for Three Women* attempted to work on these levels, as a personal story of bereavement, and as a social story of women preparing to go it alone in the world, without men, without, that is, female reliance upon men's overbearing needs. Three women confront their loss of self as they help the men in their lives to die and they begin the mourning process—in this way, the play was also prescient. If I had not known until after I left school that women could write plays, though they had done so, at least, since the tenth century when the nun Hrotswitha of Gandersheim wrote six surviving raunchy, truly S & M plays that were most likely staged in her nunnery, and women had crafted untold numbers of collective rituals before then in antiquity, I, also, could not have written a play until I had withdrawn into myself. Up until then, I was a woman in the patriarchal sense: "a thing" for the use of someone else, whether to comfort my father, who was also named Joe, or Joe Chaikin, as they shared their fears about their death, my own story was intended to be lost. Now, though, there was Jean-Claude van Itallie taunting me from across the room, "It's much easier to talk about it than to do it," and Andrea Dworkin writing feminist theory—both, unwittingly, setting me free.

In 1974, Andrea's first book *Women Hating* was published by a major publisher, Dutton, and my first play, *A Lament for Three Women*, was produced with no budget. Joe helped Eleanor and Judah assemble the cast. Tina Shepard, who was Joe's favorite female actor in his Open Theater, whose acting I admired, played the daughter. Sybille Hayn, beautiful (like my mother), a redheaded German who took workshops with Joe, was the Wife. Elia Braca, a lovely Sephardic Jewish actor who, like Joe, lived in Westbeth, was the Mother. Sybille lived with her physician boyfriend in a large SoHo loft on a high floor with windows facing west. The women wore simple dance skirts and leotards. Their movements were carefully choreographed like a living sculpture. They handled the language almost as song. The lighting effects came from the sun as it set on the Hudson River, a soft glow at first, growing fiercer with slanting shadows through the windows falling across the women performers, then nearly dark at the play's end.

"Why did you write it like that," Susan Yankowitz, who wrote the Open Theater's *Terminal* for Joe, wanted to know when she saw my play staged. I only knew I had found a voice that was mine. A poetic voice, an interior voice turned out. *A Lament for Three Women* was praised by Joe, Julian and Judith and almost everyone else who saw it. This first production had an abstract beauty about it—like a dream play. The women meet in a hospital waiting room and in those endless hours, they tell one another their stories. They gather strength from each other as they lament the sufferings of the men who have been at the center of their lives, father, husband, son, each one now a cancer-ridden relic, without will. Metaphorically, they disconnect the men's life support systems, and their IVs dripping chemotherapy drugs, while they sing a lament. "I'll hold his hand and watch his passage," says the daughter. Judith quarreled with me about this ending, which her devout Jewish faith forbade. Life at any cost was her creed. She thought my play's end sinful and wrong. But to me, the play's end evidences the desire for a good death that would guide me through Julian's and George's illnesses. Julian had no problem with the ending. He was not a religious Jew, raised in comfort on the Upper West Side—his father had been a businessman. In general, too, where Judith judged, Julian smiled.

A Lament for Three Women received a good review in an obscure downtown paper. A few months later, the production would have a short run in a tiny theater downtown and be published by a small, now defunct press, in a book called *A Century of Plays by American Women.* And it would be performed once at Cummington Community for the Arts, in Massachusetts, where Edward Ryerson saw it and became my patron for a decade, before he, too, died of cancer. Ned was an extraordinary person; a member of the Chicago Ryerson Steel family, he was a renegade, a Quaker and an educator who founded and taught at a progressive school in Boston. He was divesting himself of his personal fortune so that he could live a comfortable, but in no way extravagant, middle-class life. He remarried and started a second family. Ned responded so strongly to my first play that he gave me $10,000 annually, which I used to help pay actors for my plays.

Andrea's book, *Woman Hating,* launched her career as an outspoken feminist theorist. We were both writers now and each of us attracted older feminist mentors. I met Dorothy Dinnerstein, author of the seminal book, *The Mermaid and the Minotaur,* when she gave a reading at the Women's Salon for Literature, a monthly event held in my friend, Erika Duncan's Westbeth loft that hosted most of the significant artists and thinkers of this second wave of the feminist movement. Dorothy and I quickly became close friends. We did peace politics together. Dorothy was enthusiastic about my plays because, she said, of my "passionate coalescence of the aesthetic and political."

—

Barbara Deming, who also read at the Women's Salon, was an outspoken lesbian, and became Andrea's benefactor. Barbara was a presence in the pacifist left. A poet and writer, Barbara had been a Freedom Rider. She spent nearly a month in jail in the segregated south and wrote a book called *Prison Notes.* She was from genteel Quaker wealth. Her mother knew of and encouraged her lesbianism and though she was courted by men, Barbara never felt pressure from her family to marry. Her partner for many years was Mary Meigs, an artist and writer. Barbara and Meigs lived in Wellfleet, with the French writer Marie-Claire Blais, with whom Meigs was also in love. "I just adored her," Anna Poor, who visited as a child with her grandmother, the artist Ann Poor, says about Barbara. "She wore pants and she had long legs and she was just an extraordinary person. People were talking about what they were writing and there were hot debates. It was extraordinarily thrilling." By the time we met, Barbara had been in a bad car accident that left her permanently frail. She was living in the country in Monticello, New York, with her partner, Jane Gapen. I sat under a shade tree with her while she leaned forward intently, focusing, very much like Julian, as if I were the only person in her world, and asked me in her whisper-like voice why I "could not just become a lesbian?" She was tall, thin with a delicate beauty and an indomitable will. I told her about a threesome I had briefly enjoyed, and she suggested that perhaps I was really attracted to the other woman in the bed. Though I had several brief, and one longer and lovely, lesbian affair (with Dorothy Dinnerstein's beautiful daughter, Naomi), I was unable to pledge myself to the lesbian separatism Barbara promoted as a necessary political stance and which she believed, until her death in 1984, was the key to solving the problems of the world. In all other ways, but one's sexual orientation, Barbara had a complex and open mind. She was an epistolary writer who corresponded with a range of people from Black Panthers in prison to Martin Buber, searching for common ground. We never grew personally close, though I very much admired her and I witnessed her last arrest. Julian met Barbara Deming late in life, when both were undergoing treatments for incurable cancers. I introduced them. I don't think they ever saw each other in person as they were each quite ill by then, but they engaged in long phone conversations. Aside from their cancers, they had much in common. The influential critic Eric Bentley understood Barbara and Julian's temperamental connection. Bentley, who after critiquing their 1969 tour harshly became Judith and Julian's personal friend, wrote in his tribute to Julian after Julian died that "Julian had more in common with Barbara Deming than he had with anyone in the American theater." An astute observation. Tall and willowy both, almost fragile to look at, they exuded commitment, intellect and strength. Each knew how to listen, slightly cocking their heads, taking you in as if you were a very important person to them. Each held you in their penetrating gaze and gave undivided attention because they expected much and so one tried to be on best intellectual and moral behavior before each. Each had a will of steel. Julian with a huge actor's voice. Barbara who spoke in a whisper. Both Julian and Barbara spent months in prison for their beliefs over the course of their too-brief lives. Each, in profoundly different ways took control over their illness and deaths—and one of their shared concerns was how to be intimate with but also to spare others they loved most, all the while encouraging a great inclusive embrace of the communal circle that during their dying formed around each. When I met them, there was no sign of the cancers, which would in the next decade kill them, whereas Joe Chaikin, who outlived both, was always on the edge of death.

Joe chose three people to visit him in the hospital as he prepared for his first open heart surgery: his older sister, Shami, who had been an actor in his Open Theater, Jean-Claude van Itallie, his frequent collaborator and long-term lover, and me. Shami sat with her legs spread wide on a low stool outside Joe's hospital door, looking fierce, like a peasant doula, guarding her brother. She nodded. I entered the silent room and walked to his bedside. Joe wore nothing but a pair of blue underpants that matched his eyes. He appeared to be floating a few inches off the bed, as if he were already in angelic form. "Karen," he asked in his tremulous voice, "Am *I* going to *die*?" Here I was, and here was my chance to "save" a Joe. I answered "no", of course not. "No, Joe, no, you are not going to die." Even then I understood the inappropriateness of the question; no matter, he had reeled me in—and I had to fulfill my pledge by making him live. On the day of Joe's open-heart surgery, in 1974, I was with Judith and Hanon in the Algonquin Hotel; they had come into town from Pittsburgh and invited me to attend a private first screening of the Sidney Lumet film *Dog Day Afternoon* in which Judith plays the mother of bank robber Al Pacino. Pacino had been a Living Theatre groupie when they had their theater on Fourteenth St.; he cleaned the toilets alongside his friend, Martin Sheen. Like George, Pacino auditioned for the company several times, hoping to get in. It was one of her biggest mistakes, Judith confided much later, but she did not think Pacino, who was a Method actor from the Actors Studio, "was any good." (Judith was not good at casting, as I was to learn.) Pacino became a stage actor off-off Broadway, then on Broadway, then a film actor (in short time, a movie star) and most likely recommended Judith to Lumet for the now classic film. Judith, despite being trained by Piscator, was, in fact, a very fine realistic actor. We went upstairs to their hotel room from the screening where Judith and Al (I do not remember who else was there) nervously viewed their new, wonderful film—my mind was otherwise engaged since Joe was being operated on at the same time. Hanon phoned the hospital to find out how Joe's operation had gone and while he was on hold, I fell apart in Judith arms. I cried and cried. I howled. I could not stop myself. Judith held me while I wept and shrieked. I was safer in her arms than I had ever been in anyone's. In fact, I could not remember ever before having been held while I wept. No questions asked. She knew I was terrified and crying for Joe; she knew from my play something about the other Joe, my father, but I doubt she understood the connection. My first play had no hint of his terrible temper or of the complex and sexual nature of our relationship.

She held me tight, nevertheless. All the tears I had never shed, numbed as I'd been, needing to go on, to walk away from all that into a life that was mine—and I'd gone without thinking back, without remembering until I wrote my first play. A play that catapulted me from young and admiring critic into an artist, if young at twenty-nine, still, an artist with a first play that had won the admiration of Judith, Julian and Joe. They saw *the artist* in me, watched and helped me become.

For better or worse, for right or wrong, I knew while crying and shrieking in Judith's arms, I had to get away from Joe Chaikin. My only conscious thought as I wailed was if Joe died on the operating table, how could I live? And my outsized dependence on someone in whose life I was little more than a footnote, terrified me. How was it I felt so cathected to him? I was helplessly confused. It was less that an unfaithful gay man who enjoyed a few heterosexual flings, but could not sustain a relationship with me—he even told me as much in nearly those exact words, in an apologetic tone of voice, after we had made love in his bed, and hadn't I behaved just as he had with some women in my life—but that this Joe was confused in my mind with a father named Joe who was needy and dead, who once thought to take me in his arms, but then quickly recoiled, and dropped me, thankfully, but nevertheless, used me and dropped me and died. I wasn't yet able to write about *that*, the incestuous part, not in *Lament*. But I felt, shaking in Judith's arms, waiting for news, that I would have to die if Joe died. If he lived, I would have to wrest myself out of his emotional grasp—get far enough to be able to look back. I wept for my father, myself, and for Joe Chaikin, too, in the Algonquin Hotel room in Judith's arms, while Hanon was on hold, waiting for news of the outcome of Joe's open-heart surgery. Joe came through. He would live. So, too, would I, but only if I got free. I wrote to Joe during his convalescence—words I thought he needed to hear, a letter a day. I used all my newfound creative empathy to imagine Joe as he recovered slowly and I fancied my carefully chosen words would fulfill his every need as he convalesced. Many women spent their entire lives in this way, ministering to more famous men. It was 1974, and this is what we new feminists were learning. Women were waking up as if we'd been shocked, discovering for the first time the stirrings of a self that was ours.

So, a few months later, when Andrea Dworkin began her rampage through our world, I used her admonition that Joe was "a sexist" who deserved to be shunned to agree with her and stop speaking to Joe. It was a stupid way out, of course, as ways out often are. Joe was no more sexist than many a man, then, and he was a famous director in my downtown world, someone who had already and could do me still more professional good. We were about to publish a book together, *Three Works by the Open Theater*, with his preface and my introduction. "With a good collaboration and significant, Love Joe," he wrote in his childlike scrawl in my book. But I had given too much of myself, much more even than he had asked, and I had to cut ties, get away, with grace that I did not then possess. So, I abruptly stopped speaking to Joe Chaikin at Andrea Dworkin's behest—though we spoke, again, through the years, of course. Hugged one another when we met. Then, Andrea, on what was my thirtieth birthday, summoned me to her house, for a birthday dinner.

"I hope you rot in the gutter and no one stops to pick you up," she said. I was kneeling by that time on her floor in the attitude of a suppliant, begging to be forgiven, for what I did not know, for my essence. "Too needy," she told me I was, "too male identified" to be worthy of being any longer her friend. The two people who had directed my first play, who were set to direct the second play I was then working on, stood shoulder to shoulder with Andrea. Eleanor, very tall, with two waist-length braids, stern, wearing her Middle-Eastern-embroidered black top and, Judah, a draft resister from Israel, Eleanor's partner, angular and thin, alongside Andrea in her signature overalls. All of them very big, looming above, leering down. Me kneeling before them on the floor. Supposed to "rot in the gutter," the object of their contempt. One night, a few months earlier, in the front room of her tenement apartment, with the tub in the kitchen, across the street from my one room, we had both gotten stoned, and Andrea pushed me down on her bed, pulled down my jeans. There she was suddenly above me, large, holding my arms as she started to suck my cunt. "I have sucked the cunts of brilliant women," she wrote in *Woman Hating*, and I counted myself among them, but how, then, had I gotten here, kneeling before her on the floor, while she yelled insults at me. With effort, I got myself to my feet and out the door.

Traits I'd learned as a child, when I was supposed to pacify my father. My empathy focused on everyone but myself, doing always, what I thought the other one wished, despite myself, and earning contempt, being dropped. Eleanor and Judah would start a short-lived theater with Andrea, called Emmatroupe and they would direct her one woman play about rape. Then, they would separate. I was told by the actor who was in their production that Andrea accused Judah, an Alexander practitioner, of molesting the women he treated. Andrea became increasingly well known. Eleanor and Judah split up and both disappeared from the downtown scene.

"So your friends are mad at you," Judith said, not knowing quite the gravity of the situation in my mind—I felt *shamed* as if I had committed a crime. No matter, I was welcome in her home, in her heart forever. Julian's, too. They were never going to betray me. They were the good parents, the good colleagues, my dear friends for life. They accepted and loved.

Andrea turned on Grace Paley, who she did not think was supportive enough of her work. She yelled insults at Grace on a Greenwich Village street, which took a special form of chutzpah. Grace was a presence in the Village, held in highest regard; she with her women friends, pacifist poets and writers, stood on a corner of Greenwich Street, every Saturday for years, handing out flyers against the Vietnam war—"not your sons, not our sons, not their sons," Grace in her maternal way wrote. Ynestra King, our mutual friend, who was walking across the Village with Grace, interfered and told Andrea to shut up. "Why did you let her speak to you like that?" But Grace could not answer, any more than I could. Andrea's rage took us both by surprise. She was normally so nice, clearly brilliant, too. Andrea turned on Barbara Deming, finally, disavowing the ecofeminist peace movement entirely. Barbara loved Andrea and viewed Andrea as her successor, the next anointed leader of the pacifist, lesbian compound Barbara founded in Florida. Barbara built Andrea and John their own house, next to hers and Jane Gapin's, and she helped support Andrea financially. "I am not that person she thinks I am. I am not nonviolent," Andrea said to me out-of-the-blue, when we were still speaking. We were in a gas station rest room, driving back into town from a weekend away we'd shared with Joe Chaikin and Tina Shepard. That morning, Andrea had gone swimming naked in the small lake, and neighbors called to complain, as if they had seen a great white whale flapping near their dock. "He is interested in me, not you," Andrea told me about Joe. But I was most surprised by her disavowal of pacifism in the highway rest stop. I thought we all were all striving to be nonviolent in our lives as well as, of course, our art and our politics. I ought to have taken Andrea at her word. But, I had been raised to endure incomprehensible rages, and never to defend myself for fear of making things worse. I was unable to act in my own self-interest. I did not even know what my self-interest was, so adept was I at intuiting someone else. A trait good for a playwright, but I was rotten at protecting myself—never having been protected much in my early life. Andrea's break with Barbara Deming was long and searing because Barbara had loved her, and expected much of her, too—a tale waiting to be told in detail by Ynestra King who is writing Barbara's biography.

Andrea never turned on Judith or Julian—perhaps because of Julian's quiet remove. He, among all of us, never took her as seriously as she took herself. *Woman Hating* established Andrea as a sage among the feminists of the second wave, but Julian had been espousing his sort of feminism and gender fluidity since Andrea was a child growing up in Cherry Hill, New Jersey, with a sick mother who kept to her bed, and a father who raised her. Julian cooked, he sewed; he was nurturant and had great patience and rapport with children. He adored Isha Manna and was her caretaking parent. My daughter adored him. Though he died when she was five, she remembers him vividly. Perhaps Julian reminded Andrea of her father. And, perhaps, she confused the pacifism of the women she turned on with her mother's passivity.

In 1978, I was trying to put together a cast and director for my second play, *Rebekkah*, without my former collaborators, Eleanor and Judah. I was feeling very alone, still living in my tiny one room.

"You have to meet Burl Hash," Martha Coigney who was head of the International Theater Institute, said in her besotted, gravelly voice. "He's the only heterosexual in the American theater." Martha knew virtually every downtown avant-garde theater artist and she relished making connections. We three went to lunch. I sat with eyes downturned, staring at the watch with its wide, leather band on Burl Hash's hairy arm, to keep my eyes off his good-looking face. He wore cowboy boots, jeans and a fitted western shirt with pearl snaps.

Burl grew up in West Texas on a dryland cotton farm, the youngest child of four and the only son. Until he started community college, he had never worn a store-bought shirt; like many a farm wife, his mother sewed her children's clothing from the printed cotton of the chicken-feed sacks. Burl helped his father build their house, all the furniture in it and together with neighbors, the local Southern Baptist Church to which they belonged. At community college, the head of the theater department, a woman, took a special interest in him because of his carpentry skills. He began to build the stage sets. He transferred to the University of Texas at Austin, with its excellent theater department, continuing to study technical theater. He rode his motorcycle east for the first time, to New Haven, where he graduated from the Yale Drama School on scholarship, with an M.F.A. in lighting design. He and his new wife, a rural woman from Texas, moved to Brooklyn. Quickly, he became one of three producers at the Chelsea Theater Center housed on the top floor of the Brooklyn Academy of Music. Burl was technical producer and his partners, Bob Kalfin, a stage director of note, and Michael David, an excellent fundraiser, produced daring work, including the production of Handke's *Kaspar* I had written about and which was on Camera Three and Jean Genet's monumental anticolonial play *The Screens*, which blew my mind. They staged Amiri Baraka's explosive *Slave Ship*, not in their theater space, but in the sanctuary of the Washington Square Methodist Peace Church, run by the Reverend Finley Schaef. Decades later, in 2014, at our daughter's wedding, in fact, officiated by our long-time friend Finley Schaef, his wife, Nancy, recalled the intensity of Sunday worship when Finley's sermons were preached to a congregation sitting in the slave ship set in the nave of the church. Burl accompanied the Black actors on their European tour; they rode in a bus, he on his motorcycle, his first (and only) European trip. The three Chelsea producers had also just produced a commercial musical hit (its name long forgotten), enjoying a long, lucrative New York run. For the first time in his life, Burl felt rich. When the three producers closed Chelsea Theater, they divided city, state and federal funding among them, and they each launched new non-profit ventures.

Burl arranged rehearsal space at BAM for my second play, *Rebekkah*, about a Jewish immigrant woman, who loses her daughter in the Triangle Factory Shirtwaist fire, becomes a homeless bag lady and founds a squatters' community. *Rebekkah*, which I worked on with Eleanor and Judah, was directed by Tina Shepard who also played the title character. Gloria Miguel from the Spiderwoman Theater, the first Native American woman's theater in New York was in the cast, as were Sybilla Hayn, also from *Lament*, and Ellen Maddow, also a veteran of Joe's Open Theater, who wrote the music and went on to co-found The Talking Band. Burl arranged the venue for *Rebekkah*, at what was then a new off-Broadway theater, and is now the venerable Playwrights Horizons. I told Burl I would not have an affair with a married man. Almost immediately, he broke up with his wife. She went home to Texas with their son. (I hadn't known he had a son and was not even certain whether or not he was married.) He courted me and I so much needed to be rescued. I moved from my tenement room to his elegant loft at the far south end of pre-gentrified Park Slope. He had created a two-bedroom apartment at one end of the huge space, a dividing wall was made of the scavenged ends of packing crates used for coffins, arranged in a geometrical pattern. He built most of the furniture, a large wooden table, a couch, the bed frame. The loft was so large that he also built us an off-off Broadway theater with risers to seat 99. Burl wanted to direct my next plays. We painted the tin ceiling dark red, and the walls, pale gray; the floor was natural wood. Our New Cycle Theater was an inviting space, and it was free to the audience, funded in part by Ned Ryerson, and by city, state and federal grants Burl had taken with him from Chelsea. Burl designed sets and lights and he directed my plays, *The End of War* and *Making Peace: A Fantasy*, both of which attracted the young peace activists who just then were renovating the decrepit brownstones in Park Slope. We also attracted the Eastern European immigrants who lived in the modest row houses on our block, many of whom who had never once crossed the river into Manhattan. Because the theater was ours, we could run our productions for as long as we wished, and we got good reviews in the local press. Dorothy Dinnerstein especially loved *Making Peace* and she drove in from New Jersey four times to see it performed. The children next door came every night to see *The End of War*. "Why?" I asked them one night (aside from the intermission coffee we served which they drank loaded with sugar and milk.) "We love this play," the eldest boy, barely ten, said, and he recited the climax of every scene. Finley Schaef brought his new congregation of young Brooklyn peace activists to our theater. After his return from "reeducation" in Sweden at behest of the Methodist hierarchy, he had been exiled from his successful Washington Square Methodist Church in the West Village to a failing congregation with a small church building in Park Slope, Brooklyn, which he revived, along with his new young wife, Nancy, who had been his parishioner. Both Finley and Nancy were lively and kind, with a knack for creating Methodists from peaceniks, and their new church became a neighborhood hub. Explaining the reasons for Finley's theological disgrace, and Brooklyn exile, Grace Paley said, "Sometimes it is impossible to do a lot of politics without doing a lot of sex."

I became pregnant by mutual consent, but when I told Burl the good news, he replied, "I don't want this relationship anymore," and I ran crying from the room. It was the first serious crack in our relationship, though, as the child grew inside me, we made efforts to work it out, and once she was born, he fell in love. When I was six months pregnant, Karl Bissinger and I saw Judith and Julian off at the dock. It was 1979. Judith was still unwilling to fly. The Living Theatre was returning to Europe to live and work. The huge ocean liner in the background, Julian bent down and kissed my belly, "a girl, let it be a girl," he sang into my womb. It was Karl's idea that I, with my pregnant belly, do the press conference for an anti-nuclear action on Wall St. "It's safer to be here with my unborn child, than to be home waiting for the bombs to fall," I said to the cameras, standing sideways so my pregnant belly looked even larger. Burl had gone off on a sailing trip with a friend so he never knew the risk I took "You're pregnant! You could have gotten hurt," the police officer taking our names on the arrest bus said. "But who would have hurt me," I laughed, "surely not you." I was sitting next to Dorothy. She was calmly slicing a green pepper she carried to rehydrate using a paring knife. The police officer looked at her, smiling, "she's armed and dangerous." In fact, the police in New York agreed with our anti-nuclear stance, which, after all, affected their families, too, and were gentle with us.

The night before I gave birth, I sat on the floor reaching over my belly to collate the scripts for a large new play with a chorus of (dancers as) crows, the Celtic bird of prophecy. *A Monster Has Stolen the Sun*, is based on the myth of the Celtic goddess Macha who, when nine months pregnant, is made to run a horse race against the king. She wins and puts a curse on the king that he will never ride into battle again without becoming as overwhelmed as a woman in childbirth. I thought it a wonderful, pacifist feminist tale. In my play, the hugely pregnant goddess wrestles the king on stage. In a highly physicalized scene—pregnant woman against man. She pins him to the ground, delivers her curse, and he never rides into battle again, becoming instead as Dorothy suggested in her book, the nurturant caretaker of his own child. When Carrie Sophia was born, Judith and Julian sent a congratulatory telegram. "Dear Wisdom," Julian called her. We celebrated my daughter's first birthday in the theater with the actors in our large cast on a rehearsal break with a cake I baked.

We were invited to become the theater-in-residence at a new arts venture, The Arts at St. Ann's, housed, then, in a large Episcopal Church downtown. We presented a revival of *The End of War* in 1982, to coincide with a massive anti-nuclear march of a million or more, and we staged the premiere of *A Monster Has Stolen the Sun*, both of which Burl directed. X, our producer at the Arts at St. Ann's, took to stopping by our loft every night after dinner, just hanging around, playing with our small daughter and flirting with Burl. Did she and he have an affair? He denied it. But I was confused and upset. I did not believe there was nothing between them. Our home and my professional life both felt violated. "I want her plays, the child and him but I do not want her," X said to our leading actor who repeated the comment to me. Burl's and my relationship was permanently frayed. We continued to live together in the big loft, increasingly strangers, raising our child and his son who lived with us some of the time.

While the Living was away in Europe, which was much of the time between 1975 and 1984, we wrote back and forth, Judith typed long letters on onionskin, and Julian sent colorful post cards crammed with news in his tiny precise hand. "Dearest beloved Karen, comrade," he wrote of their triumphs in Europe and of the heightened political consciousness there, which energized him. "USA seems such a prison, such a repressed area. Here there's so much political alertness, that all—well, some anyway—of dreams seem PRACTICAL & REALIZABLE, Love, Julian." From Pompeii, the Villa dei Misteri, the red room, which I would later visit with George, he sent, "an ancient painting of a sister being whipped—a rite that helped her understand the mysteries (of life, of life) to which she was initiated. The benefit of the masochist syndrome is that (it) engenders feeling, feeling which makes it possible to understand the pain—and therefore to understand ½ of the reason why to change the world: ½ #2 is what to change it into, love Julian."

From Naples, "This card of lovers (male and beautiful) is another painted message from the past. What did I say that implied somehow that I had whipped you? (whipped your consciousness perhaps—but only in sense to urge it on?)" Julian considered himself a masochist, and he identified me as one; it was part of our bond, preferring suffering in love to inflicting pain, though inevitably we did that, too, like all of us who engaged in serial love affairs in those sexually liberated years, when birth control and abortions were readily available.

I took a job as guest lecturer at Smith College and was in North Hampton three days a week during spring semester for the next four years. At Smith, I co-sponsored an anti-nuclear weekend festival. Judith and Hanon came to campus to teach Judith's stylized processional techniques, which the Living used for their plays on the streets. My students created a ritual procession through the campus, picking up participants as we went, ending in a tunnel underground where they performed dream-like images of their nuclear nightmares mixed with their mother-daughter stories. The ritual event was inspired by our studies of the Homeric Hymn to Demeter, goddess of grain, therefore, of life, and the Eleusinian Mysteries, practiced for centuries in ancient Greece—whose initiates lost their fear of death. I was a faculty advisor to students who occupied the administration building in support of divesting from the apartheid government in South Africa. I taught standing among them as they sprawled outside the President's office. These student protests resulted in a daylong teach-in at each of the five colleges in the region, followed by significant divestment. In the summers, I was given the Hallie Flanagan Theater at Smith to workshop new work. Flanagan was a personal hero; director of the Federal Theater during the early years of the New Deal, she created federally funded theaters in every state, in rural and urban locations, presenting daring, new plays and classics at low cost. Her book, *Arena,* is a classic of America theater history in its own right. In it, she tells the story of Federal Theater's many accomplishments in just four years, and of its demise at the hands of a conservative Congress, heralding the start of the McCarthy anti-Communist period. Before being tapped by Eleanor Roosevelt to head the New Deal's theater project, Flanagan ran the experimental theater at Vassar College; she spent her final years teaching at Smith.

In their last extended residence in Europe, the Living Theatre toured their anti-torture play, *Seven Meditations on Political Sado-Masochism*; they also presented it in New York, in the nave of the Washington Square Methodist Church where I first saw it, stunned with the rest of the audience by its intensity. Decades later, on the tenth anniversary of the September 11, 2001 attacks, which caused the United States government to initiate its own torture program, under George W. Bush, my anti-torture play opened on September 11, 2011, in the Gerald W. Lynch Theater at John Jay College, part of a festival, Performing Justice, funded in part by the Soros Foundation. For the play, I interviewed many lawyers who were defending torture victims and prisoners at Guantanamo, and many of them, from the Center for Constitutional Rights and elsewhere, spoke to our audience after performances, in what we called "A Festival of Conscience," during four productions of the play in Manhattan, Brooklyn and London, between 2011 and 2013. *Another Life,* is a darkly surreal satire about the so-called Global War on Terror (GWOT) and the US torture program. George played a mogul Handel who runs a private contracting firm, Deepwater, (a.k.a. Blackwater, the actual firm run by Eric Prince that provided contractors for the governments' hidden torture sites in Afghanistan and other countries and at prisons like Abu Ghraib in Baghdad, where enlisted soldiers also tortured Iraqi inmates). Handel is a malignant narcissist who bears a striking, if unintentional resemblance to Donald Trump (yet to appear on the national scene). Handel begins the play with an eleven-minute tongue-twisting, monomaniacal monologue justifying his rise to power, (an impossible feat for an actor, which perfectly suited George, who loved to do on stage what no one else could) while we see the twin towers collapse outside his loft windows in SoHo. Judith, by then using oxygen and confined to a wheelchair, saw the second production of *Another Life* at the Irondale Theater in Brooklyn. "It's a brilliant play. It's too brilliant for the culture. It should win a Pulitzer Prize. It won't, but it should," she quipped. In fact, its early scenes were published in the Kenyon Review, with exactly that sort of rave from its editor, David Lynn (but we were afraid theater critics would not understand and we did not allow them to review). Torture as both the Living's *Seven Meditations* and my *Another Life* dramatized in such different ways is never about getting accurate information since victims will agree to anything to make the pain stop. Torture, as practiced around the world, and in our prisons, is about brute force and sexual sadism, brooms up the ass, underpants on heads, electrodes to the genitals, that sort of thing—as the US torture program showed—torture is simply sadism let loose. Handel maintains an Eastern European trophy wife, Tess, who is his sex slave, along with an immigrant Arab taxi driver he imprisons as his personal servant in his home. She ends up in chains in a box; Abdul is humiliated with underpants on his head (as were prisoners in Abu Ghraib). Tess and Abdul escape as Handel dies and is refused entry to heaven. Abbas Noori Abbood, a recent refugee from Iraq, played the captured cabdriver Abdul in the four productions of *Another Life*.

My generation grew up taking "shelter" under our school desks, covering our heads from radiation spreading from the atomic conflagration, much as school children today are trained to take shelter from mass shooting events. Complying with these mandatory drills for the end of the world, it occurred to me as a child (and to others, of course, we were the sixties generation) that the grown-ups were idiots, offering us up to be incinerated. The adults did not have our best interests at heart. Riding our bikes under the canopy of elm trees, (before Dutch elm disease wiped them out) whose branches reached to touch from opposite sides of the street, forming a leafy roof above our heads on Hartzell Street, in Evanston, Illinois, we talked back and forth about the imminent end of the world. When my aunt and uncle, she one of the first women cartoonists in the United States, Cissie Peltz, and he, Richard Peltz, a philosophy professor, considered building a bomb shelter in the backyard of their Whitefish Bay, Milwaukee, suburban home, my family made fun of them. We were not into self-protection, obviously. "Whenever you didn't call, we assumed you were dead," my aunt said to me much later about my father's violence. At the same time, building a bomb shelter to "protect" one's own family seemed hardly the answer to nuclear terror. We four, my mother, brother, father and I, ridiculed Cissie and Dick for believing they could survive an atomic war in their backyard bunker underground. There was public discussion in those years about whether or not you should have a gun and would be justified shooting your neighbors if they tried to enter your bomb shelter when, obviously, they would also eat your limited supply of canned foods. I do not remember when I first thought war was ridiculous, that violence solved nothing and was terrorizing. It seemed I'd been bred to be a pacifist.

As my relationship with Burl continued to fray, I desperately needed passionate commitment. I found it among the women in the antinuclear movement. The Women's Peace Encampment at Seneca Falls of 1983, like the two Women's Marches on the Pentagon in the fall of 1980 and '81, and the Women and Life on Earth Conference between them, were feminist responses to the nuclear threat. At this time, the US was planning on deploying nuclear missiles on trucks that would drive around Europe, pointing at the Soviet Union—a strategy for Armageddon, and one that terrified the Europeans. There were large anti-nuclear demonstrations in Europe and the US. I missed the first Pentagon action, about to give birth. I went to the Women and Life on Earth Conference with my child in my arms, so small, I bathed her in the motel sink. I accompanied Dorothy Dinnerstein, who was one of the speakers; Ynestra King organized the event and both of the Women's Pentagon Actions. In November of 1981, I joined a silent procession of women with puppets and banners walking through the rows of graves at Arlington National Cemetery to the steps of the Pentagon close-by. Symbolically, using yarn, like weavers in so many myths, we wove the Pentagon doors closed. We planted a cardboard cemetery on its lawn—for victims yet to come. I expressed my breast milk into a Pentagon public toilet underground in the basement, feeling this, too, an ironic ritual action of sorts (my baby was safely at home with her father). We were ecofeminists in the 1980s, quite aware of the catastrophes of deadly wars and of climate disruptions in the post-World War II world as petrochemical products were repurposed for domestic use, like the herbicide my father sprayed on his roses, inhaling the poison, and the Soviet Union and United States stockpiled quantities of nuclear weapons. The collectively devised Unity Statement for these actions, edited by Grace Paley, in her voice, as pertinent today as it was visionary then, began:

> *We are women who have come together to act on a common hope in a fearful time. We enter the eighties with alarm for the future of our planet. The forces that control our society threaten our very existence with nuclear weapons and power plants, toxic wastes and genetic engineering. A society and world economy organized for the profit of a small number of white men has created the conditions for widespread unemployment, violence at home and in the streets, oppression of third world peoples, racist attacks, inadequate food, housing and health care, and finally, the ecological devastation of the earth.*

Dorothy and I spent hours at her dilapidated summer home on the North Fork of Long Island, side-stroking in the bay, face to face, talking as we swam. She was struggling to articulate the central ideas in a second book to be called *Sense and Sentience*. Her first, *The Mermaid and the Minotaur*, published in 1976, became an instant classic, when feminist Vivian Gornick recognized its brilliance in her front-page review for the *New York Times Sunday Book Review*. Making a strong psychological case for the equal parenting of babies and children by women and men, Dorothy's book changed the way children are raised. (Before *Mermaid*, men were seldom seen carrying small infants on their chests in snuggles or caring for small children in public; after *Mermaid*, nurturant men became cool.) Dorothy was attracted to my plays, because in them I often showed men as nurturers and women as doers. But Dorothy could not find a similar simple and profound explanation for human beings' conscious and willful destruction of the natural world we profess to love and which sustains us. She was in the early stages of memory loss, and terrified, but because she was brilliant, it was easy for her women friends to ignore her complaints about her failing mind. But her writer's block went deeper than that, and despite her best efforts, no one—not Freud or Marx, or any of the great thinkers to come after—has truly been able to understand in a way that would cause us to change, why humankind is so bent on the violent destruction of its own kind, and of the living world.

Dorothy Dinnerstein and Grace Paley were beautiful, full-breasted women, lusty and lively, brilliant, each in her way. Grace was a master of quick wit, Dorothy of deep thought. They wore their hair long and wild and wore dresses, not pants. Dorothy dressed often in bed sheets she had sown into caftans of sorts and walked barefoot at her country house. She was intellectual and sexual; she loved the natural world with a passion—snorkeling was a hobby and she hoped to visit many more coral wreaths before their destruction by rising sea temperatures. Like me, she tended toward depression. Grace was wryly funny; a writer of masterly short stories, she had keen insight into people and could sum up their salient character traits in a sentence or phrase. Judith, Grace and Dorothy, each older than I by nearly two decades, had borne children; each took me aside when I was pregnant and as if reading from a shared script, each one told me in a confidential voice, "this is a wonderful time for creative work. You are so busy making a new life, you don't give a fuck what your critics say." Grace was married a second time to her great love, Bob Nichols, who wrote the summer street plays for George Bartenieff and Crystal Field at Theater for the New City, until Bob quarreled with Crystal one last time and decamped permanently to Vermont. Grace divided her time between her apartment on 11th Street in the West Village and his land. Grace died of breast cancer in Vermont in 2007, attended by Bob and family. Dorothy was less lucky. Her second marriage was also to her great love, chair of the psychology department at Rutgers, in which she taught—and the reason she got tenure, as feminist women were regularly being denied permanent jobs despite their brilliance unless they slept with the department chair—but Danny was vastly overweight and he soon died. She told me he was so fat, they had trouble, at first, figuring out a position in which he might penetrate her. When I first met Dorothy at the Women's Salon where she read from her book, she had recently married an African-Jew who was her tour guide in Kenya. She took a trip to flee her grief; she came home with a new husband, handsome, dark and kind. As a young Mau-Mau in the war of liberation, Benny was badly tortured by the British. He escaped execution only because his fellow prisoners knocked him unconscious and chopped off his chains. They threw him into the sewer, hoping the filthy water would wake him and he could swim to his freedom. It worked. But American feminism was a freedom fight of altogether another sort. Benny became alarmed when arriving in Leonia, New Jersey, with his new American wife, he found she had a full life comprised of independent women. He demanded she stay home. She went out, complaining to us all. Culturally unmoored, he became increasingly domineering and threatening. Finally, he decided to go, or was sent, home to Kenya, for he was a gentle soul. Dorothy was free but alone without a love as her memory failed.

In the summer of 1983, Julian Beck was diagnosed and operated on for metastasized colon cancer, and he was preparing what would be his final play script, *The Archaeology of Sleep*, in Nantes, France. In a way, his final work sought to realize Dorothy's question how can we become fully sentient beings, protecting the natural world. It did so by showing on the stage that in our dream lives we experience vivid sights infused with wishful imagination and thoughts that might, if remembered when we woke, enhance the development of the human race—or so Julian wished to believe.

In July 1983, Barbara Deming, fragile with terminal ovarian cancer, was arrested with other women trying to walk over a bridge and imprisoned for five days in a makeshift jail in an elementary school, in Waterloo, New York. We were camping out, with our children if we had them, that summer at the Seneca Women's Encampment for a Future of Peace and Justice, in upstate New York. The women-only community was on land women had bought for this purpose. We were there to protest the scheduled deployment of Cruise and Pershing II missiles before their suspected shipment to Europe in the fall from the Seneca Army Depot we surrounded during the days. A neutron bomb was also stored at the military base in rural upstate New York. We were putting our sentient selves on the line to avert nuclear destruction. Dorothy and Grace were there and I was sharing a tent with Dorothy's daughter, Naomi, and my three-year old child. During the long summer days, we talked about peace, life, and disarmament through the fences with the young soldiers guarding the bombs; we danced and sang, and symbolically wove the gates closed with yarn so the missiles could not pass.

We had a Women's March planned from our encampment through the town of Waterloo to Seneca Falls on July 30, the anniversary of Elizabeth Cady Stanton's 1848 Women's Rights Convention. A scene was about to unfold on a bridge that prefigured what the country was to become in the twenty-first century with Donald Trump's ascent to power after coming down the golden elevator in 2015. We intended to walk peacefully to Seneca Falls where women of the previous century had advocated for women's rights. This upstate New York land we marched through was the ancestral home of the Iroquois Nation and was where the tribal women gathered in 1590, to form the Iroquois Confederacy, a union that successfully put an end to the tribal wars devastating Iroquois life. The Native women leaders forced the Iroquois men of different tribes to come together to form a federation that, while preserving each tribe's individuality, united them under a single rule (the Iroquois Federation influenced the new United States when it formed a federalist government comprised of semi-independent states). We had a permit for our march, which was simply a nonviolent walk in support of the Equal Rights for Women constitutional amendment (unratified still). It was a bright, sunny day with trouble ahead. We were met on the bridge in Waterloo, New York, by a large citizens' brigade of white men carrying guns. Twenty miles away was Harriet Tubman's home, a stop on the Underground Railroad. This march of women through "their" town of Waterloo in 1983, was considered dastardly provocation by the white men who shouldered their guns to intimidate, block, and make us submit to their show of force. Women, evidently, were not supposed to walk in a group. The Congresswoman Bella Abzug marched among Grace, Dorothy, Ynestra and Barbara Deming, who was fragile, ill, and undaunted.

Blocked by the armed men, we women sat down on the bridge, in nonviolent defiance, while the men taunted us: "lezzies," "communists," they called us. One line of women formed on the bridge facing the men. Behind our front line, the rest of the women sat down in a circle to better discuss what to do. The sun was glinting fiercely off the white t-shirts of the white men, turning bright the dark, curly hair on their muscled arms that pointed their hunting rifles and handguns (before the AK-47) in the ready position, directly at us. The sun was so bright I could not see the looks on their faces. Had they thought we would turn and run, or beg, or renounce our ways and submit to their show of force, give in to those who "knew best" for us? Martin Luther King had called for the marchers to kneel on the Pettus Bridge to avoid being beaten. Many of us knew the story. Certainly, Barbara Deming did; she'd been a Freedom Rider. I do not know who gave us the signal to sit but we complied as if we had pre-agreed, yet none of us could have imagined this sight, a militia of white men facing off against women, some of us with our children, walking peacefully for an end to nuclear terror, for the right to love whom we chose, and for the environmental integrity of the living world.

My blond three-year-old, dressed in a red, white, and blue striped bathing suit, and I quickly wiggled away from the seated women and blended into the watching crowd. I put my little daughter on my shoulders. We had been warned that women with children camping out against nuclear proliferation could have our children removed by child welfare services and sent to live with local white families who disapproved of our actions. Standing among mainly the wives and families of the armed men (though at least one or two women, the wife of a banker among them, spontaneously joined the women's sit-down on the bridge), my child and I watched while a flatbed truck pulled up to arrest the nonviolent women still being held at gunpoint by the men. I watched with my child as the women on the bridge, who had committed no crime, who had simply sat down unwilling to move, were marched up a ramp into a truck to be carted away to their prison in a school. Barbara, ill with cancer and weak, had her fist in the air in a Black Power salute, as she walked the ramp and I told my daughter who she was, "a great, pacifist woman," I said. "You will read her work someday." Barbara had recently published a new book *We Cannot Live Without Our Lives*—she was referring to Catherine Earnshaw's plea in *Wuthering Heights* that she cannot live without Heathcliff, in Barbara's reading, the necessary masculine part of herself. Barbara, from her perspective as a lesbian, and Dorothy, an avowed heterosexual, were in agreement that to be whole we had to become androgynous beings.

The women arrested on the Waterloo Bridge remained jailed inside a local school for nearly a week. The men most likely returned home with a sense of satisfaction of a job well done to dinners prepared by their wives. I made my way with my child and Dorothy, Naomi, Grace and her friend, Sybil Claiborne to a motel room that had been occupied by Grace and Bella Abzug the night before and now was a welcome respite after our days camping outside—though many of our friends were in prison. Bella Abzug had left her nightgown behind and we had fun trying on the flimsy, flowered, feminine thing, so unlike her powerful voice and words.

In a video interview Barbara gave shortly after her release, one week after her arrest, she remembers the scene on the bridge: "Go home commies. Go home Jews. Nuke the lezzies," were the chants of the armed men. They perceived, very accurately, we were a threat to patriarchy," she leaned forward and said in her voice like a whisper. On the bridge, seated in their circle, the women discussed what to do. They came to a collective decision not to leave the bridge but to allow themselves to be arrested. "What gave me so much hope for the future," Barbara says, was this way of "slowing down time," witnessed by the men on the bridge and then by their jailers, a commitment to deliberation maintained even in their schoolhouse prison so that each woman had a chance to speak and be heard. In this way, reminiscent of a Quaker Meeting, the entire group could think things through. Early one morning, two women made a jailbreak from the school, climbing out through a window. The other fifty-three prisoners were marched into the cold halls and threatened with being strip-searched. The guards made a show of pulling on rubber gloves. "Do you think you will find the missing women in our vaginas?" a woman had the wit to ask. "What thrilled me," Barbara repeats, both about the debate on the bridge and later, the earnest discussions in the school-turned-jail, is how, "as the police observed it, I could see them begin to respect it" –this slowness, this shared deliberation that took everyone's voice into account was at the heart of Barbara's view of nonviolent action.

"Nonviolence is androgynous," Barbara liked to point out, a word much in favor among us at that time before "they" and "them" pronouns became used to denote much the same thing, a mix of "female" and "male" attributes, a nurturant strength. The unarmed women sitting down in nonviolent defiance threatened the system's male supremacy in every way. The women's insistent respect for each voice, their willingness not to do until they had thoroughly discussed, had, Barbara is certain, an effect. Going fast is a waste, she says. To achieve nonviolence, time has to be slowed. Only then does perception have the time in which to change, only then is there the possibility for true inclusion of every person's voice. Slowing down time is a tactic the Living Theatre frequently used in *The Archaeology of Sleep*, Julian's final play, in *Seven Meditations on Political Sado-Masochism*, in *Mysteries and Smaller Pieces* and in other works. Making us sit and take in, making us watch, wait and contemplate. Nonviolence, Barbara says, is an act of *invention*, sitting down on that bridge in Waterloo was a form of street theater, in fact—an improvised action intended to teach. And although ill, Barbara was strengthened and heartened by being in this way in jail, because the women's decision to take the time to hear and value each voice, and to make decisions collectively, no matter how long that took, released a deeper creativity of the sort she felt certain was of instruction even to their jailers. Barbara walking up the ramp into the truck, her fist in the air, was my last sight of Barbara alive. After her days in prison, she returned to her lesbian commune in Florida, where she would create a stunning, communal death ritual, but not yet.

The autumn before the encampment, Burl and I had gone to the Hamptons for the weekend. "Put that kid to bed, I want to have sex." He did not normally speak to me like that. He told me he would not make theater with me, again; it was too hard. He was turning all his attention to the summer festival he had started in Prospect Park, and for which he had funding from the city and state. A few weeks later, the word "Sappho" came into my head in a dream. I began researching and writing a play that I could do without him. Though we shared the loft and he fully participated in raising our child, we had little in common. He was without the need for emotional closeness I craved. Sometimes I wondered if having grown up on a farm in the bare flatlands of west Texas, as a Future Farmer of America, raising pigs for slaughter, had shut down his desire to feel. Pigs are highly intelligent, communicative animals; like dogs, they come when called and bond with their humans. What was it like to care for creatures, walk them and make noises to which they responded, to look in their eyes, then slaughter and eat them for dinner? I had wanted to stop eating meat when the pet lamb at my horse trainers' farm appeared on the table as chops. I became a vegetarian in my early twenties out of my love for animals. Though we still lived together, Burl and I were increasingly distant—with separate work and without shared interests. I was lonely and estranged from the man with whom I still shared a bed and sometimes had sex, but I did not know how, when or with whom, I might change my life.

In 1984, I finished my play *Sappho and Aphrodite*. I read it aloud one night at a weekend gathering of women at Dorothy's summer home on Long Island Sound. Her beautiful daughter, Naomi, was there and after the reading, we began a brief love affair—we were both living with others. We workshopped my play at Smith College, in the Hallie Flanagan Theater, the summer of 1984. It was directed by Lois Weaver, who was about to found Split Britches, a lesbian theater, with her longtime partner, Peggy Shaw. In Northampton, we all lived together in the large country house of two women science professors. The original score was by a lesbian composer, Roberta Kosse. Sappho was played by the Black lesbian actor Beverly Wideman. The drummer was the wondrous, fierce, Edwina Lee Tyler, one of the first out lesbian Black drummers to emerge on the New York music scene. In my notes to the published play, I state that the play must always be staged with a mixed-race cast, and that a Black actor always be cast as Sappho. The isle of Lesbos is not far from the African continent, but more than that, I wished to acknowledge the role Black women have played in the struggle for equal justice. I dedicated my play to Barbara Deming.

Julian had a part in a major Hollywood film. He was to play the gangster, Sol Weinstein, in Frances Ford Coppola's *Cotton Club*, and the Living suddenly had cash. They came home to New York in 1984, to present three new, large works at the Joyce Theater. They hoped to revive and secure their reputation in the United States as they had done on their electric American tour, in 1968-'69. Judith was tired of constantly touring in Europe. She wanted to base the company permanently in New York, but the times were different—Ronald Reagan was president. Julian had been diagnosed with colon cancer in France.

New Cycle Theater, now run by me alone, was still a resident theater of The Arts at St. Ann's, which was still located in the large church in downtown Brooklyn. But my lesbian play deeply upset the Episcopalians. And, of course, X could hardly wait to get rid of me; she was still pining for Burl. After negotiations, I was allowed to present three performances in Brooklyn—then my city funding would be pulled. But the play had won the attention of a lesbian music producer, Virginia Giordano, who moved it into Manhattan. In 1984, the *New York Times* would not run an ad with the words "Sappho and Aphrodite", nor would a single male *Times* theater critic come to review it. "You can't write like that," a male dramaturg angrily told me. "You cannot use the word, vulva in a play."

"But I already have," I replied. "Vulva like folds of the sea."

Jennifer Dunning, the *Times'* dance critic, and an admirer of Virginia's producing skills, wrote, quite favorably about the play under the guise that my poetic text was actually a dance drama. "She's nothing but a chicken hawk," a white-haired lesbian, in jeans, said in disgust as she walked up the aisle during intermission, speaking of Sappho and her affair with her young, favored student, Atthis, and I wondered if she were right. Judith took another view: "Such tenderness as you deal with so tenderly is hardly permissible in our ice-hard culture. And what great homage to your skill that one can't tell where the ancient poet ended and the living poet takes up," she wrote in her introduction to the published text. Erika Munk, theater editor and critic for the *Village Voice*, sat next to Julian on opening night; she whispered a nonstop screed of insults about the play into Julian's ear. At intermission, he changed seats with Judith; he couldn't stand what he'd heard. "Don't pay any attention to the press," he gently counseled me. Erika damned the play in the voice. The producer and I made love in her car on opening night. We were very stoned. The sex was a big mistake on my part, as I was not attracted in any way, but my gratitude to her made me feel I "should," and the location, a car, had submissive sexual resonance. I still did as I was asked, but, when I could not continue our affair, she was furious. She had planned on a hit production and a great fling with me. In 1984, *Sappho and Aphrodite* was controversial. So was Julian's final work, *The Archeology of Sleep*.

(An aside about theater critics: Years later, I was at a party with Erika Munk; she complained to the host, our mutual friend, that I had been rude to her. Erika brutally slammed two of my plays, *Rebekkah* and *Sappho and Aphrodite* in the *Village Voice*, I explained. Erika told the host she had never reviewed any of my plays. "But I have the reviews in my file," I said. She had no memory of them; they must have been written when she was "an alcoholic," she said.)

In an interview Julian gave two weeks before his death in September 1985, he describes his reaction to receiving the cancer diagnosis:

> *I am sure I turned pale in the doctor's office. We got into the car and just talked for half an hour. Judith said right away, "you've got to fight this." I said, "I'm going to." We talked about ways to do it. We had been commissioned by the French government to do a new play we were going to take on tour. So, I worked on writing, putting together the collective ideas of the group, creating* The Archaeology of Sleep. *I battered away at the typewriter and finished the play about one o'clock in the afternoon one day. We all drove into Nantes and went to the theater. I read the play to the company and there was great enthusiasm. Then I picked up my bag and went to the hospital for the operation. The company went to work on the play by themselves with Judith there to direct.*
>
> *A curious thing happened then, and I should preface this by saying Judith and I had never been sick a day in our lives. Well, Judith*

had been having a pain in her side and had gone to male doctor after male doctor and each of them told her, it's just a neurosis; it's not anything real. Well, we finally found a doctor in Nantes who said, "oh my god you have to be operated on immediately. Your gall bladder is about to burst." So, she went to the hospital, too. We had adjoining rooms.

Meanwhile the company rallied marvelously. They would come to the hospital for advice and go over staging with Judith and the scenic appurtenances with me. It was a kind of heroic period. We got out of the hospital with about five or six days to go before opening, and the opening was marvelous. The play was beautiful and extremely well liked.

The last works of major artists are sometimes hardest to comprehend, as people on the edge between life and death break their own forms. Edward Said focuses on the confounding brilliance of last works of composers like Bach, playwrights Genet, Ibsen, and Euripides in his own last work (written while he was dying of leukemia) *Late Style*. Julian describes his intentions for *The Archaeology of Sleep*, in the prologue to the published script: "I wanted people to see that we go to bed full of hope, because I think that in our sleep-life we have these immortal urgings that begin to be expressed. It is my theory that we try every night, as an evolving species to figure out how we can go on to the next step, the development of humankind." If only we could remember our dreams. In dreams, we have wished our fulfillment, not as individuals so much but as dreamers for the collective whole. Julian might equally have been describing the final works of the playwrights Said writes about—*The Screens, When We Dead Awaken, The Bacchae*—each substitutes vision for reason, each haunts the realms of the dead, each astonishes. Written on a precipice, as Said says, last works abandon formal restrictions. If last works are not easily understood, that is because they are not entirely of this world. It is pure Julian to assume that we use our dreams to advance the development of humankind. How good it would be if it were true. In any case, the thought makes it worth suspending disbelief to engage with a challenging theater piece.

The Archaeology of Sleep is a meditation on sleep science, as the monitoring of brain waves during rem sleep was just then, in the 1980s, emerging, and it is a phantasmagoric trip through the dream imagery of company members Julian interviewed. "One is love," is a repeated refrain. In our sleep we might leap. Individuals and the human race might evolve and advance from knowledge gained in our sleep. Gathering dreams from a collective of artists who lived and worked together to advance shared ideals ("the beautiful, nonviolent, anarchist revolution"), Julian created a series of vivid, visual meditations that made us see and experience dream life as one, the collective audience. If sleep is the shared portal into the unknown, which we enter unconsciously but from which we might wake in possession of new understandings—then who knows what leaps of understanding might happen, if we are allowed to dream collectively in theater works like this one he was making. His was a completely audacious last work.

While Julian wove together the dream images of Living Theatre company members for the play he was creating in France, knowing he had a potentially terminal disease, I was in a dream group in New York with four feminist women. Convened by Dorothy Dinnerstein, our group included Ann Snitow, Eve Merriam, and Sybil Claiborne; all three feminist writers would die too soon from cancer. Dorothy was rattled because, as her memory began to fail, she could no longer remember her dreams. In a way, she called us together so that we might dream for her. In our group, one person described a recent dream and the rest of us took turns stepping into the dream as if it were ours. "If I dreamt this dream, I would feel … think … associate …" we filled in the blanks, improvising. Each of us made the dream ours, and by sharing images and thoughts, the dream came to represent a relic of our collective unconscious. The dream work enlarged our own imaginative capacities and deepened our sense of solidarity. We all had recurring dreams of ever-changing, expanding, increasingly luxurious, or tiny, constricting, decrepit "homes." Homes that became larger or smaller, more elegant or more rundown, depending upon the state of our waking minds, of our work and love lives. (The five women in the group had had fifteen husbands, and I still had one husband to come.) I still have recurring dreams of living in unfamiliar spaces that are barely tolerable, or large and expansive, and I still dream of struggling to find my way home to unfamiliar, hostile or welcoming neighborhoods. I am the only member of our dream group left alive. Dream work was on many of our minds in the 1980s—when we were metamorphosing as women, and Julian, too, was looking, as always, for transformative knowledge. I used Dorothy's shared dreaming techniques with students at the Tisch School of the Arts for several years—at the end of the semester, they were required to make a work of art (anything they chose, and though they were all studying acting they painted or wrote, sang, played music, or improvised). Each of the students found their imaginations freed and enhanced by the semester's shared immersion into their own and the other students' dreams.

Sleep is an audacious study on the part of a man who has terminal cancer. His final work, not, of course, about his own death, as final works seldom are, was nevertheless like other perplexing far-reaching last works, written on the precipice where one sees both ways at once, into the origins of self and beyond, to Julian's dream of collective leaps that would propel humankind past the violence holding us back. The idiosyncratic nature of his vision included the wry humor of his fascination with Egyptian temple cats who, played by sinuous actors, become central characters in his drama. He created a sleep train, on which dream imagery created by actors in space moved slowly into our view, and out, again. His willingness to slow stage time into a meditative trance with moments of stunning visual shapes, forced the audience to abandon our thinking minds and become part of the meditative rhythm of the play and, perhaps, in these lapses of time marching forward, to reach more deeply inside, and to experience perplexing dream-life together. His sleep play was unique and brave, and not easily intelligible by intellect alone. It truly demanded we suspend disbelief. Unlike 1968's *Paradise Now*, which demanded audience action—take off your clothes, burn some money, have sex on stage, take the revolution into the streets—the 1984, *Archaeology of Sleep* sought collective introspection, by putting on stage the shared dream experience Like most late-style plays, *The Archaeology of Sleep* asked its audience to do some serious imaginative work.

While in Europe, the Living had abandoned their *Legacy of Cain* cycle of short street plays in order to create large works funded by and suitable for performance at the big European festivals. For their return to New York, they would present three new works premiered in Europe, each created by one of the now three Living Theatre directors. Hanon Reznikov Judith's long-term lover had become an equal partner. Hanon conceived and directed *The Yellow Methuselah,* based on Shaw's wry *Back to Methuselah,* and the work of the abstract painter, Kandinsky. Judith reached into her German artistic heritage to translate and direct a production of Ernst Toller's *Masse Mensch (The One and the Many),* an expressionist play about revolutionaries from between the two world wars. Julian's *The Archaeology of Sleep,* was not an adaptation of a classic, but an original work. These three made an ambitious program. But hope for a repeat of their American success in '68-'69 was bitterly crushed when all three plays were brutally panned in the New York press. Julian's *Archeology of Sleep* was particularly despised by the critics. He was told he was "passé," "ridiculous," "out of touch," "a druggie," and worse, that the Living Theatre had been fraudulent all its life—by the all-powerful critic of the *New York Times*. Their past successes were nothing. They deserved no reverence. Beck and Malina were frauds who had put something over on gullible audiences for decades. A young Frank Rich, then lead theater critic for the *New York Times*, later, a liberal political commentator on their op-ed page, led the attack. After the premiere performance of Julian's *Sleep* play, Jack Gelber, standing outside on the sidewalk, overheard Rich leading the other critics who had been in the audience in a discussion about how they all would damn the play. They agreed on the sidewalk to shared condemnation. During the performance, Julian had touched Rich somewhere on his body, as he passed through the audience with the other actors, asking gently, "are you afraid if I touch you like this?" Frank Rich was.

"Though Mr. Beck and his partner, Judith Malina, are still turning their old tricks, their gimmicks look tacky now. In 1984, we can see the Living Theatre's sexual assaults for what they are: pathetic and impotent attempts to camouflage the troupe's far cruder assaults on our brains."

In 1998, unrepentant, Rich added this note to his review: "The Beck-Malina troupe had almost no resemblance to the company that electrified the theater with Frankenstein some fifteen years earlier. It now seemed instead like a demented cult that had lost its way after too many years abroad and too many drugs. This was, however, the only time that I was actually molested in the theater—an experience so weird I was more stunned than angry."

—

Garrick Beck, who happened to be standing upstairs in the mezzanine, had a clear view of the scene. He watched while Julian put his hand gently on Frank Rich's thigh—hardly a sexual assault. Competing narratives, no doubt, but it is difficult to imagine Julian "actually molesting" a man seated on the aisle with a notebook on his lap, obviously a critic. Though, one wonders what made Julian touch Rich at all—perhaps his attachment to Sacher-Masoch.

Julian was used to respect and praise in Europe, as due an artist. He was friends with intellectuals like Michel Foucault and with Jean Genet. The Cultural Minister of France had commissioned, funded, and praised *The Archaeology of Sleep*. In his hometown of New York, in his hometown newspaper, he was described as a demented drug addict and a sexual predator who "assaulted" Frank Rich. George remembered Julian standing alone and forlorn in the lobby of Theater for the New City. Julian could not understand the hate, nor the personal assaults. The New York critics had also brutally attacked Judith and Julian's daughter, Isha Manna, then a new graduate from the Tisch School of the Arts (where she was a student in my Ibsen class) and performing, again, with her parents' theater. Julian asked George, in a tired voice, "What is wrong with New York?" He looked thin and beaten.

Surely the trauma caused by the hate-filled reviews, collectively decided upon in a sidewalk huddle so that no one critic would be "wrong" but all were united, and the premature closing of all three plays, ending any possibility of a tour, did no good for Julian's health. There would be no triumphant recognition, as there had been the last time they returned home, in 1969, at the height of the antiwar movement. Yet Julian, ill with cancer, had no choice but to rise above, and after the initial shock, which was severe, we did not speak of those events again.

He continued writing his last book, *Theandric*. "In this book we are watching the wrestling match between Death and the Poet," Judith wrote in her afterword to the published volume. Julian continued to act in film, television, and on the stage, creating masterful performances in *The Cotton Club, Poltergeist II*, and in Samuel Beckett. The community around him strengthened. We were the bulwark against the disease. We gathered around him at Mount Sinai Hospital and at 800 West End Avenue, always in celebratory fashion. We'd been summoned by Judith at Julian's request to form the loving community. He would share with us his life with cancer as he'd shared every part of his life with artists always.

It was silent and still when I opened the door to his Mount Sinai hospital room, which was usually crowded with friends, hangers-on, old company members, poets, musicians. Judith would be telling stories from her chair next to Julian's bed, stoned. The sounds of chants, laughter, song. Julian sitting up at the center of it all, his beatific smile on his wan face. But now he lay, alone, curled, a chrysalis about to change form, in the hospital bed, the bars up, a crib, his long form dissolved into a series of yellow-gold circles, like one of his abstract expressionist paintings, knees into chin, arms looped about spindly legs, feet fallen at sharp angles. Head on stretched neck bent to the side. Eyes closed. He did not know I had come. I reached down to touch some part of him. A bony shoulder, a limb. "Whither thou goest I will go. Your people will be my people and your god my god," I whispered. A sudden, sharp turn of the head, bright, angry eyes staring up, a voice, not quite his but from deep. "I am *not going* to die," he hissed. He had a gorgeous, full voice, the voice of a man in command. These words were barely audible, but enraged. Quite clear. I said nothing more. I removed my hand from his fragile flesh. Took a breath and a step back. I stayed at his bed.

So, he would not be dying. I understood. Though we each understood dying was exactly what he was doing and would continue to do until he was dead, all too soon, of the cancer that could not be cured. But death was to be no concern of ours. I had overstepped with my words. I vowed, silently, never to speak of death again. I never did, a pledge I know he received. In this way, we were comforted. Death would come, but we would not stoop to acknowledge the fact. Never stop living long enough. Love is what lures us to stand in the shadow of death. Only those who haven't dared love can refuse death's siren call. And I loved both of them. Judith Malina and Julian Beck were as close as any family I have. My mother, when we grew closer, after Julian's death, looked upon Judith as a close relation. But what also brought me to Julian's side during the final years of his life was an unstated, selfish need to remake my own. I was living then in a strange situation, still with the man, Burl, with whom I had started New Cycle Theater in Brooklyn, and with whom I had a child. But he had moved on to creating and producing Celebrate Brooklyn, a large summer festival at the Prospect Park Band Shell. I was on my own with my theater work, and very much on my own emotionally as well, as he was decent but extremely removed. Worse, Burl's whatever it was with the woman X, who was becoming an ever-more-powerful producer in Brooklyn, had also queered any hope I might have had to continue making theater in the borough where I lived. I was blacklisted, so to speak, while her power over funding and arts producing grew. I was at loose ends, without professional or personal focus.

So often, by giving to someone else, we receive back an essence of ourselves, uncovered, unrecognized, perhaps not fully formed, an essence we'd misplaced long before, or never had known but without which we will never be whole. By sinking down into another, by giving, we reseed ourselves in more fertile ground. Nothing was consciously done. I was drawn by my love for Julian to a place at his side where even though he was dying, while he died, we'd made a pledge to share our devotion, not in grief, but in joy, and, here, in his hospital room life was happening—vivid, unpredictable, nurturant. The communal life in which he and Judith always thrived. In ways I could never have guessed, attending to Julian brought me the rest of my life. I would enter into a mad, sexually ecstatic, emotionally draining affair and emerge hurt to the core, my life in shreds, but would then write the play that would bring me to George. Grief is a furnace in which we are melted down like raw ore and we ooze into new shape as the fire in the life that we mourn goes out. Or, at least, that is what happened, then, when I was just entering my forties.

1984. The Seder:

All night. I am tongue-tied about the illness and (recent) operation. As we leave, Carrie Sophia goes up to Julian. She speaks for me when I cannot.

"Julian, don't you get sick ever again," she commands with all the authority of her four-year-old self, her bright green eyes looking up, pretty in her new green and blue holiday dress.

"I won't," Julian promises, smiling his radiant smile. "I won't." She is comforted and we leave happy.

May 14, 1984:

Yesterday, Allen Ginsberg and I visit Julian at the same time. When Allen tells Julian to "let go," tells him that when his father died, Rinpoche (his guru) told Allen to just "let go of him" and that when he did so, he felt immensely better, Julian replies sitting straight in his hospital bed, "but you don't understand, it's *me* I would have to let go of and I'm not ready to do that." Allen has no response. He says his good-bye. Later, as I leave his hospital room, Julian whispers, "it's going to be all right."

June 25, 1984:

Changing every plan, in fear for Julian's life and wanting to be with Judith, I rush home from my artists' residency in Minneapolis, pick up child in Chicago, see mother, aunt, grandmother briefly, arrive, drop my bags and run to the hospital uptown where Julian, sitting up with a prayer shawl around his shoulders, is surrounded by several handsome men. S. is there from Vermont and Andy Nadelson (a gifted composer who soon would die of AIDS). S. is an acupuncturist. He has been working with pressure points on Julian, hoping to build him up so he can tolerate acupuncture needles in his hurt flesh. Julian's eyes are clear; his voice is strong. He looks much better. He is clearly happy to see me and says, "I enjoyed your letters. Your writing has improved." I'm mortified.

S. was beautiful and wounded, like my father. He was dark, like him, with large, dark eyes that contained the wound. He was French-Algerian, child of mixed parentage and of the French-Algerian war. He spoke with a lovely accent. He knew how to flatter, how to please. He smelled of, moved as if, smiled like after sex. There was nothing else a woman could do with such a man but be fucked by him. But I could do something else, too. I would write my second cancer play, the play that would change my life. Much later, after I was living with George, S. would return, lurking about at a book launch I had, coming to the production of a play. He wanted to write plays himself. He did write one and it was staged, but S. was not a playwright, as he claimed to be but a hurt poseur. I thought when we met a few times, years later, meetings I hid from George as I hid little else, that S.'s fascination all along had been that he wished not to love me but to be who I was: a writer, a theater creator. But when we met at Julian's bedside, I thought of S. as a magical healer whose considerable powers would benefit my friend. S.'s long fingers were dancing lightly on Julian's bony body. He had the air of calm confidence associated with healing. He made his living as an acupuncturist. The mother of his son, with whom he lived as a family unit in Vermont, was a physician and homeopathic medicine provider. (Which means that S. was, then, taking his identity as a healer from her, as he spoke with seeming authority of the arcane world of disease.) Like many a wounded person, S. had scant access to his own sorrow; he did not want to dwell on his own pain, which was considerable; he would rather inflict it on others. He was a user because he had no idea who he was, hiding his pain with a winning smile. (He was, in fact, an accomplished gigolo. But, if so, what, then, was I? Captive of desire, a home wrecker, wrecking his home and mine.) He had the finely chiseled face Living Theatre men shared, like little Julians—they didn't eat much—a lithe, just slightly stooped frame. I thought he was gorgeous. Dark and mysterious. My Heathcliff. My demon lover come to life. He always wore a suit jacket with a dress shirt open at the throat. He spoke softly and was polite. I was about to become unthawed after two decades of grief, locked tight. Two decades in which I had given myself to many men and women, often, unfeelingly, because I thought I should, without love because I did not know what love was. I had married the man my father targeted on the asphalt driveway, left him, then settled down with a decent yet closed-off fellow who, though he knew Julian was my dear friend, refused to visit him even once while he was ill. If he had come with me to the hospital, S. and I never ... I would now betray him with S. Neither of us could stop ourselves. Drawn together by our love for the man who watched us aghast from his Mount Sinai hospital bed. Drawn together by our own sorrows. Julian had been madly in love with a younger, gorgeous Italian who left him, as S. would leave me, and I needed to be left by S. Even at the start, I knew I could not live with such a person. We inevitably would leave each other, but Julian was especially concerned. Trauma and cancer were connected in Julian's mind:

> *When I first found out I had cancer, in March of 1983, I asked how long the cancer had been growing. The doctor thought anywhere from two to three years. I immediately calculated that three years earlier there had been three very significant events in my life. The most significant of which was the loss of the person I had been in love with who said to me one day, 'it's over, I'm going away.' (italics added) Then, just one week later, my mother died. We had had a very good, solid relationship. Then when I returned to Europe, I began working like crazy on* The Yellow Methuselah. *It was five months of the most strenuous work imaginable: building and painting the set and making 150 costumes. I hardly slept at all. I didn't eat. My body was under enormous stress. Finding out I had cancer, I made the connection between that stress and my health. I realized immediately that I had to change my form of life. I had abused myself, and felt abused by the world, so I simply had to take better care of myself. And that has been part of the therapy.*

The second time S. and I met in Julian's room, Judith was distraught; she had dropped an amethyst somewhere in Central Park someone had given her as a charm. She feared her lost luck. S. and I volunteered to go back to Central Park at night to look for the crystal. This was the perfect chance to be alone. It was raining lightly. When we returned to Julian's room, it was too late for any warning. All was written on our faces. We found the crystal, picked it up in the wet and we had kissed in the rain in the park. We made love at 800 West End Avenue, that same night.

"He's a vile seducer," Julian told me, thinking of his own gorgeous Italian lover. He and Judith had seen how S. treated our friend Rain House, who had become sexually enslaved. S. entered the Living Theatre in Europe by sleeping his way in, as many people did. There was a company rule; one's erotic love was always allowed to join the troupe. S. seduced the lovely Black person who went as a woman named Rain. "I thought she was a woman," S. said. He picked Rain up in a bar. It didn't matter to S. what sort of genitals Rain had, Rain was his ticket into the fabled theater then passing through the French town S. wanted to leave. S. had no moorings, no money, and he ran away with the Living, as many looking for adventure had done. Rain assured Judith and Julian, he could not live without S., and Rain was a beloved company member. Not too much later, Judith and Julian watched Rain crawl across the floor begging for sexual contact while S. smiled and stepped back. Judith described the scene to me standing at the Mount Sinai elevators. A warning. By then, I could not stop myself. "She is an exquisite lover and we are having a great time," S. told Judith when she asked him to leave me alone. Sometimes, it's impossible to be around a lot of sickness without doing a lot of sex, to paraphrase Grace.

We met frantically and furtively. We had sex where we could. Outside behind a bush. In Isha's bedroom in Julian's house, when Isha was away. In borrowed lofts. I climbed a rickety fire escape one dark night—he was not answering the bell at our appointed time in the loft where we would have a just few hours, nor was he bothering to answer the telephone when I called from a booth on the corner, but the light was on. He knew I was there. Was he sitting in an easy chair, smiling? Climbing up, my leg was caught in the bent and unstable ladder-like fire escape steps and my knee was badly swollen and scraped by the time he opened the window on which I knocked and he helped me to climb through, with a satisfied look. He liked to play small torture games. He put arnica cream on my wounds and took me to bed. Nothing was said. I did not ask why he hadn't just opened the door. Needing to be loved so much, or, rather, fucked as I'd never been fucked before. I was with a man who pleasured me, his orgasm, when it happened, was after I had had many, rolling, rising, yelping like a delirious puppy. We were just learning, then, in the eighties, how women's orgasms worked. I was feeling my body thaw. I was feeling deeply in a way I had never before. *He* was an exquisite lover. He pleasured me. We were, together, champions of erotic sport. His long, slender, purple cock reached farther inside than anyone had. His large, heavy balls were made to coddle, to suck. His fingers danced deep in my cunt. His gave tireless attention to my insides, so that his touching my flesh released me to myself. I was coming alive. "Should I buy the instruments," he asked me one night. "If I can use them on you," I said. He did not buy the handcuffs or chains, or the slender knife. Our sex in that way was pure. Pure delight. I'd never known I could respond like that. "Is it all right," I asked the night he first sodomized me. I had no idea what was happening. "It is all right, Kareen," he crooned in his French accent. I came and came again. Though I had had good lovers before—Burl, Jack Gelber, of course, more than a decade before—S.'s attention to my physical self was revelation. His stamina, and, yes, his gentleness, after all. Gentleness that was hard and relentless. There was nothing separating us, it felt. Our wounds meshed. We were so hurt, I needed to be hurt again, and he needed to inflict emotional pain, if I would not allow him to do the physical S & M thing.

When there is death, there has to be sex. Fucking to keep him alive. Julian, whom we loved. S. had been a child in the French-Algerian war. Hiding on the floor as the bombs fell. I, too, had been a terrified child— curled in my bed, during the domestic battles. My parents, like his, from different ethnicities and classes. I would use all of this in my play, *Us*, writing my way into my new life after S. I knew all along that I did not want S. for any extended length of time. What I did not know was that S. would heal me, or rather, that I could heal myself by writing a play. But not before I gave myself over to the sorrow of losing S., whom I assumed I loved since we fucked so well, and to the real sorrow of Julian's imminent death. Writing was the farthest thing from my mind. If someone had said, you must stop this now, or you will never write again, I could not have extricated myself. I did not extricate myself until I began to write. I had no idea if the affair would kill me as Julian thought his affair had. As someone said, "all S. can give you is AIDS." Never mind, I could not stop. S. and I were fucking so Julian would live. Fucking for love of him. Eros is all that we had. Flesh. Incantatory. Transformative. Magical. His long purple cock. My muscles closing around him. I got pregnant against my will on a night Julian nearly died, but he lived. We fucked death away, so it felt. We chased Thanatos and we won. Got pregnant because I convinced myself I had to remain unprotected, open and entered. (I thought it was a "safe" time of month, as we always think.) I was frantic. I left my diaphragm in its case. There could be nothing between us. Death would triumph if so. There could be nothing in the way. Julian was so close to dying this night while we fucked in his house, across the park from his hospital room. When we left the hospital together, we wondered if he would live until morning. Got pregnant because by opening myself to new life, death was sated, passed Julian by. Nothing made sense but desire. Delirious with fear, with hope for an impossible cure. More time. Hope for more time. Julian was alive the next morning. So, there! I am stuck with a child no one wants. Bearing that burden. Julian never knew I was pregnant, nor Judith. She might have opposed the abortion. Fucking to keep him with me, not the one that I fuck, but Julian. I am not in my right mind. I am in an incantatory space, between love and loss, and the screams when I reach orgasm will scare death away, welcome life. I can scare death away with my joy. We can. As if, *this is our death. We will have it here, now, so Julian can stay.* In joy that is grief, I will lose myself. Like my father, my lover has suffered wrongs I do not know. He is badly hurt, so badly he cannot speak of it, though he croons to me all the time, in his French accent, his voice a balm. Sense goes. I am screaming with what seems like joy, the pleasure of terror. He was a child in a ball on the floor, holding his knees, making himself small. Bombs falling around him. Child of colonial violence, of liberatory war. His mother was a pied-noir, his father, an Algerian, a revolutionary, so I fantasized. They were bound, therefore, by attraction and rage. Bound by impossibility. Like we, now. Bound as my parents had been. Across fault lines. The lineage, hurt people using sex. Hurt people from enemy camps. Loving Julian as we writhed on a bed in Julian's mother's home while Julian lay across the park on the cancer floor at Mount Sinai, fighting death. Death, which we called, attracted and caught, like a wild bird, in our net. There is nothing I would not have done. Crying in pleasurable pain, "Is it all right," like an innocent child, "yes, yes," as he pushed his cock further up my ass, and I howled. Let me die this little death. Let me offer myself. But Julian does not like this man. He does not approve. He expects me to be hurt. We all expect that. He will hurt me because he cannot help himself. He must seduce and betray. His power lies in his ability to wound. As must have been done to him as a child, many times. What was done to him he cannot recall, does not want to know, and must act out. I will make his story up when I come to write the play that will heal me from him. But, now, I am actually in danger. In my belly will root his child. I will be tossed away, as surely as Julian's beautiful Italian lover tossed him. Let it happen to me. Let me take into myself the sorrow, the hurt. No longer numb. Sorrow is better. I have been numb for too long. And we triumph. Our spell works. Julian lives the night through. He slowly recovers some strength. Death is vanquished. "I am not going to die," he said, and I heard him, stepped in; I sent death away, accepted, instead, the fertilized egg. There will come a mini-death of a creature I made whom I will not let live. A sacrifice. Mine. I am the sacrificial lamb. The knife raised over my throat. I shall rupture and bleed.

I have become a creature of the night. Leaving his bed at 5 am, making my way home through the empty city streets, fetid garbage blowing across my path, hitting me in the face. Getting to where I live, but can't live for long, in time to get my daughter to school, and endure the wrath of the one who'd betrayed me first. I existed like that. Lying and sneaking, pregnant. In the days at Julian's bedside. The nights in a spell. No, not death, not death, not yet. The greatest sensual pleasure I'd yet known, the worst pain. Awake. Alive. In a delirious state. Throwing my flesh against death.

I'd read Fanon and Genet; I'd seen *The Battle of Algiers*. I had empathy for the hurt boy, my lover in those days. For the Algerians fighting for self-determination, blowing French people up in cafes. For the French pieds-noirs, also victims. For the boy child, S., born into war to parents on warring sides. Many years later, S. said to me, quite casually, "oh, I forgot about the abortion." I looked at him across the table as if staring at an alien race, one that forgets what a woman can never forget. Women had been killed for doing what I did in the night. Or killed on the way home. Killed for getting "themselves" pregnant. My life was at risk in the only way I knew.

Sex. Julian need not have feared for me, though he did. I was bound by a translucent thread to a life I had yet to live. A happiness few people know, a perfect, deep love, just a few years ahead. Just a few years after Julian died. I would just have to write the play, *Us*, about S. and me, and our parents before us, that would bring me to George.

July 1984:

Judith says, "Julian's spirit is so present it's hard to think about how sick he is." Yes, the other day when he told me he was not going to die, I believed him. His spirit shines like an eternal flame. One almost believes in an afterlife. Where such spirits dance, forever, exalted. Except that Julian says, "If the body is not the soul, what is the soul." He, himself, cannot imagine himself disembodied. Who can? We are Jews. We know no idea of an afterlife. We have no choice but to commit to life, to hold to life, love life, find our messiah in our ability to hallow this earth, for there is no paradise Judith says, "where I cannot have coffee with my mother."

July 1984:

He is completely the autocrat in his hospital bed. Julian sits, directing us to direct all of our energies toward him. He accepts whatever a mere healthy human offers, whether orchids or daisies, healing waters, herbs, crystals, an ungraceful comment or good conversation. He cannot eat. Has eaten nothing for weeks, he is kept alive by intravenous feeding, but he is voracious for the health we bring.

August 1984:

We have come slowly and carefully to the hospital roof, pushing the feeding machine to which Julian is attached. We sit cheerful now in the sun, looking down at Central Park, while Julian recites his lines from *The Cotton Club*, which will have to be dubbed in his hospital room. When Coppola let him keep his long hair pulled back in a bun under the fedora hat, he knew they agreed he would play the gangster Sol Weinstein as a mask so that we might learn to see violence as the mask, which has fallen down across the human form.

September 1984:

"Imagine wanting to die," Julian gasped at Barbara Deming's memorial service. He would outlive Barbara by just over a year. She did what was nearly unthinkable, then, and hard for most to contemplate now. Against her physician brother's wishes, she insisted upon taking herself off chemotherapy treatments, so she might "dance toward her death" as she said, naked each night to drumbeats and songs from her close friends in her Florida lesbian compound. She struck me as brave and wise, and Julian, while appalled, perhaps thought so too, though his choice appeared the exact opposite. Each chose to walk their path accompanied, calling upon their communities to surround them. Conscious deaths. They had lived for and with like-minded others and bound their communities together by their passion, and in Barbara's case by her generous funding of women in need. Each sought to minimize sorrow, though the sorrow at their deaths would be greater precisely because of the care they took to include and to protect the rest of us. To let us bear witness. All their lives they had been uniquely present in a world they seemed to see, call forth, and inhabit, a nonviolent world that did not yet exist and perhaps never could for lack of sufficient people like them. Who believed above all in transformation. Who practiced change from within. Who exhorted others to change. And made us stand firm against violence. Who, with each act and word, defied what was, and lived instead for what might yet be. There is a Hasidic tale Julian and I particularly liked from a book, *Hasidic Tales of the Holocaust*, I gave him, about the thirty-six righteous ones who keep the world on course. They do not know who they are and neither does anyone else, but for lack of those thirty-six, we would be lost. Julian and Barbara were among these thirty-six Tzadiks. Making their way, carefully, shedding light. Always at the edge of the possible. Tipping the balance toward the good.

Julian was aghast when he learned of Barbara's decision to stop cancer treatment and begin her "dance toward death." He was dying, too, but his way was different, though each approached their deaths with eyes open, with concerns not just for themselves but for all who loved them. Each evening, the women would gather, drumming and singing, while Barbara, naked, and ever weaker, would dance in the middle of their circle. They played and sang music from the Civil Rights Movement. Aretha Franklin. The nightly ritual bringing Barbara closer to the inevitable. Dancing. Naked. Surrounded by a circle of love. On August 2, 1984, Barbara died in her sleep. Karl Bissinger called to tell me. Those of us who were not with her in Florida would receive a parting letter, typed on her typewriter, on the thin, yellow student composition paper Barbara always used, dated July 21. Mine arrived after Barbara's death, sent to me by her bereaved lover Jane Gapen in response to my condolence note:

To so many of you:

I have loved my life so very much and I have loved you so very much and felt so blessed at the love you have given me. I love the work so many of us have been trying to do together and had looked forward to continuing this work but I just feel no more strength in me now and I want to die. I won't lose you when I die and I won't leave you when I die. Some of you I have most especially loved and felt beloved by and I hope you know that even though I haven't had the strength lately to reach out to you.

I love you. Hallowed be (may all be made whole). I want you to know, too, that I die happily.

Bobbie (Barbara) Deming

Now I sat next to Julian at Barbara's memorial service, at the Quaker Meeting House off Gramercy Park where Judith had found me in a crowd in 1972. In Quaker fashion, people rose at will to speak to the wonders of Barbara's life. I wept quietly through the whole service. Not just over Barbara's death, though, yes, of course, for her, and for Julian, too, but also for the bad love affair I felt stuck in, and for my abortion to come. I was mourning the not-to-be-a-child I carried. I could not bear it. Could not bear not to bear it. Could not stop crying. I had not yet conceived, much less written the play that would be actual fruit of this mad affair. The not-yet child that was to be unborn was still in my womb busy in the very first weeks with cells dividing. I felt terrible grief for the life I was going to deny, for myself, and my impending losses, the home I lived in with my child and a man with whom I now merely coolly existed, he with me, in mutual domestic animosity. I wept for life lost. For my foolish, irrevocable choices. Julian sat erect and silent next to me. I have no idea what Julian thought was the source of my weeping. He asked nothing. He did not comfort me. He allowed my grief, which surely, also, was his, and perhaps he took comfort from my public weeping. Perhaps, he thought I was crying tears for him he could not cry. Perhaps, I was—weeping for all that could not live.

"We are members of one another," Barbara said often, quoting the Apostle Paul from the Bible, quoting other spiritual leaders who quoted the same six words: "We are members of one another." Such a simple, significant concept. The "I" and "thou" of Martin Buber, which Judith and Julian quoted often. We belong to each other, we are members, as in sentient flesh, one of the other, we feel with, and for one another, if we can imagine. I feel as you. If I wound you, I wound myself, too. And the child whose life I would willfully stop was part of this too. Though I felt no lasting guilt about the abortion, I felt sorrow. If I thought I could have made a family with S., but I knew he had not the character I was looking for. He had two children already, with two different women. I could not have been with him, had he asked me. We are like the mycelium under the earth, linking the trees in the forest, shooting them messages when danger advances. We are one. Bound. The child I would not let live was proof of the hurts S. and I had inflicted, that I had yet to inflict when he came back to me and I turned him away, several times. And the child I would not let live meant I would have the time to write the play that would heal me but not S. How selfish I was. Selfish as an artist is. As male artists always have been. Now, me, at last, putting my work, myself, first before sex. One doesn't go back. Hard won as this freedom was. The lesson learned at Julian's bed. When it came time to die, when Barbara made the decision to end further treatment and prepare herself for death, she knew that although the decision was hers, she owed explanation, and invitation. She could not die alone as she, too, was a member of the community she had formed, and a member of the living, sentient world. Ritual, her communal dance toward death, and writing, the letter she sent, were methods she had employed all her life to create understanding and which she used now, not so much to explain, but to gather-in those who loved her. "I am not leaving you when I die." No, she was lodging herself in us, as a member of our imagination, our flesh, with her message, with her chosen approach to her death, her public acknowledgment. We would not forget her when we needed strength. "I want you to know, too, that I die happily"

"For Karen Malpede, With a kind of translucent love, Julian," he wrote with an ink pen in his elegant script on the thick brown paper, next to a black and white image of his face, in the small book of his poetry, *Semi-Permeable Membranes: Twenty Songs of the Revolution,* he gave me on the 25th of December, 1984—a Christmas gift. A gift Ilion had made for Julian, multiple copies of the elegant book he might give as gifts. Likely, he inscribed a number of the slender volumes for his friends this last Christmas of his life. I am looking at the image now. Julian staring straight at me, intense and beautiful; at the same time, there is a deeply private expression on his face, as if looking in. He was seldom still, though he was becoming so. In health, he was more often flailing his arms, raising his voice, but he became inward looking at the end, quieter. "Translucent love" emanates from his face. A shimmering silken thread, nearly invisible to the eye, strong, which never knots, breaks, or binds. From the evening we met in the Brooklyn kitchen until his death, this translucent love between us would remain secure whether he was far away in Europe on tour, or we were across the table at Schraft's, in New York eating pie, or in his Mount Sinai hospital room, or sitting together on the couch in Mabel Beck's, now his, living room, my hand resting lightly on his naked foot.

Never lovers, though we once spent a naked night on a futon in his room in Pittsburgh feeling each other's sexual parts, we referred to this as our "mutual fascination," we were joined by translucent love from the start.

Julian loved many people, none more that Judith, Garrick and Isha, of course, and Ilion Troya, his lover of many years, who endured the young Italian flame who broke Julian's heart, and who spent nights with him in his hospital bed at Mount Sinai, giving Reiki massage, or sexual pleasure, or holding Julian from behind while he retched from the chemotherapy treatments. Julian's and my love was chaste. The first man who did not expect I give to him. "You need someone who will let you live." He wanted me to become.

January 22, 1985:

Last night to St. Marks for Julian and Judith's poetry reading. He is nearly translucent now, radiant in his weakness, in the glory of life departing which clings to him as pure spirit. He is beautiful in a pink and red sweater given him by Garrick, and strong, though his voice is weak. The reading takes place on Ronald Reagan's second inauguration night. Julian greets us, "We need these gatherings of poets to let in a little light in these dark times … I begin with a warning," and he reads his poem "The State Will Be Served Even by Poets," a long list of male poets serving the needs of the state. Later he reads love poems and he says to one who was faithless, "The beauty, dear one, was never you, but in me, the lover."

April 1985:

Julian sits in a yellow sweater, backed by his sensuous paintings, peering at me through a flowering branch, a bright white rug on the floor. "Found on the street," he tells me proudly. Once, years ago, as we walked through the Village, he plucked a half-bristled broom out of the garbage. "People are so wasteful," he said to me sternly. How good it is to see him glowing this spring. And we speak of theater all afternoon. When I go, he says, "that was good." I'm pleased to have pleased him with talk that pleases me, too.

Last Seder, 1985:

The room is full as always at Passover, the extended family of the Living Theatre, company members and friends. Julian and Judith sit together on the couch at the head of our improvised, long, winding circle. We sit on the floor at low tables, which are made of long pieces of board set on milk crates over which tablecloths have been draped. We read from Judith's feminist "Haggada for the Seder." We read, as always, Allen Ginsberg's long incantatory poem, *Holy*. Then Julian then goes around the entire room, saying each person's name: Holy Garrick, Holy Isha, Holy Amber, Holy Carrie Sophia. He smiles into each person's eyes. Holy each one of us in turn. It takes a long time; there must be fifty people or more. He does not forget a single name.

August 1985:

Julian sits in the bath sucking on ice cream from a bowl he holds, a spoonful at a time, until it melts in his mouth, the door ajar. In the adjoining room, Judith sits at her small writing desk, Hanon and I on the big bed. The talk turns to Martin Buber. Judith and Julian heard him speak in 1959. She reads from her diary, her voice vibrant, her words and Buber's intertwine, filling the rooms, catching us up in their spell. It was to have been a holy place, Buber says of Israel, a place where the most holy went, it was to have been an experiment in living, and that necessarily meant community among Jews and Palestinians. But, then the war happened and after the war the most wretched came to Israel, those who had been most badly hurt, those who had lost everything, who were weakened by cruelty, by hate. Judith's voice breaks, and Buber's. But she picks up again, about his sadness on that night, about the loss of hope violence always brings. Her words are beautiful, and her voice, though their content is only despair. When she is finished, Julian, naked and beaming, comes into the room.

"That was a zap," he says, ruddy from the bath and aglow with delight in the moment. He settles himself cross-legged on the bed.

—

In the interview two weeks before his death, Julian speaks about touch and the importance of friendship to those who are ill:

I've always been a lover. I love people. I love to embrace and to hug. I love the sensuality. After I found out I had cancer, I felt tremendously inhibited, suddenly, but now I am able to express more in the house, in the family and with friends. I sense a much greater openness than ever before. Many people don't realize how important family and other means of support actually are to the person who is ill. I really hope the importance of home-based support can be proven in a scientific way.

He would perform in one final serious theater work, a Beckett play, *That Time*, at LaMama, directed by Brazilian Gerald Thomas, who was making his mark in the downtown theater world and created a significant event by bringing together three well-known actors of the avant-garde, Julian Beck, George Bartenieff and Fred Neuman, in three short American premieres by Beckett. "Old white face, long flaring white hair, as if seen from above, outspread. Voice A, B, C are his own coming to him from both sides and above," Beckett describes the actor in *That Time*. Julian was perfect for this part. A spectral image, speaking in three different voices, each one himself, coming from where? From beyond the grave? Beckett does not say. Julian leaned against a slanted black platform that supported his weakened frame, his feet on a ledge, he was hoisted high. Only his face was lit. He appeared to be floating in space. As Beckett asks. He pre-taped Beckett's words as the text demands, his hiccups edited out: "that time you went back, that last time to look was the ruin still there where you hid as a child." He acted the emotions with his beautiful, ravished face while the tape of his three different voices played. A glorious performance. George Bartenieff, whom I did not yet know, Fred Neuman, and Thomas Walker, in a nonspeaking role, were in the two short companion Beckett plays on the bill, *Theater I*, *Theater II*. Julian's play haunting. George and Fred, eerie and comic.

For each of his acting roles in the final year of his life, whether on film, television or in the theater, Julian received high praise. No longer doing his own radical plays, he was recognized, at the end of life, as a consummate performer in other people's works. His face and form ever more chiseled as he approached his death, he occupied a liminal space. As cancer eats the flesh, the frame appears, the shape of the self, there is no longer anywhere to hide. The eyes pop from the face. The bones protrude. Nothing extraneous remains. The skeletal form looks both as if it might break at any moment and pure, and indomitable, as if made of metal, like a Giacometti sculpture. Julian went on, through the great disappointment of the critical reception of his final creation, *The Archeology of Sleep*, which brought the end of *his* Living Theatre, using his failing body and voice to create memorable villains on film and television, since the market would pay. He was trying to leave behind as much money as he could for Judith and Hanon, so they could restart the Living Theatre in New York after his death. He was the maniacal villain in the film *Poltergeist II*, Sol Weinstein, the gangster in *The Cotton Club*, and a villainous banker in the television cop show Miami Vice.

On the stage, one last time, he created Beckett's questioning everyman. Samuel Beckett seems to me, now, the playwright emerging from the resistance in the Second World War, as the playwright of the buried trauma of that war generation, inarticulate trauma acted out as riddle, vaudeville turn, game, rambling tale, "that time, that time" is the repeated refrain in this play, but what happened "that time" is never voiced or understood; only its impact not the event itself is seared into consciousness. War trauma. No one spoke of war trauma, then, when so much of the world had been fought over. PTSD was not a concept until soldiers returned pot heads and worse from Vietnam and the rap groups began. After World War II, people were silent about what they had suffered, what they had done. Characters unaware of what has happened to them once, *in that time*, dominate Beckett plays. As if he, consummate poet, could not write a description of what happened to so many incinerated, tortured, bombed, displaced, hunted. Beckett worked underground for the French resistance. Only the impact of a terror inarticulate, often reacted to with gallows humor, remained (as it did for decades among the survivors). So many people who never spoke of what happened to them, then, as soldiers, refugees, resisters, collaborators, were haunted by inarticulate feelings of fear and terror. Inexplicable explosion of rage or of grief; a stony, implacable silence. "That time," of collective destruction. How insignificant any single person seemed amid global suffering. Stuff it down and forget. How contrary to Julian Beckett was. Julian, himself, thought so. (Julian had avoided the draft by coming out as homosexual.) He lacked patience for Beckett's inability to explain or exhort. Yet, they remain complementary artists. Both gravitate to the extreme, the unknown, the leap, or in Beckett's case fall, or pratfall, the confusion that masks the forgotten essential event. Julian said to me that he did not share Beckett's worldview, and yet, there is something in the poetic extremity of each, their purity and the position of the characters they create who are always on the edge, so it seems, of finally arriving at some great understanding, ever eluding them again. In their theaters, both manifested Artaud. George, who directed *Waiting for Godot* twice, with his students, argued that Didi and Gogo committed suicide, jumping from the Eiffel Tower before the play began. I argued back, impossible. There would be no play, then. He insisted, "The entire play takes place after their death." I disagreed vehemently, "they are refugees." We liked to argue about work. Each of us had a point. Beckett does seem always at the end, final words, last testimony, inchoate, and perhaps all of his characters *are* already dead, and this is why they can no longer remember their traumas, in which case George was correct, and Didi and Gogo had already leapt. Or, as I thought, the terrible events of today have their roots in the past traumas not yet fully understood and never expiated that must be relived over and over again, "that time" without knowledge. The Godot waited for with such eagerness, the revelatory presence, is absent in the afterworld and in this. The savior does not exist. And *That Time* is a man recollecting from the grave, or from just before, on the turning points of his life. He remembers each consecutive moment well, *that time, that time, that time,* again, but he has no idea what happened to him, then, though each time he changed unutterably. But why? Perhaps, he is trying to recount the moment of his dying. We write from what we know and what we don't know yet and the unknown speaks through the known words that we choose. Beckett was one of the first writers to be able to touch and record the unspoken horrors of World War II, nightmare annihilation for which we have no words. He broke theatrical form, as did other post-war artists like Judith and Julian, to reveal history's nightmare and the poetry that might yet be found in the extreme—in other ways of perceiving, of being. *That time when that happened to me* is the call of the one who cannot recall the event too terrible to know.

Julian went, emaciated, to Europe to perform one last time in Beckett's *That Time*; unable to eat, he had refused anymore to be hooked twelve hours a day to an intravenous feeding machine. He, too, like Barbara, therefore, renounced essential treatment, but he never confessed to this. Instead, he said he hoped his appetite might return on this tour with George, Judith, Tom, Fred, and Ellen Stewart, to Munich. George took photos of Julian at the airport, beaming his smile, beneath large dark glasses. No one could guess from the happy face in the photo how close he was to death, though the tour was cut short. They returned home from Munich, the performances in Venice abandoned. He would die the next month. Yet, he went on, unable to stop. The life force burning into death, stronger as the flesh vanished, a continuous transformation. Julian lived in his final months what he was searching to convey in his last play about dreams. He seemed always exalted in those final days. Always on the verge of wish fulfillment. The insult and cruel dismissal of his *Sleep* play had been left in the past. Julian was a man looking forward—peering into the unknown as he always had been. He was acting, and writing. Around him in his last year, a community of the self-elect stood, determined to live with him as he died. We understood our privileged place. We have no choice but to continue to transform, until we are lifted from this world.

September 10, 1985:

Last night, Hanon reads Julian's new poetry at Theater for the New City, the theater George co-founded and he must have been there, though I don't remember. Julian is in the hospital and cannot be present. I phone him today to compliment him on his writing. "That's good to hear," he says and we speak of a fall and winter spent writing. I am on my way out of town for a reading of my play *A Monster Has Stolen the Sun*, at Smith College. I tell him I cannot come to the hospital. "Oh," he says, disappointed, but then, "you will only be gone a long weekend."

Julian died Saturday, September 14, at 6 pm. I was in rehearsal in Northampton and had not the heart to call until we finished at 9:30, but I knew and my heart was heavy. "Don't come home, Julian would have wanted the theater work to continue," Judith said. "Julian was not about being brought down."

When we spoke the day before I left, he had said, "I'm a little nauseous," but when I praised his poetry, I made him happy. We spoke of the cancellation of the Beckett tour. "Venice will still be there when I am ready to go," he said.

"How did he die, mommy?" asked Carrie Sophia. "He went into a deep sleep, and god came and took him." He had a cerebral hemorrhage.

When I return on Monday, I pick up my child and we go straight to the apartment on West End. Julian's spirit seemed and seems still everywhere and we, all of us, half expect him to arrive. Burst through the door, smiling. "Holy" each one of us. But other people now sit in the corner of the living room on the couch where he sat so often, and often I had sat next to him there and reached out and touched his soft feet. Never to touch those feet again. Never to hear that voice. Never. Never. Or as Judith says—"forever"—the meaning of the word coming clear to her. People come in and out, Andrea Dworkin, Andre Gregory, Allen Ginsberg, company members from now and before, friends, hangers on.

I leave the Shiva to walk with Carrie Sophia in Riverside Park. "Don't cry, mommy," the five-year-old says, whom Julian loved who loved him back, "We can still talk to Julian but Julian can only talk to god."

Rabbi Schlomo Carlebach, the guitar playing Orthodox rabbi upon whom Judith relies, leads the packed service at Riverside Memorial Chapel.

But it is of the cemetery that I must write. For never in my life have I experienced a parting such as this. The day dawned soft and hazy, a warm fall day, with the death of the year in the air, the leaves heavy and already beginning to turn, and all of growth being pulled by the force of renewal down toward the earth. Julian, like the Tzadik he was, died between Rosh Hashanah and Yom Kippur. (My father had died, then, too; his Catholic high mass held on the high holy day of the unobserved faith of his Jewish wife, with his unbaptized twins sitting next to her.) When I saw the plain wood coffin at the front of the chapel, then I wept for the glorious body bereft of spirit that lay in that box. The spirit hung in the air, Julian's spirit, freed from the body, taken from us, but not lost to us, loose in the air as if looking for places to settle, in whose heart, in whose soul, in whose mind-body does this part of him fit, and there was felt among the many of us in the packed Riverside Chapel a general opening up, an expansion of inwardness, a making room for the new spirit to enter, to dwell, the indwelling begun.

The light at the cemetery was clear, noonday light, with an autumnal haze. Almost immediately, the coffin was lowered into the ground, but then the grave diggers stepped back and Shlomo began to daven and speak. He said that when Garrick recited the Kaddish, Julian's soul would enter the body of his son. The sound of the Kaddish rose, the men in the circle speaking in their deep voices the Hebrew words I have just begun to learn. Garrick threw the first handful of earth down onto the coffin and the sound, the sound of soft earth hitting the wooden box, which holds the body of our beloved friend, was as if some bell had rung, or that some gates had been opened.

We are being separated. He is being taken, but not taken, we are giving him over to a higher reality in which none of us believe. We each throw earth upon the coffin, sending Julian away from us, sending his body back to the earth and his spirit up into the ether so that he may return, an essence alive and living on in the world, so the flesh becomes spirit, that comes back into us, even as we send him away, casting him out, with our handfuls of dirt, casting him out of life. It was the hardest work any of us had ever done. Who dares throw dirt upon the beloved. Judith says later that when she picked up a handful of dirt, all the Antigone performances she had ever done (hundreds of them) flashed through her mind in one continuous picture. Burial of the beloved. A necessary ritual.

I took handfuls of dirt and bent low over the grave. I wanted to see, to see the coffin. I bent low, throwing the dirt slowly, hearing the sound, more final than any other, harsher than a bomb, softer than words of love, and I whispered "I love you" as the earth fell on our beloved.

Garrick picked up a shovel and began the even harder job of shoveling the earth into the grave. A handful of dust seemed like nothing, then, though it had been so difficult to throw it. Now the work began. I was startled and thought, the men will do this, but broken-hearted Serena took a shovel from one of them and then the women knew it was our task, too. I watched Erika with the shovel. Erika who had been with him at the last. Erika with her weak back and her large heart. I watched Mark, and Luke and Elaine and Joni and Renfrew. I shoveled dirt into the grave across from Allen Ginsberg, in rhythm, his shovelful, then mine. As we had stood once in his hospital room, together, across from Julian in his bed. I could manage but three or four shovels, my heart gave out, and I handed my shovel over to Mark's father. The earth kept rising. At first one could see the coffin and I felt we would see the coffin, that all of us would stop here with the coffin exposed and the few piles of dirt on its top. But the earth covered the coffin and then the earth began to rise. And we were doing this. We covered the grave. No one spoke, except Elaine whispered to me that the workers were delighted we were doing their work, four small gravediggers who stood to the side of the crowd.

It was the hardest thing I had ever done. Julian exacted a certain discipline always from me. He expected me to get better, my writing, my discernment in love. Schlomo began to daven—or perhaps he had been doing so all along. Judith, wrenching herself from her grief, for she had wept and called out *"Julian, Julian"* as the earth fell, Judith began the chord, we held hands, and our voices rose then in unison for a long time. The chord, the Living Theatre signature piece, all of us, our voices rising and falling together as we tune in to each other. It is wordless, the chord, like a very long Om, rising and falling. And if Julian had left anything unfinished it would be finished by his friends, Shlomo said at the service. When the chord quieted in our throats, Shlomo said, "we do not turn our back on a grave," and we began to back up, a widening circle, away from the grave of our beloved, back into the world of the living whose work we resume as we can.

For I cannot explain how the dust stayed on my fingers and I felt the earth seep into my veins. I cannot explain the weight of that shovel, far heavier than anything I ever lifted yet light as a feather, the hardest work I have ever done, like giving birth, the concentration total. I cannot explain the sound of the earth in my ears.

Judith and I, arm in arm, walk on Broadway the next day. "Oh" she cries, "to pass by Cohen's," the local stationery store, "and not to be able to tell Julian what is on sale."

I accompanied Judith to Shlomo Carlebach's shul on Shavuot, the Jewish holiday that celebrates the giving of the Torah to the people. The place was divided, men on one side, women on the other, but on this year for the first time, the Torah was allowed to be carried by the men (god forbid women who menstruate should touch it) through the women's section, so that it might be kissed by female lips. This was a very big deal for the observant. Judith kissed the scroll and began to wail. She fell to floor in spasms of agony, shrieking her grief over Julian's loss in loud, tortured cries. We knew none of the women around us, dressed in black, who witnessed and swayed, as Judith railed on the floor, crying out against the unfairness of death. But they stood and watched. No one attempted to comfort her. "She's going to have a good year," someone said, "She is letting it all out." Theirs was a ritual action, as was hers. They witnessed. Judith shrieked. She was not commanded to be silent, to calm; rather her grief further sanctified the moment. We stood silent around her in a circle, making with our bodies the container to hold the unbearable.

What held us all together in those days, an electric current running through our lives, was the idea of transformation, through art and in our own lives. Joseph Chaikin and George Bartenieff, the two finest theater artists to work with the Living Theatre, were, like Julian Beck, transformational actors, each in his way. I mean instead of "putting it out" (current fashion) by getting "bigger," "louder," "jumping about," they opened themselves up and allowed us to witness their depth, vulnerability, and their wonder. Joe and George followed the Living. Both their esthetics were based on the major tenet of the Living Theatre, the belief that the world *Does Not* have to be as it is. That the actor in the theater might show what can be and by doing so, bring the unknown into being, giving the future form. Transform, Change, Become. Beneath the violence, the hurt, there is a beating heart. And a world of possibility inside of each one on earth. "One is as important as one million," Judith used to say, speaking of reaching into the audience in a way that caused someone(s) to change. The idea, the certainty, that people could change (after all, we had all become artists) drove all of us in those years. Julian, Joe, George each believed fiercely in theater as a means for transformation, as a way to bring the news to others. Each had a different embodied way of manifesting their belief through their acting. If Julian was the prophet come down from the mountain bearing the news, Joe was the individual epiphany, opening himself before us, revealing the fragile inner life. George was the man who became someone else. His was the humanity, the gift of entering and materializing the other. The Other become Self.

Each of these men—Julian, Joe, George—advanced their idea of a theater. They were not just actors, they were auteurs. They created; they nurtured. They partnered, often with women. Julian is impossible to imagine without Judith, as is she without him. They were the most tightly wound together and yet each one more fully realized themselves because of their unique collaboration, their artistic union. Susan Yankowitz wrote *Terminal* for the Open Theater; Joe's sister, Shami, and Tina Shepard, were main actors in his company, and Joe had many women friends (sometimes lovers), Kristen Linklater, Susan Sontag, others. George founded a theater with Crystal Field, in part to produce the new plays by women he felt essential for the culture and that he knew would have trouble being produced elsewhere. Our partnership, the last half of his life, was based on his desire to act in my plays and on my willingness, eagerness, as it turned out, to write good parts for him, anticipating his desires as he aged. Each of us practiced nonviolent resistance to war and injustice in our lives and each used nonviolence as an aesthetic principle in our art—seeking to visualize the intricacies of nonviolence on the stages and streets where we performed our work. True nonviolence is *androgynous*—a term of equal balance between assertive and receptive actions that Barbara Deming used to define lesbianism and a concept Dorothy Dinnerstein popularized among men and women raising children together.

Julian never lost his fascination with the radical potential of dreams. He had continued to work on *Theandric*, a compilation of radical poetic exhortations. In Mount Sinai Hospital, July 11, 1984, two months before he died, he wrote the last full entry in his final book:

My Lens
The lens with which I observe, my opera glasses, binoc-
Ulars, telescope, microscope is no casual invention
And I didn't buy it cheap in a flea market, I've been
Polishing it for years, developing my eyesight, sharp-
Ening my equipment because I knew when I first began
Going to the theater and looking at the world that
Everything was covered with the fine dust of illusion,
And things were in a disastrous condition because
Nobody could see what was going on. Naturally at a
Certain point in organizing our theory of revolution-
ary process Judith and I declared that the first thing
that needed to be done was to change perception
so that need for change could be perceived. I want
to change everyone's vision. Those with their eyes
bent to the ground or focused on TV or on public
statues, those in Nietzsche's mud, are locked out of
their own paradise, tho any of us at any moment
is capable of seeing the face of god, experiencing
satori, flying straight up from rung I to rung X.
I give this lens to you now, what has been observed
Constitutes the substance of this book. The lens,
Like most lenses, had its origin in Holland.

The luminosity and courage of late-stage cancer patients, as the flesh pulls taut to the bone, the only word to describe this is awe—they exude awe for the tortured life they are still fiercely living, and we, awe for them. Certainly Barbara, Julian, and in years later, George. They were all so alive in their dying. Of life so fully. Even as the cancer grinds on, relentless, now. Only their nearest ones witness the physical agony that exists grueling alongside the luminosity they exude.

Ilion Troya, Julian's lover, recalls vividly after all these years: "I was there to sleep beside him and to hold his back when he was having convulsive bouts of vomiting. Chemotherapy was exhausting, and so was the IV (feeding machine), the hiccups, and yet Julian continued recording Beckett and going to Europe with Nam June Paik to the 1984 Locarno International Film Festival, then the tour with George in Gerald Thomas's Beckett production to Frankfurt." When too weak to tour, he finished his book.

I read my diary excerpts at Julian's memorial service held at the Joyce Theater, November 25, 1985. Among others on the program along with Judith and Garrick Beck were his friends and colleagues, John Ashbery, Amiri Baraka, Eric Bentley, John Cage, and Ellen Stewart. S. and I make love for the last time, in a borrowed apartment. I look out the window and think, never again. The sorrow of the last time. Our affair had always been about Julian. Julian's dead. I will give myself the new play, *Us*, very different from anything I have written, my first mature work of the second half of my life, my seventh play. *Us* will bring me George. To his credit, S. said to me, years later, "I am glad you are with George. He is marvelous man." He also said, "One of us will die first and I will be there for you." S. died one year after George, though he was younger than us both.

I wrote a published tribute to Julian in the magazine of the War Resisters League:

"Our beloved Julian Beck, co-founder with Judith Malina of the Living Theatre, died after a long struggle against cancer on Saturday, September 14, in Mount Sinai Hospital. He was sixty years old. Founded in 1947, the Living Theatre is recognized worldwide as a major artistic and pacifist force.

The last year of his life, knowing he was terribly ill, he worked as hard as he had always worked. He wrote fifty-one poems and the day he entered the hospital, finished his book, *Theandric*. It tells of how the theater reveals the divine in humankind. Also in that year, through acting jobs in Hollywood and television, he supported plans to relocate the Living Theatre back in New York, after many years of residence in Europe.

Two weeks after his death, he was seen in "Miami Vice," playing a (corrupt) New York banker. He gave a speech about money in which the actor's longing to be free of capitalist restraints upon the human spirit shone through the banal words he spoke. He simply could not help turning everything he touched to art.

His work as a theater actor, designer, writer, and director inspired several generations. His literary work will inspire many more. He showed us that theater is a sacral place where through daring acts of the imagination, through brave image and delight we might first realize our dreams of human justice, human love. He knew that creativity is the only antidote to violence.

He was proud. I've never met a man more proud. And gentle. With Judith Malina and members of the Living Theatre, he was on many picket lines and protests and many times in jail for acts of civil disobedience. He faced death with the same defiant nobility with which he faced all cruel situations in this world. He held death in disdain. It was not a topic upon which he wished to waste one moment of precious life. The theater he leaves to Judith and to others, after all, is called The Living. And since life was of such inestimable value to him, he had a gift for enormously enriching the lives of others, making us care that much more dearly for ourselves and one another. In this way, as in all others, he was preeminently as man of peace."

The Nonviolent Activist, Nov/Dec 1985

Chapter Two:
George Bartenieff, "That was good."

He came running through my dream naked and carrying a torch, his shape-shifting actor's body well-muscled again, all signs of cancer and age gone, loose flesh hanging from jagged bone, which I'd come to find stunning and luminescent. It is one of few sightings I've had for he seems to have left me quite alone. "You will not be alone," I promised him, many times. In Nazi Germany, he had been an abandoned and hidden child. He feared being left, as he feared death. Feared leaving life by himself, unaccompanied. So I promised I would, and I did, walk with him to the edge.

In the spring of 1987, I read the opening two scenes of my new play, *Us*, at a women's bookstore uptown. Judith Malina grabbed the script from my hands. "Gangbusters," she said. I was thrilled. I'd had no idea what to do with the play—a stark a departure in form from my earlier work.

Judith would direct *Us* in New York that December, her first new scripted play since *The Brig* in 1963, which featured George Bartenieff as Prisoner #6. She took my play to Theater for The New City, founded in 1971 by George and his wife, Crystal Field. The two actor/producers were a fractious pair, bound together in a simmering rage by the theater they ran, which provided downtown theater spaces to hundreds of young and experimental artists. As rents rose, Theater for the New City moved three times from the West to the East Village, remaining always a destination for new and daring theater work. As Second Avenue gentrified, putting their lease in jeopardy once again, George, along with a board member friend who knew the real estate, scouted the East Village for a permanent space.

They found a city building for sale, an old market, used as storage for the Sanitation Department, occupying most of the block on First Avenue and Tenth Street. They mounted a campaign and raised the money for a down payment. The city reneged. They staged a large public protest, with stars of stage and screen testifying to TNC's importance. The city relented. With some fanfare, Mayor Ed Koch helped push the piano around the corner from Second Avenue, and they took possession. *Us* was one of the first plays produced in the new building. The theater spaces inside it were raw. Chairs were on rickety risers; the stage was the floor.

Both George and Crystal wanted to act in my play. They still shared an uptown apartment, with separate beds, and George still paid the bills, but Crystal had fallen for someone else who worked at their theater in a technical capacity, and George had begun having affairs. Their son, Alexander, was in college. I knew neither of them. I admired George's acting but I did not like hers; it was too broad, too caricatured for my play—a multi-scene erotic poem. Judith felt Crystal would not let the play be done at her theater if she were not cast in it. We had no budget. Still, I resisted. Judith arranged a reading uptown in her apartment at 800 West End Avenue, where I had spent so many hours with Julian. We sat in the living room around the same small table. I was in a chair, directly across from Crystal, who read in a low but intense voice, with few histrionics. Then, she leaned toward me and said softly, "Do you see what I can do? And they never let me." I relented.

Crystal and George would play six characters, themselves and their parents as lovers in eleven scenes of psychosexual dynamics. Each couple fused across class and ethnic barriers. *Us* was what I knew and imagined of S.'s childhood in Algeria during the French-Algerian war and mine in the American Midwest under the shadow of the bomb and my father's rages. Michel's character's mother was a pied-noir; his absent father, "the man who comes in through the window," was an Algerian freedom fighter or terrorist, depending upon one's point-of-view. Hannah's father's incestuous behavior was extreme, so was his violence. The French kiss I got in the car would be reenacted, as would my father's fears of his cancer, and my mother's meekness. The beatings she endured (he had thrown her down the stairs while she was pregnant, among others), were enacted by a woman dressed as a man throwing a large, stuffed rag doll against the wall and swearing at "her." As she turns back into herself, she pulls a baby doll from the belly of the beaten dummy, holds her "daughter" out and asks, "Someone come take her from me. Take." There were sudden transformations in every scene. Scatological and sensual, obscene and lyric, *Us* was a deep dive into ecstasies and the sorrows of these six characters bound by inescapable desire and intergenerational trauma. I dedicated my play to the memory of Julian Beck and his friend, Jean Genet. French critic, Rosette Lamont, who helped introduce both Eugene Ionesco, with whom she had an affair, and Samuel Beckett to American audiences, and who was a staunch admirer of my work and of *Us*, in particular, wrote a long Sunday *New York Times* feature article about the coming production, focused on Judith's return to the New York stage with her first new American play in over twenty years, and the theater couple, George and Crystal, who would act in it.

Judith directed by telling stories. A compulsive diarist, she recorded much of her life in detail. Her dark eyes lit up as she punctuated her words with broad gestures. She expected to, and usually did, enchant her listeners. She had taken a job in a laundry as a young woman. The workers' clothing clung to their sweating bodies in the wet heat, outlining nipples and genitals; they found all sorts of sexual detritus as they unwound dirty sheets, "including a fetus," she leaned forward and whispered—this was the sort of sensuality she wanted, dripping, terrifying, intoxicating, addictive. She staged the play on a set that was sixty-feet long, thirty-feet high and barely a foot-and-a-half wide. The structure was made into separate rooms by the designer, Ilion Troya, with furniture he found on the street. He went out early in the mornings to scavenge. The wooden assemblage was three-dimensional and hazardous. The actors were always on edge as they transitioned from scene to scene, climbing up and down, from room to room, acting on a ledge, at risk of falling. *Us* was to be hot and dangerous. Its characters vulnerable, caught, fierce, tender, furious and lost. A set of swings came down from the ceiling for the lovers' duet. George jumped for and hung with one arm from a heating pipe before landing on the floor to transform into a stallion, while Hannah relived a scene from her youth of horses mating. At one end was a window to climb through when the Algerian fighter visited his French lover. There was a double mattress plastered high on the set, up against the wall where the Italian-Catholic father compulsively rolled between his baby daughter and his Ashkenazy-Jewish wife, touching both, unable to stop, while his wife in a little voice, pled, "What have you done, Tony, what? The child's in bed with us." I had not actually experienced this, only in my unconscious, but the scene visualized in a shocking way an incestuous emotional legacy, which also separates girl child from mother, turning them into rivals. There was an oversized dressing room mirror for the boy's mother. George played her in blonde wig, clear plastic mask, silver high heels, a slinky gray dress. She admires her frozen face while her son desperately tries to tell her he has been abused by his brother. All six people in the play were wounded and bound by violence—political, social, inter-generational, economic, religious. There was no way out but through; each couple compulsively fused by desire that might heal or drive the wound deeper, as S. and I had been, my parents, too, and as I imagined his were.

But Crystal was having none of it. Once rehearsals began, she grew angrier day by day, at George and Judith. She ignored me entirely. The play she had so wanted to act in was stirring emotions she could not control, and, perhaps, had not known she felt. She came to rehearsal in a short skirt; spread her legs wide on the chair so the view was of pubic hair bubbling behind panties. "I'm garbage," she said to Judith in a menacing voice, leaning forward, "and anyone who works with me is garbage, too." It became difficult to rehearse. Crystal would demand George clean the theater bathrooms before the scene work could start. He would do so to avoid an altercation, while Judith and I waited. No doubt, the fact that the husband she had already abandoned for someone else, but still relied upon for financial support and as a business partner, was soaring, no doubt she could see George and I were being drawn to each other even as we barely knew what was happening, no doubt both were having a wretched effect on her, too, but something deeper had been touched, some original terror she could not face—exactly what the play is about. Judith coddled and cajoled, never raising her voice or losing her temper. Blocking was laboriously figured out. On the swings for the lovers' spoken aria, as erotic as I could write it, Crystal pulled at the ropes, kicked her feet in rage at George while he tried to make love to her with my words, "without shame, without shame in your arms." *Us* was being torn in two. George striving to fulfill each lyric and sensual moment, Crystal frightened, furious, bellicose. And I watched, silent, admiring the man's consummate acting and despairing.

"How are you feeling," I asked him at lunch, our first ever. We were on break He took me to an Italian restaurant he frequented across the street and down a few blocks from the theater.

"No one has ever asked me that before," he answered, and we leaned closer. In those days, his face was permanently creased, as if he had turned in on himself to hide who he was. He wore secondhand ski sweaters in garish colors. His blue eyes were so sunken the light hidden there was all but extinguished, except when he was on stage, which he rarely was. Raising money and running the theater meant he had nearly given up acting. *Us* was a play George insisted upon not just producing but acting in; like *The Brig*, he got goosebumps when he read the script. He was in love with my language before he met me. *Us* was a play he'd been "waiting for all his life," he told me at lunch. It expressed his feelings about Eros. He asked me questions about his characters. I answered as well as I could. No one had ever asked me to speak about my work with such keen attention. He was teaching me what actors needed to know by asking. I was learning how to approach what I'd done from the outside looking in. He told me that I should direct. That I "knew how to talk to actors" in specific ways they could use. We would collaborate like this for the next thirty-five years, talking over together every aspect of each new work. He never told me what to write. But, once the idea was formed, we would discuss. I would write whatever I wished for him to act. Thinking always, of course, about what he wanted to do and of what he hadn't done yet. He would embody my words in ways far more visceral, elemental and full than I could imagine. He taught me how to direct. He was the better director, I thought. But he thought I was.

Closer to the opening night, when it became clear he would need sexy underwear—that the grayed, baggy jockey shorts he wore would not do—I went to a fancy store in Park Slope and bought three silky bikinis in pastels. When he went behind a set piece that just covered his groin and stepped into a pair in front of us all, director, estranged wife, me, crew, the deal was done. He emerged as if transformed. In bikini briefs, his beautiful, sculpted body and his sensual movements became apparent. He had changed from harassed and betrayed husband into the ardent love object he acted in the play and was becoming in real life. We had not so much as held hands when he put the new underwear on, a costume for my play and a brazen public proposal for a life we would share. It was to be mutual devotion for the rest of our lives, to our work, to each other, and to my eight-year-old child whom we raised together.

George had longed for such sensuous language on his tongue. He delighted in the many physical transformations *Us* demanded. Along with the stallion, he became a boy swimming through seaweed and fish between the thick flesh of Arab women's bare legs, their skirts pulled up, in the warm Mediterranean Sea. He became the boy-child's narcissist mother, a sated male lover describing sensations, a father torn between wife and daughter. He was becoming better and better—he would win the Village Voice Obie Award for Sustained Excellence in Acting that year—while Crystal was becoming more shrill. And watching my play be ripped apart in this way, one half being coddled and brought to fruition, the other, the female, being trashed, was made bearable only because George and I were falling love. Fell in love, perhaps, at that first lunch with my question and his answer. *Us* would be denigrated in the press, though admired by those in the full audiences, there were lines around the block to get tickets, who could see and hear past its flawed production. But the anti-sex feminists in attendance, led by Andrea Dworkin for whom all intercourse was rape, would trash the play, too. Judith, heartsick, called a few downtown critics and asked them to phone me to apologize. Some did. Dworkin phoned, too, saying she did not "intend to hurt" a new work coming into the world. "Can you say anything nice about my play," I asked. She was silent. Yet, the word on the street was good and audiences kept coming; *Us* might have been extended for some weeks but Crystal refused. Performing the play she had so wished to be in had become unbearable for her.

One night after we closed, I sat on George's lap in my writing and sleeping room, at the back of the loft I still shared with my daughter's father, who was out on a date, while my daughter slept. I looked out the window at a lone streetlight on the dark commercial street and felt torn between despair over the fate of the play for which we had both hoped so much and a terrifying joy with which I was shot through, trembling, knowing I had been damned but blessed, holding hard to the glow on the black asphalt. Our life together would again and again be this way. Plays in which we believed would be met with derision in the mainstream press while lauded by audiences, activists, intellectuals, and younger reviewers. Soon after *Us* closed, Judith gave me a present she had made, a 5 by 3 ½ inch, hundred-page paper book with cut out drawings and photographs of paintings and sculptures of proud women in rebellion or distress, Käthe Kollwitz, Frida Kahlo and the like, pasted page after page. "The book of wise women: Kassandra (who is on the front), No one believed her, For Karen Malpede from Judith Malina," was the book's cover. Yellowed with age, its pages wrinkled, the glue coming off at the corners, I keep the handcrafted, little book on my desk, next to Judith's ink line drawing of Julian's face on a stone and her mezuzah. But Judith and I never spoke directly about what had happened to my play or why. Though we remained close friends, we never worked together again. George and I would live, work, and love together until he died in my arms thirty-five years later. The "death" of my erotic play on the New York stage met with the birth of our selves intertwined. And *Us*, too, found a future. The play became something of a feminist landmark, going on to productions in the UK, Australia, and Los Angeles. It was published in a collection *Women on the Verge: Seven Avant Plays*, edited by Rosette Lamont, before being revived in 2001, directed by a former student turned colleague, Yana Landowne, staged in an old porn house on 42nd St. as part of the reclamation of the area before it moved to HERE Performing Arts Center in Soho. *Us* has just been republished.

George was fifty-four, I was forty-two. He was physically delicious, well-muscled and stunningly graceful at the same time, masculine but only in form because he radiated, not anything particularly female, but the healing force of a man unafraid to give, who believes his duty to be enhancing life. Gentle and unfailingly kind. Brimming with a joy that increased as he aged. There is a photo of us taken from that year, 1987, when we met, by Ira Cohen at an opening of a show of Ira's photographs. I have hung my arm around George's neck and am looking adoringly into his face. He is leaning into me, his arm is around my back but he stares straight into the camera, like an actor, looking rakish and so happy, his black and white tie crooked, his white suit jacket rumpled. His deep-set blue eyes impishly sparkling, as if his inner life had revived. He was in his prime. "Mom, now we have our clown," my eight-year-old daughter said when we all moved in together, and he loved her unconditionally, as if her spirit and his were kin.

How to run the theater they co-founded became an issue for George and Crystal once George and I were living together, and wished to marry, and I was writing plays with large parts for him that we still produced at Theater for the New City. For several years, they continued their increasingly hostile relationship as co-executive directors. He continued to produce and promote the work of artists he admired. George had an unerring eye and he filled Theater for the New City with many of the best experimental artists around. He was the first in New York to produce the wildly inventive, hilarious and elegant English drag group, Bloolips, founded by classically trained Bette Bourne, who became his close friend and was one of the few people whom George turned to for acting advice. He produced *Crystal and the Star Fish*, the first play of the now world-known Anohni, then an undergraduate and my student at the Tisch School of the Arts. Both George and I were great admirers of Anohni's clear genius, and of their lovely, unassuming manner. George acted with and produced *The Talking Band*, the company founded by Paul Zimet and Ellen Maddow, who were part of Joe's Open Theater, and he produced the Brazilian, Gerald Thomas, who had directed Julian and George in Beckett. He produced Lee Breuer, JoAnne Akailitis and Ruth Malezech's Mabou Mines, whose *Dead End Kids* he was also in and which transferred to The Public Theater, where George often acted. The producer Joe Papp was George's admirer and friend. George commissioned and produced Sam Shepard's Pulitzer Prize winning play, *Buried Child*, and seven premieres of plays by Maria Irene Fornes, most of which won the annual Village Voice Obie best play award. He continued to produce the work of Judith Malina as she reconstituted the Living Theatre. TNC produced the first part of Harvey Fierstein's *Torch Song Trilogy*. He continued to raise money for Theater for the New City, again putting his acting career on hold. Night after night, George stepped forward after the final curtain call of each of the four plays that were running simultaneously in the four spaces. Night after night, he gave the same speech four times, "If anyone knows anyone who knows anyone who wants a theater named after them, please let me know." Indeed, eventually, someone in the audience introduced the sculptor Seward Johnson, of the pharmaceutical family, to TNC, and the Johnson Theater, the largest of the four theaters in the building, was named and with the endowment had its roof raised. George wanted to return to acting, more or less, full-time, but he was also committed to the theater he co-founded and to the artists he produced. He did not leave TNC until he engineered the sale of the roof rights to the building, ensuring that the theater's mortgage would be paid. Without George and his belief in his own artistic judgment, so many, many artists of note would not have been discovered or supported, would not have had a theater in which to produce their plays. I count myself among them. Once George committed to an artist's vision, he believed completely and he never wavered in his belief. If I leave myself out of this equation, though I can hardly do so, I can say his taste was uncommonly good. If I include myself, I can say without hesitation that without George's unwavering belief, and his wondrous performances in my plays, I do not know what would have become of me and whatever talent I might have possessed. He was surely one of the most eccentric and committed producers the American theater has ever known. He is certainly, also, the finest American actor who ever devoted himself so wholeheartedly to supporting the work of so many avant-garde artists whose work he prioritized often over his own. This "beautiful man," Judith called him, had been beaten down into nearly unrecognizable shape by TNC's endless demands. "You gave him back his life," producer Linda Chapman, who worked at Theater for the New City in those years, said.

George was my muse. How did that work, exactly? There was no one he could not become. So much of writing is wordless. Feeling one's way in.

This man I was learning to love, like learning a new terrain, this consummate actor, with sweet underarms, anus, and groin I was nosing around, was full of possibilities for story and character. He could play good or evil, funny or not. A wealth of possibility lay within body and self and in his early history which we would excavate together over the years, so much he had forgotten, pushed far down, out of mind, he would end up revisiting his past as we worked, his story and mine mingling, opening the way into many other stories invented. We fell into each other's lives. Flailing there, in the throes of our new love. The imaginative world became fecund for us both; better understanding ourselves we could also better sense our way into others imagined. George was first a giver of great gifts to others: he gave his enthusiasm, support, the theater space he created, and, then, the theater spaces we were able to find for my plays. But most of all, he gave to me as a playwright his ability to transform himself into another being, human or animal, so completely, with such a deep sense of manifesting who that other was that he, himself, metamorphosed—he was a true shape changer. And he loved those he gave physical-emotional birth to on the stage, loved his characters completely. His compassion for others was boundless; whether characters imagined or in his dealings with people off the stage, he was without malice; he was a sharer of joy and of love. He saw into and embraced others, and he saw always their highest selves, calling them through seeing them to transcend, to become. The experience of being with him was to be constantly opened, to be constantly asked to respond with delight to that which had suddenly become more splendid through his gaze.

The next play I wrote, my first with George in mind, could not have been more different from *Us*. *Better People* is a surreal satire about genetic engineering and reproductive technologies—both subjects of much excitement in 1989. The play alternates between scenes in genetic scientists' labs as they race to map the human genome and scenes that take place in their dreams. It was based on a great deal of research and interviews. I found scientists eager to talk. I interviewed an elder woman scientist who showed me into her lab, filled with the cages of hundreds of rats upon which she did genetic experiments, because she said, she "liked mice." A geneticist at NYU painstakingly explained how to map genes, drawing on a yellow pad in his small office under fluorescent light for several hours. Then, he escorted me to the elevator bank and began inexplicably to rant about how nature must be controlled by genetic science. The renegade mystic, biologist, Rupert Sheldrake invited me into his London home. He poo-poohed the importance of genes, preferring to believe in morphic fields outside the earth that determined organic form. He was a staunch ecologist who did not believe in messing with nature.

I was, also, fascinated by George's upper-class, renegade mother, Irmgard, who died in 1981. Though I had not known her, I knew she had been formidable. I modeled Haila Gudenschmartzer on my image of her. George's mother was a choreographer, and the creator of the field of movement therapy, but in my play she is refashioned as a brilliant, domineering scientist, who in a dream sequence also speaks as a beleaguered Mother Earth. Made to do medical experiments on Jews in the concentration camps, Gudenschmartzer escapes Nazi Germany with a vial of sperm she uses to impregnate herself and give birth to a son, Edward Chreode, played by George. A chreode is the name for the pathway that individual cells, all of which are genetically the same, "choose" as they differentiate in form to become discrete organs, blood, and bones. It is as if each cell is magically endowed with something like "creative spirit" or "mind". Edward Chreode begins the play as a scientist mapping genes, meekly working under his mother's domineering personality. His "love interest," Theodora Forensic, was created in a petri dish from the sperm of two Nobel Prize winning scientists. Like the goddess Athena, Forensic is born motherless, and, therefore, becomes the most brilliant woman in the world. The three work in the lab run by Philbert Wallace, named after Walter Gilbert, then head of the government's effort to map the human genome, until he resigned in disgrace over economic malfeasance. Philbert plans to use his sperm, and, by harvesting hundreds of Theodora's brilliant eggs, to create a new super race, birthed by surrogates—a plan that might appeal today to someone like Elon Musk. Into this "rational" world of genetic experiment, a large, rare Yak-like animal ambles into Edward's lab. The only survivor of her species, she speaks one word, "Rendezvous." She refuses to be cloned. Instead, she dances with and swallows the scientist. The beast then expands, so that a dream love scene between Chreode and Forensic can be played inside her web-coated belly. Then, Chreode is vomited from of the belly of the beast, a changed man—a holistic climate scientist and a fierce environmentalist protector of endangered species. "Rendezvous," is the necessary meeting of mind and nature.

Along with his intimate scenes dancing with the huge animal, George played a dream sequence as a bodiless, talking head, rolling around on the seat of a wheelchair, beneath which his body was bent pretzel-like and out of sight. I did not know how to end my play, but George did. He improvised the ladder of evolution beginning as a praying mantis, ascending into a bird, becoming a stealthy lion, and, then, a man, who settles down in front of the large beast, while a baby beast (my nine-year-old) in fur costume with sweet human face, settles in front, a peaceable kingdom. The amazing Yak-like beast was the first New York work crafted by the master puppeteer, Basil Twist, a young man whose talent George recognized immediately and who now designs and creates all over the world. *Better People* was the first premiere I wrote and directed, and the first of our plays in which we invited panels of experts to speak about the play's themes for interested audiences, a practice we often continued as a way of placing our topical works within the larger frame of current intellectual and activist discourse. We even performed the play in front of an audience of genetic scientists, including Walter Gilbert, at a conference at Harvard—where it caused quite an intellectual ruckus with its audience staying up half the night to debate the efficacy of the play's conflict between mechanistic and environmental science.

George's mother died in 1981, so I never knew her, but, now, as George's new partner, I entered the Euro-American world of her good friend, Ursula Corning, a patron of the arts. George visited Ursula alone to tell her he was living with me. I was introduced to Ursula at a private lunch in her Upper East Side apartment with Maria, her lady's maid and companion, who served and ate with us. Though lunch was gracious, it was clear I was being vetted. Ursula gave large Christmas parties in New York. I, in thrift store black velvet, followed my child as she swept through the crowded living room in a fifties prom dress, its black skirt crisscrossed with pink ribbons, which on her reached to the floor, so that she looked the part of a small princess. "You have done rather well for yourself," Edna Gurewitsch commented to George. "So have we," I shot back. Edna was the widow of handsome, charismatic Dr. David Gurewitsch, personal physician and close friend to Eleanor Roosevelt. My mother idolized Eleanor Roosevelt; interviewing the former first lady, on the radio program she created and hosted, *Something for the Girls*, was a high point of my mother's life. (In my mother's secular family, the Roosevelts and their New Deal were deified.) Edna and I began to talk. She and David had lived with Mrs. Roosevelt in their Upper East Side townhouse, during the last years of her life. He attended her faithfully and when she died, he accompanied her body by train to her grave at Hyde Park. Edna wrote a book describing their threesome and the uncommon devotion Eleanor Roosevelt felt for her husband. "I love you as I never loved anyone else," the former first lady wrote to Dr. Gurewitsch. George told me his mother, perhaps, Ursula, too, had had a crush on the handsome Jewish émigré doctor, who was a noted polio specialist. George's mother used her innovative physical therapy techniques to treat polio victims in the 1950s and she worked with him. Now, in Ursula's living room, Edna Gurewitsch laughed with me about trying to keep Mrs. Roosevelt out of her kitchen while she was preparing dinner, as she "could not even wash the lettuce without making a terrible flood."

Ursula's family was in possession of an Italian castle. George, Crystal, and Alex vacationed there every year in June. Now, my daughter and I would vacation there, too. We landed at Fiumicino and took the train north from Rome, a rickety thing that circled up and down and around the Tuscan, then the Umbrian, hills. We were met by a car at the station in Umbertide, a nondescript town in a valley. Crystal was already at the castle with their son, Alex. They had always stayed several weeks while Crystal and George wrote the text for the street play they produced later each summer. Now, Crystal would write the script by herself. She and George would maintain a cordial silence and I was expected to behave myself. We drove up the road through rolling country past the tenant farms, once the feudal outposts of the castle. In the thirteenth century, this was the land of the warring Guelphs and Ghibellines. The Ranieris were Guelphs, and, therefore, loyal to the Pope. The Ghibellines were fighting to unite Italy under the Holy Roman Emperor. Mary Shelley made these brutal civil wars the setting for her novel *Valperga,* in which she wrote about the Ranieri castle, which we were headed to now. We drove past fields of yellow sunflowers, their large blossoms facing the sun as if in salute, their petals reflecting sparkling light. We passed fields of low red poppies, on roads lined with wild golden broom, and bluebells. These could not all have been in bloom at the same time, but I see them all flowering wildly in my mind. The castle sat at the top of a hill surrounded by a stone and brick wall. There were gardens outside, thick with roses. We drove through the open archway and now could see the castle directly in the center of our view. A real castle, large and square with huge, leaded windows and tall turrets at its corners. Its light brown stone shone in the sun. A castle as if from a picture book, or Mary Shelley's novel. We followed one fork of the split gravel road past a worn stone statue of a noble Ranieri, exactly in the center of the manicured castle lawn. The car entered the castle's inner courtyard through another archway in the close wall and stopped in front of massive stone steps; there were not many of them but they were very wide and not quite level because they were handmade and worn, centuries old, leading to the archway of the castle's entrance, its heavy wooden doors with iron hinges, thrown open. Ursula greeted us on the steps, smiling. Inside, all was cool, quiet, and dark, punctuated by streams of golden light from the high windows, cutting across off-white stuccoed walls, falling like shards on deep red tile floors. There was a Ranieri family tree painted on the wall in the entranceway. We were shown to our bedroom with its high, domed cathedral ceiling; down a short hall was my child's simpler room. Coming from a fractious Italian family that had disowned its unbaptized Jewish children, this was my first acquaintance with the refined Italy I would come to love, having nothing at all to do with my Calabrian peasant past in a rocky southern village whose name was lost to memory as my Italian relatives were lost to me.

This was the green heart of Italy: Perugia, Gubbio, Assisi, Monterche, the Italy of Piero della Francesca, who grew up near here in Sansepolcro and painted frescoes on the church walls, the Italy of rich agricultural tradition but also of cultured and accomplished people who lived for centuries in castles such as this. The Italy of dressing for the evening and of refined conversation over drinks before dinner, of sumptuous meals served by Valentino bending slightly with his heaping platter before each guest as he worked his way around the long table in the castle's huge dining hall. Of fabled lunches. We would cut excursions short and race back so as not to miss the fresh pasta with its succulent sauces and pitchers of the local red wine, served at midday. Mischievously, Ursula, who arranged the seating each evening, had put me directly across from Crystal on my first night, while Theresa, the cook with coal dark large eyes, peered from the kitchen door to assess and see if I behaved myself. (It helped that I looked Italian, of course.) This was the castle that had been in the Ranieri family since the tenth century, destroyed but built up again in the thirteenth century, destroyed, once again, during the harrowing tales of love and betrayal narrated by Mary Shelley, and rebuilt again in the fifteenth century. This was the Ranieri castle in which we were guests. In the towers, there were holes so that boiling oil could be poured down to scald any raiders climbing up. Ursula Corning, sturdy, white haired and handsome, was in benevolent control. If Mary Shelley's heroine, Euthanasia, had grown old, instead of being lost at sea, she would have looked like Ursula. She sat at the head of the table, and spoke little, but she beamed at all her guests in turn. She was so glad to have us. Our only duties were to be happy, well exercised, stuffed and polite. Therefore, I smiled at Crystal, across from me. She nodded back. Ursula wanted most of all that we, her guests, come to love Civitella and its surrounds as much as she did. She wished us to know the stories of the towns, to admire the churches and to hike the hills. She had been a mountaineer in her youth, climbing in the Alps. Now, she hosted car tours from town to town, to Gubbio for Sunday dinner, so the staff could have a break, to Assisi to see the church of St. Francis, and the monastery, to Perugia for market day, to San Sepolcro, where I saw my first hummingbird, and Monterchi, to view the frescoes of Piero.

"It's a friendly castle," Ursula used to say, and she peopled it with her friends, and friends of friends, children of friends, cousins of friends, first wives, second wives or husbands, everybody's children, and those who arrived she did not know, who were camping out and had been given directions by someone who had stayed at the castle. Once, the story went, there were tents on the lawn outside and four people slept on the pool table for lack of beds. No one who behaved themselves was turned away from this paradise in the Umbrian hills. At meals in the vast dining room, the long table hummed with conversations in French, German, English, Italian. There was the unfriendly castle we visited once or twice, also in the Ranieri family, where several unfriendly Ranieris lived in isolation, without guests. George had been to a formal affair there once, before my time; the dour servants with white gloves served canapés. The unfriendly castle was made of a forbidding dark gray stone, with dark cavernous halls, guarded by large Great Danes with saliva dripping from their jowls, as if they'd just finished gnawing on a leg. Ursula was from the other branch of the Ranieri family. She smiled almost all the time, a beatific, kindly smile. She wore flowered dresses in muted colors and sturdy shoes. She loved cats. There were always several fat, orange tabbies in the parlor she crooned to who slept in her room at night. There was often a new litter of kittens tumbling about, delighting the children on their knees.

In the mornings it was good to walk up Elsie's Road, named after a castle guest long gone, past the pig farm to the top of the hill, and then stop for ripe cherries hanging on the tree half-way back, or cut across the sunflower fields for a swim in the pond below. Or join an excursion to a nearby site with the driver, Jeremy, a law student from Ireland, who would marry a relative of Ursula's and live in London. In the evenings, we could watch the sunset from the castle roof, or play a game of Happy Families with the children in the parlor, or scrabble, which Ursula always won, have a piece of chocolate and a sherry or cognac. There were to be no fights between Ursula's friend who had been a Reagan appointee, her right-wing doctor, and those of us who held opposing political views. I would regularly say to George, "This is the most beautiful place I've ever been, but I cannot stand these people." Then, a new carful would arrive, Communists from France, the son of one of Ursula's good friends, with his wife and daughters, or a classical pianist from London and his lively therapist wife with their children and we'd have our clique of friends.

We had time to work on our artistic projects, and George and I did so over the years. I conceived *The Beekeeper's Daughter* at Civitella, in the summer of 1994, when the astonishing beauty of the land was in such dire contrast yet so close to the destruction of the war in Bosnia, that I felt I could hear the terrible rumbling of the guns through the green earth. The castle was the sort of place where the distance between reality and imagination often collapsed. One walked in beauty opened, deepened and enriched. We could share our work after dinner. George performed sections of the diaries of Victor Klemperer, which we worked on next. Ursula, like Ned Ryerson before her, funded these productions. Smiling, she simply wrote us large checks. The concert pianist would play the grand piano in the music room. She was his patron, too, paying for his solo recordings. A string quartet would mysteriously arrive. Sometimes, on a Saturday, there would be a wedding: a couple from the village below would marry in the castle chapel, their family and friends with children come up the hill dressed in pastels and ruffles, and we, the castle guests, would watch the ceremony from the chapel balcony. Sometimes, after dinner, we would drive down to Umbertide to eat gelato and join the families promenading around the square, pushing baby carriages.

We made pilgrimages every summer, sometimes more than once, to stand in the small chapel and gaze on her, The Madonna del Parto, painted by the local early Renaissance genius Piero della Francesca. Two angels, one dressed in green with reddish wings and one in red with green wings, pull the curtains back, revealing Mary, no older than a girl. So perplexed she looks, her hand on her swollen belly, her eyes so wide. Can she really be pregnant with the son of god, but who, after all, is not? Ursula liked to come to the chapel as often as she could, every time new guests arrived, and she would tell us each to make a wish, to ask for something from the pregnant Madonna. It was an extraordinary pleasure to stand before this beautiful fresco where it had been painted, behind the altar directly on the plaster wall of the small, rural church, were Piero's mother worshipped; a painting to honor his mother, as he imagined the young Mary. Painted in just seven days after his mother's death, before her funeral service here in this chapel. There was no glass, no frame, just the fresco of the pregnant Madonna on the wall, rough stone underneath, sun from the round window above. Perhaps, the only painting that shows her big with child. The chapel empty but for its wonderful fresco. An old guard asleep in a plastic chair in the sun outside. In later years, the pregnant Madonna was cut from the chapel wall and taken to Monterche, to be imprisoned in a museum behind plexiglass alongside Piero's other masterpieces, the beautiful boy angel's head, that came on loan to the Metropolitan Museum. She was not the same in the museum but this is what we now had, plus the memory of her on the wall. George loved the humanism of Piero, the distinct characters visible in all his work, the personalities of his angels, and the precision of his perspectives—all new to painting, then.

There was a rustic feeling to the castle life for all its understated elegance. Ursula expected sturdy guests, ready to climb a mountain to see the sunrise and the wild horses, or walk miles through the Piano Grande when it was miraculously alive for a week or two with varieties of wildflowers. We were warned to shake our shoes upside down in the mornings before we put them on for fear of stepping on a castle scorpion. At dinner, when bats flew in through the open windows and dive-bombed the guests, we were expected to sit up straight and continue the conversation unfazed. There was once a scandal: a minor scholar, forever writing his book on John Updike, and his wife were caught by one of the maids with some of the leather-bound books from the three-story library packed in their luggage. We were all shocked that such nondescript people had dared such a crime. They were forbidden ever to return. But mainly, everyone behaved, Ursula's hospitality being prodigious. It was our honeymoon of sorts, and became a yearly honeymoon where we fell ever more deeply in love surrounded by the beauty of the Umbrian hills. I walked to the top of the hill where a dozen trees were planted in a circle, like a fairy ring, and imprinted the view of the rich valley below so I might recall it whenever I wished. George and I would say to one another, "you die and you wake up in Umbria, at Civitella," just like the Renaissance painting by someone or other we saw in a museum somewhere in which decayed bodies from earth clamber through the clouds to emerge in heaven, young again, their muscles tuned, their hair thick.

This was Civitella before grief. Everyone was then alive. Maria had not gotten cancer and become so afraid. Ursula did not yet have dementia or need to wear diapers to dinner. The woman who replaced Maria and was now in charge of meals had not yet served hot dogs at lunch. George could still hike the hills. Although nothing seems now to have come before grief. Not even Civitella. Its stunning beauty shot through with feelings. We are born into this world already having forsaken a paradise. We are born into this world as refugees on a hard journey to a place where we might feel safe, born longing for a nonexistent world already lost to us, a place not of our making, perhaps of our dreams, perhaps the earliest moments of consciousness, perhaps the womb. Perhaps Civitella as imagined by angelic Ursula. We are born into a world from which just minutes ago we were absent, about which we have no idea; we, you, the us we long for, are born astonished and already bred for grief. Nothing lasts. Not even Paradise. We have lost it before we knew it and will forever lose it again before or whenever Paradise dares appear. Everyone in those ten summers at Civitella was Alive; there was no death in those golden days. There was light, the dawn, the day, the sunset, the moon, the stars, the barn owls screeching underneath the eaves. We were tanned, with bright eyes; our dark skin shone. We dressed in soft reds, violets and yellows, in flowing garments that revealed breasts and legs. "You must be careful of Peter Marengone," Ursula warned George about the local Lothario, who drove up after dinner in his green Ferrari to seduce the female guests. We laughed. Peter only liked blondes. We were always on good behavior for Ursula in the Eden she made and which she stocked as one might stock a fishpond, with so many varieties of persons—all of whom knew to behave, quietly, gently as if on holiday at a castle with the queen. Today Civitella Ranieri is an international artists' colony, in memory of Ursula, but when I went there with George, year after year, it was our love-soaked fantasy.

We opened our own not-for-profit theater, Theater Three Collaborative, in 1995. Our third partner was the dancer-creator-painter, a large, eccentric Lower East Side presence, Lee Nagrin. Lee moved and spoke very slowly, as if channeling visions. I wrote major roles in my new play *The Beekeeper's Daughter* especially for Lee and George. Her character was called Sybil, as Lee was sibylline and he, her brother, played by George, was Robert Blaze, a famous, Robert Gravesian poet who sought refuge on an island in the Adriatic after his wife's suicide. Conceived at Civitella the previous summer and set during the Bosnian war, which was still in progress, my play was accepted at a new international theater festival, the Dionysia World Festival of Contemporary Drama, whose director came to George looking for new American scripts. It was all quite posh. There a press conference where the festival's six writers from six countries spoke about our plays, held in the City Hall in Rome. We toured the Vatican, and ate a superb gelato at George's favorite spot, outside the Vatican walls. He fancied himself a gelato connoisseur. Then we moved to the Tuscan hill town of Veroli, halfway between Naples and Rome, where the festival took place. I staged *The Beekeeper's Daughter* outside at sunset on the stone piazza of the old Church of Our Lady of the Olives, against a view of the Tuscan hills, with swallows swooping and the light changing. The production was sparse yet beautiful and the story was especially meaningful, as Bosnian women were still being raped and impregnated a few hundred miles away, as a means of cultural genocide. The play was a trip to a magical world where such unbearable wounds might begin to heal. In four scenes, House, Bee Hives, Forest and Sea Storm, its characters move deeper into the wildness of nature and their own unconscious, emerging seeing self and other in new ways, and, most important, being seen. Traumatized victims of violence often believe that what has happened to them, through no fault of their own, casts them apart from the human community. They feel polluted, unclean, alone, isolated. When Christen Clifford, who, at age twenty-three played the raped and pregnant Bosnian woman, walked through the town wearing her big belly underneath a blue jean maternity dress, boys and men cried out "Eh, Madonna!" Christen had been raped twice in high school; she worried she had not suffered enough to understand women tied to beds, repeatedly raped by battle crazed Serbian forces, but she had. The haunted look on her face, her stony silence, her arms held at odd angles from her pregnant body so as not to touch her own flesh, grown large despite her will, made clear the suffering captive Bosnian woman were going through right then, just several hundreds of miles away from the Italian hill town where we rehearsed in the golden light of the summer sun.

The women of the town gathered to watch us rehearse the birthing scene. Admira, unwilling, frantic, comforted by Sybil, unable to look at or touch the child implanted by force. And the town's women smiled when the poet, Robert, falls in love with the unwanted child, begins crooning to him, and carries him everywhere. The men gathered to watch the fight scene between father and daughter, in which he slaps her. Artists from Slovenia, the first nation to secede from the former Yugoslavia, felt *The Beekeeper's Daughter* spoke directly to what people were going through right at that moment, and thought our play and production the best in the festival. George would play the poet, Robert Blaze, over the course of twenty-two years in four productions, 1994-2016. As the actor aged, the character took on force made bolder by experience, and by our evolving culture. Everyone in the play changes, but bisexual Robert most of all as he redefines ego-driven masculine genius into the wisdom of nurturant caretaking—and becomes a better poet and father, happier, too, in the process. Each time George approached the character, he deepened the stakes, until in the final production—at age eighty-three, white-haired, bearded, and vigorous—he had the force of a prophet who fiercely embodies the virtues of caretaking love and poetic truth in a role I had fashioned on him over two decades earlier. Creativity and nurture were no longer in conflict; commitment to one strengthens the other. And this is how our relationship worked. We were made better artists by our love.

"To me, Homo sapiens are only 'good' when all their individual ingredients aspire to realize the best in themselves coupled with a desire to benefit self-realization *in all other living creatures*," George wrote in his diary at the end of his life. I find similar exhortations about how to live replete with his generosity in the diaries he left on tables and in drawers. He lived as he wrote, taking as much if not more pleasure from the creativity he nurtured in others as he did from his own gifts. He was loved and admired by many hundreds of artists he shared the stage with, whose work he produced, or whom he taught. No one as lucky as I, who lived with him and received his humor, his insights and generosity first. When he died, Christen Clifford gave me a note, folded many times, that, unfolded, revealed, "George is love. You are love. Thank you for showing me a good life."

When we met, George had pushed so far down, he had "forgotten" he was a hidden child in Nazi Germany. By the time George died in my arms at 2:08 am on Saturday, July 30, in 2022, at the age of eighty-nine-and-a-half, of side-effects from multiple myeloma, a smoldering, hidden cancer and from its treatments, which he could not tolerate, he had come to elegant understanding of how his first six years in Hitler's Germany formed him. He lived an invented life, becoming a uniquely poetic actor, producer, rebel, pacifist, nature lover. Joy mixed with terror was his métier. He remained always something of a precocious, curious, rambunctious, beautiful boy, full of impetuous delight, with deep-set blue eyes that sparkled until he died. "If you want to be taken care of, you don't want George," a couple therapist who was also enchanted by him told me early on. He was impractical to a fault, realizer of impossible dreams; he co-founded two New York institutions, Theater for the New City and the Greenwich Village Halloween Parade. He worked for five years with the artist Danny Simmons, to convince the New York Metropolitan Transit Authority to allow five large public art murals they curated from neighborhood artists to be installed in the then-derelict G train station in our Clinton Hill, Brooklyn neighborhood—where they remain over twenty years later, graffiti-free. Together we made plays set in the future, the past, in torture sites in Iraq and Afghanistan, on wilderness estates and enchanted islands, plays that addressed violence but showed nonviolent change happen. Our shared aesthetic was transformation. Conflict is not the essence of drama, evolution is. He played villains and poets, unfaithful husbands, flawed fathers, human rights activists, environmentalists, a Noam Chomsky-like linguist (Noam and he admired one another and looked alike when they wore beards), and he played many animals; he was swallowed by a large beast to emerge an ecologist; he assisted "live" stage births, as thrilled and disorganized as any of us; after his death his prerecorded voice animated a talking fish, choking on plastic: "If I cannot breathe neither can you. That is tragic irony. I'm just a fish. Get used to it," he said on tape from his place out of this world.

George liked to play historical characters, and he did copious research, learning to think, walk, gesture and speak as they had. He played UN weapon's inspector Hans Blix in David Hare's daring and important play, *Stuff*

Happens, about the lead-up to the illegal invasion of Iraq, at New York's Public Theater. He came home many nights enraged because some in the audience, seated in a circle around the performers, put their fingers into their ears, showing their displeasure at the Palestinian lawyer's final speech, which was her plea for justice for the Palestinians. He played Sigmund Freud in Willy Holzman's *Sabina,* about Carl Jung, Freud and Sabina Spielrein, a protégé of each. Jung's mistress and a major contributor to psychoanalytic theory, she was burned to death by the Nazis with her children when they took refuge in a church. George did much research as always and reading in Freud's prodigious writings, he slowly transformed body and voice, until I had the uncanny feeling I was going to bed with Sigmund Freud. He played German philologist Victor Klemperer for many years, in our adaptation of Klemperer's hidden Holocaust diaries *I Will Bear Witness,* the most personally consequential role of his long career.

George survived two near-fatal sepsis attacks before he was diagnosed in 2019 with multiple myeloma, an invariably fatal bone-marrow cancer, whose most prominent effect on him was not the breakage or weakening of his bones, nor cancerous tumors anywhere, but the weakening of his immune system. With the onslaught of sepsis, he shook uncontrollably. I learned, after his first attack on a midtown street, to get him to a hospital as fast as possible. So when he began to shake after breakfast, I said, let's go to the hospital in Brooklyn, instead of uptown where his heart specialist was. "It's his immune system," friends said while I was shopping in the Park Slope Food Coop, and so we asked for a comprehensive blood test. After the results, we were sent by the infectious disease specialist to see the hospital's new head of oncology-hematology. In September 2019, George began cancer treatment. He could not tolerate the Revlimid he was given, and we were opening *Other Than We,* a climate change play, at LaMama, so he took himself off treatment. He was back on treatment with thalidomide on September 11, 2020, when he became very ill with sepsis again and nearly died; again he survived, his life force so fierce. It was the midst of the COVID pandemic. I left him that night, lucid, when after many hours, he was moved from the ER to a bed in a private room, but he was incoherent an hour later when I phoned him from home. I asked if he wanted me to come back. He mumbled something that sounded like "yes." It was nearly ten o'clock. I texted his doctor the news. His doctor replied, "I'll be there." I arrived first. Stopped by the stern guard on a high stool, like Gabriel guarding the gate, I pleaded and begged. Very ill … I must … Doctor coming. The guard didn't believe me (I wasn't certain myself the doctor would appear; what doctor comes back to the hospital at 10 pm to see someone? Unless, of course, he thinks they might die). There was absolutely no way the guard would let me pass. I was loud and creating a nuisance. "But …" I tried. Again, the guard told me to get lost, visiting hours were over; he would not let me in. I stood wedged into a corner of the hall trying to make myself small while attempting to phone the nurses' station, too upset to dial correctly, when the doctor sidled up to me like a stealth lover. Shoulder to shoulder we passed the angry guard and entered the elevator without speaking a word. How I needed the cancer doctor to be my special other and, he, too, perhaps, needed me to be the same for him—we were each enchanted by George. Together, our healing powers increased, or so we thought without, again, ever saying anything about how we felt or what we meant to one another, until much later, after George died—while George lived, we forged a bond, intellectual, emotional, which we nurtured between ourselves. We needed each other to keep George alive—together we bonded over playing God.

We both thought George might be dying upstairs. When we got to his room, I sat on his bed, took his hand in mine, and kissed him gently. George was unable to form a coherent sentence. He did not appear to recognize who I was. "Where were you on that day?" meaning September 11, 2001, the oncologist asked. "En-en-et to du …(with great effort) *pah.*" I had no idea, but George later laughed and reminded me that we had gone to the Brooklyn Promenade with hundreds of others to watch in horror as the towers smoldered and ghostly survivors covered in pasty gray ash began to make their ways home. (In the following months, I would work with survivors, taking their testimonies for the Columbia Oral History Archive.) "Promenade" was what he was trying to say but could not. "Pah," he sputtered. I had never heard George unable to articulate. His diction was perfect, his voice resonant, but not now. I looked into his eyes, hoping for recognition I wasn't certain was there. I kissed him again. No response. The doctor stood next to the bed. He swabbed George's mouth with a lemon-flavored sponge. He would do that again one day, when George really was dying. We stayed until we were both certain, without speaking to each other directly, that George was not going to die, not that night, anyway. We left his room shoulder to shoulder without exchanging a word and parted at the hospital door. It was pitch dark. I found a cab. I could not have stood it had I not been able to get past the guard into the hospital to see George that night. I was surprised a doctor would be so devoted, but he has a reputation for being so. Soon enough, we all called each other by our first names. The next morning when I phoned, George was lucid. I texted his doctor. "That's good news," he answered immediately. Sepsis, often fatal, takes a long time to recover from, and many antibiotics. The doctor took to stopping by George's room on his morning rounds with a strong cup of Sumatra coffee, George's favorite. They would have morning coffee together and chat. I gave the doctor an anthology of four of my plays in which George starred, with photographs of each production, in thanks. He, in turn, invited me to come to his administrative office to see his first wife's watercolors. In the midst of the pandemic, I would help the doctor conceptualize and place an Op-Ed for the *New York Times*, and later, in 2021, he would become my confidant as I directed the final play in which George would act. And we flirted with each other, catching one another's eyes, looking each other up and down. "You have a thing about____," George would say, using the doctor's last name. I did not disagree. Eros drives Thanatos away, and we were both, the doctor and I, determined that George should live.

George began his professional acting career on Broadway in 1947, at age fourteen, in *The Whole World Over*, written by a Russian, Konstantine Simonov. Set during the post-war housing crisis in Moscow, the romantic comedy follows a group of people billeted in the same crowded apartment at the command of Stalin's government. It shows Russians, our allies in World War II, as dimensional characters. Harold Clurman directed the Soviet play in a commercial production on Broadway. Clurman, with his hat and cane and his booming voice, was a theatrical legend. He co-founded the influential Group Theater in New York in the 1930s, and wrote a classic of American theater history, *The Fervent Years,* about the Group's socially conscious, ensemble work, and his collaboration with Clifford Odets, whose plays the Group Theater produced. Clurman interviewed George in his apartment and cast the fourteen-year-old as the understudy, but in out-of-town tryouts, George went on for a night, and the original boy actor was fired. George would open the play on Broadway. This is the play in which Herbert Berghof, who also came in as a replacement, met Uta Hagen—they would become a noted theater couple and found HB Studios, where George taught Shakespeare, play-creation and directed late in his life. George played a war orphan rescued in the Polish forest by Russian soldiers and brought to Moscow to live in the communal apartment. It was a more autobiographical role than George, at fourteen, consciously knew. A child immigrant to the US in 1939, George was forbidden by his parents to speak his native German, even at home, so he would learn English quickly and not be taunted at school or beaten up. But the loss of the German language at age six also meant the repression of his earliest memories, memories that would return with force as he was dying.

"Uta, I fear Herbert does not have honorable intentions," the blond boy actor said, standing awkwardly in her dressing room door; George had a crush on Uta himself. She remembered the moment so clearly. She quoted the remark to us, laughing, at her book party, shortly before she died. On stage in her role, she took special care of the orphan, brushing his hair and fussing over him. The production was a hit, at first, but it closed abruptly when the Cold War began. As anti-communist hysteria swept the nation, audiences stopped coming. In 2019, in a staged reading at HB Studios commemorating Hagen's centennial, George played the lead, a wise elder architect, slyly opposed to Stalin's Five-Year Plan, who urges the young people in the crowded apartment *not* to do what the Soviets dictate but to follow their dreams. Because by then, George had macular degeneration and could not read a handheld script, I printed the script out in forty-nine-point bold type—it was over four-hundred pages. He memorized the entire long part, word by word, tracing each letter with a magnifying glass. He sat on a stool in his bathroom, where the light was bright. He would come running out and find me at my desk or somewhere else in the apartment to share his newfound admiration for the script and its lead character, with the excitement of a teenager. And because he learned his full part, the other actors, too, had to step up, learning their lines and the reading became quite like a full performance, with George energizing a much younger cast. It was like him to do the seemingly impossible with excitement and grace. On stage in his last years, no one could tell he was legally blind, though he had a bad habit of falling down on the sidewalk on opening nights. Once we had to go to the dentist to glue together broken teeth and he opened the second production of *Extreme Whether* at LaMama in 2018, with a band aid on his scraped nose. Two years after George's Broadway debut, in 1949, at age sixteen, he was on Broadway again, in *Montserrat*, written and directed by Lillian Hellman, her metaphor for the McCarthy hearings.

At age nineteen, George returned to Europe to study at the Royal Academy of Dramatic Art and the Guildhall in London, but, first, he went to visit his Tante Irma on her war-ravaged estate near Düren, from which she had been forced to flee under Allied bombardment, with the family members who remained, as the US soldiers advanced. George's cousin Brigitte drew her memories in what we now call a Zine, which George was a given a Xerox copy of late in his life. Brigitte's first sight of a Black person was the American pilot who was strafing the German refugees below, flying close enough to the ground she could see into the cockpit. Nevertheless, Tante Irma, even post-war, had more money than George's mother in the US (he had worked on a farm that summer to pay his passage and would work as a fishmonger in London to pay his bills, while studying acting on scholarship) and his aunt bought him a new set of clothes. He also went to Bavaria to visit his old headmaster at the Steiner school he and his brother attended in 1938. At age nineteen, he did not yet remember the full story of why he felt compelled to visit these two who had kept him safe during the Nazi years until 1939, when he escaped, but he knew he had to go see them both, and to sit, tongue-tied, at their feet. He wanted to become a Shakespearean actor and because ticket prices were cheap for West End shows, he could see Gielgud, Olivier and other great actors perform. At the Guild Hall, he directed Milton's *Samson Agonistes* to good notices. He made plans to stay on in England. After completing his course at the Guild Hall, he worked in a summer theater with Eileen Atkins and Alan Bates, both wonderful actors and lovely people who became quite famous. Decades later, when they were performing together in New York, the two came to our rented, big Victorian house for a very drunken, post-theater dinner. Alan was bisexual. In London, as a student, George was in a serious homosexual relationship with a handsome man named Stanley, who was of half Arab descent. This is why his parents, who since their divorce were seldom together, united in a trip to London to bring their son home to New York, with much cajoling, to "save" him from homo- or bi-sexuality and why, in the end, George became neither a Shakespearean actor (though he always loved to act, direct and quote Shakespeare) nor continued his homosexual life. Stanley made a trip to New York a few years later to win him back, but George by then had fallen in love hard with the American avant-garde, in which he became a key player, and he had married, as he promised himself, at thirty, the second woman to whom he proposed.

In 1960, he was cast in the American premiere of two landmark avant-garde plays, first as the understudy but then he played Peter in *Zoo Story*, by Edward Albee, back-to-back, with his Krapp in Beckett's great *Krapp's Last Tape* at the Cherry Lane theater in Greenwich Village, directed by Allan Schneider in a production that ran from 1960 to '63, and opened again in 1965. When George's brother could not tell whether he was Peter or Jerry in the Albee two-hander (he was Peter), George thrilled to his confusion. Proof he could do what he always wished—disappear completely into character. George would continue to work with Albee periodically, the last time in the revival of *The Sandbox* and *American Dream* directed by Albee, in 2008. He performed two of Beckett's late short plays, *Theater I* and *Theater II* on the same bill with Julian Beck at LaMama and on the European tour cut short by Julian's ill health and he performed at Lincoln Center's tribute to Beckett upon the playwright's death, along with other respected American and Irish Beckett actors. Late in his life, he directed *Waiting for Godot* twice with his HB Acting Studio students.

Also in the early 1960s, George found and helped to create the American avant-garde, his great love, at Judson's Poet's Theater, where the actors were often dancers, poet, or amateurs, the plays were wildly poetic and inventive.

He made Judson his artistic home. No one was paid, but he loved the mix of dance, music, and poetry. He performed in *Promenade* the first musical by a new young writer, Maria Irene Fornes, a playwright he would later produce many times. He committed himself to the downtown experimental theater scene, the dancers and poets, the gay and female playwrights, the whole New York avant-garde just then burgeoning. He began to balance a potentially lucrative commercial career with his love of creating the unknown. Often riding his bike (which he rode through New York until a fall when he was eighty years old) from uptown after a Broadway curtain racing downtown to perform late night off off-Broadway. His fancy agent dropped him when he co-founded Theater for the New City, in 1971, because George became permanently burdened with producing, management and fundraising duties and was often unable even to go to auditions. He gave up his professional acting career to produce and perform in plays by unknown writers. TNC was a center, a force for "new theater", as George called the avant-garde, including the writer Bob Nichols, who wrote TNC's early summer street theater plays. George loved to tell the tale of Bob's first street play, *The Expressway*, a public debate about the proposed four-lane highway right through Greenwich Village, which would have destroyed it. When Joe Papp saw the play, he insisted it open his new Public Theater, and *The Expressway* was staged outside the Public's doors on Lafayette Street, in the building Papp reclaimed that had, in the forties, been used to house Jewish refugees. People walking by on the street thought the actors were actual New York politicians and citizens debating the newly proposed highway plan. They stopped to watch when, suddenly, a car ran into the stage. The platform shattered in front of them—and the play stopped as the audience watched amazed—was this real or fake? The destruction of the stage and disruption of the debate were a potent example of what would happen to Village life if the proposed highway were built. It was not because of continuing protests. The simple-but-astonishing stage magic, the stage that shattered, was made from cardboard packing boxes and duct tape by Bob Nichols, the play's author, and a carpenter. When the car hit, a strip of duct tape was pulled by an actor and the stage simply fell apart.

George, the great storyteller, the enthusiast for life who danced through our golden-yellow living room, the sun streaming in, playing an ancient Greek line on his wooden song flute, naked sometimes, like a sprite, saved for the last half of his life his dive into his own earliest memories—they were too frightening until he felt safe.

"Why are you always reading all that Holocaust stuff," George asked me, annoyed. I was deep into Robert Jay Lifton's *The Nazi Doctors*. I was a member of Lifton's Center on Violence and Human Survival at John Jay College, a think-tank for activists and intellectuals.

"You are a Holocaust survivor," I answered.

"No, I'm not," George shot back. His silence was broken by the vehemence of his denial. He began to realize, at that moment, I think, that he needed to excavate his own repressed past in order to live a fully examined life. As he aged, he worked to recall and to write more about his early life in Hitler's Germany, and this journey into his past had the effect of making him seem ever younger as he grew older, more spontaneous, surprised and braver.

If the rising cancer rate is exacerbated by the petrochemical pollutants our naked bodies are ever more fiercely subjected to since the end of the Second World War, and, also, by the social stresses and emotional traumas we carry with us, passed down generation to generation from that time and before—and why wouldn't this be the case—then cancer, whether survived or not, presents us all—as we all may acquire the disease at any time, and more so as we age, and we all have close others who already have cancer—the extraordinary challenge and potential of living a self-examined life. As we understand more about where we have come from, we also can work harder to end war, pollution, and social inequities. Which always were George's desires. To say George continued to become a more consummate and luminous actor as he grappled first with his repressed past in Nazi Germany as a hidden child, then with his hidden disease, is so.

When George and I met, his brother, who had changed his name from Igor Bartenieff to John Barrett, was still alive. (He would end his life by suicide in 1991, during the First Gulf war.) Early in our relationship, we visited John (we called him Igor between ourselves) and his wife in their large Connecticut home, furnished in part with antiques inherited from George and Igor's mother's family, which were shipped from Germany towards the end of her life when, at last, she received her inheritance. Rowena Barrett, whom I had just met, took out a large family album; we sat together on the floor while she showed me napkins used on the table when the Kaiser dined at the family home and medals the Kaiser had bestowed on the family Dombois, George's mother's maiden name. It was to be understood I was marrying into an old and prominent German-Huguenot family. This was news to me, because George and Igor were raised in poverty in New York by their working mother. They ate diners from cans, and moved often, seldom seeing their mother because she worked so hard. She was, in fact, making a name for herself, developing innovative movement therapies. George had a habit of carrying his worldly belongings—scripts, business receipts, rehearsal clothes, whatever else he needed—in paper bags. For the last decade of his life, he used a red paper wallet he had carefully constructed from a bright red envelope held together with wide layers of clear packing tape. He repaired this "wallet" many times, carefully layering on tape which grew thicker over the bright red paper. Inside this construction, he kept his bills. He never used credit cards. He had none. These were frugal habits he'd acquired from his mother, who had died five years before George and I met. She carried her notes for the classes she taught, her musings on physical therapy, her choreography, in two large paper bags almost reaching the floor, as she was small, while she hurried between jobs, from dance studios to hospitals where she treated polio sufferers, psychiatric patients and others with her innovative movement analyses, extending each person's range of movement through exercises she designed especially for them.

Irmgard Dombois Bartenieff was an innovator in her field. She brought Laban dance notation techniques to America and virtually created the field of movement therapy, teaching many young dancers at the Laban/Bartenieff Institute she founded. She came home late and exhausted. They moved often. For a while, they lived in a basement apartment owned by an Irish family with four beautiful, redheaded daughters. Young George's job was to stoke the furnace with coal. Irmgard owned a small house in Queens for a few years and the boys kept many cats who went in and out on a ladder that reached a window left open a crack on the second floor.

They moved to an apartment next to the elevated subway on the East Side. On hot nights, George and Igor, like many sweltering New Yorkers before air conditioning, slept outside on the fire escape while the trains clanked by.

If I imagine his brilliant, obsessed mother looking something like a harried, aristocratic bag lady, I can say with certainty that George was a combination of European gentleman, good-looking, well-spoken and gracious, and a vagabond, in baggy cargo-pant shorts, socks falling down over scuffed sneakers, and ragged t-shirts, with an old white dress shirt worn open thrown on. In this outfit, he auditioned for and got the role as a replacement for the rabbi in a Broadway revival of *Fiddler on the Roof*, starring his friend, Harvey Fierstein as Tevya, who teased him on stage as George struggled, without much rehearsal, to learn the movements and songs. Late in Irmgard Bartenieff's life, after her children were grown, she received her inheritance from her family in Germany and the furniture I saw in George's brother's house, the medals and napkins, were shipped to America. She undoubtedly used some of this money to found the Laban/Bartenieff Institute of Movement Studies in New York, as George would use a chunk of his inheritance from her to support Theater for the New City, and some to fund plays we did. Her book *Body Movement: Coping with the Environment* is the classic in the field of movement analysis and movement therapy she pioneered. When she died in 1981, she was renowned among legions of dancers who studied with her.

Irmgard Dombois was born in Berlin in 1900. Her maternal grandfather, Prym, was the inventor of the ubiquitous snap fastener; the factory was run by the family, and for a short time, in the 1980s, George's brother was its president. Irmgard studied dance and dance notation at Rudolf Laban's school in Munich, where she became his best student, personal assistant and friend. She was married, soon, to a professor of classics named Berve. Someone approved by her family, but unfortunately for her, homosexual. She met the Russian émigré Mikhail Bartenieff in the Laban Tanzbuhne, for which she danced and choreographed. Bartenieff taught her Russian ballet, lofting her high, leaping with her across the stage. A Jewish refuge from a Russian family of accomplished actors and musicians, some of whom also immigrated to New York, Mikhail was a passionate, handsome fellow, irresistible to the brilliant young woman starved for physical intimacy. Their first child, Igor, was born out of wedlock while they were on tour in Stuttgart, in 1929. In 1931, Irmgard and Mikhail left Laban and founded their own dance company, which exclusively performed her choreography, made for the company that featured the two of them as its stars. There are many photos of the lead dancers, Irmgard and Mikhail, smiling in mid-leap in each other's arms. One such photo sits on George's mother's inlaid antique desk, which he inherited after her death, along with a set of heavy sterling silver, perhaps once used at the Prym table for the Kiser that we used for large dinner parties. Theirs was a folk-inspired company, comic and broad, energetic, crowd-pleasing. The tall, handsome Russian dancer spun her and twirled her, swept her off her feet, spirited her away into a romantic fantasy of her making. For him, a talented, fearless woman from a wealthy German Huguenot family must also have seemed like a fairytale ending. No wonder they named their new dance company Romantisches Tanztheater Bartenieff. Quickly, Irmgard was disinherited by her father Dombois, and grandfather Prym, perhaps because Mikhail was a Jew, or because she became pregnant with his child while she was still officially married to someone else, probably both. Never mind that the classicist Berve had not yet given them an heir, and seemed to have had no intention of ever doing so.

Perhaps none of this mattered very much to the two young lovers dancing wildly in their own world because they earned their living by touring Germany with their dance company and they received good reviews. Irmgard divorced Berve and married Bartenieff. The couple kept an apartment in Berlin and continued to tour. Their second son, George Michael, was born in Berlin on January 24, 1933. Six days later, on January 30, Himmler appointed Adolf Hitler Chancellor. Almost immediately, Irmgard and Michail's Romantisches Tanztheater was targeted. Their bookings were cancelled. Their dancers were forced to resign or lose their membership in the German artistic union, now Nazi run. The two founders officially disbanded their company. One night Irmgard watched from her 13 Berliner Strasse apartment window while a neighbor and friend was led away by the Gestapo. She began trying to convince her Jewish husband to emigrate. He refused. He could not bear the thought of leaving behind his beloved, adopted Germany, where he found success and had felt so welcome. (George's father would return to Germany two decades after the war ended, without bothering to wait until George's son Alexander was born; he would marry a German woman and die in Germany in the 1960s, of melanoma.) In 1933, their dance company closed and Hitler in power, the young family began to take refuge at least some of the time on the estate of Irmgard's aunt, Irma Hasenclever. Tante Irma, as George always called his great aunt, defied the family's ban on the renegade dancer and her Russian-Jewish husband and welcomed them with their children. In 1934, at a nearby bathing resort, blond, blue-eyed George was voted "the most Aryan baby on the beach." The parents' argument about immigration would last three years as Hitler continued to consolidate power: Mikhail refusing to budge from Germany. Irmgard increasingly insistent. Until, at last, in 1936, Mikhail agreed to go with his wife on visitors' visas through Cuba to the US, to see if they might earn a living in the new country. Irmgard found them a sponsor in Pittsfield, Massachusetts. The rebellious, prescient Irmgard had finally wrenched from her passionate, misguided husband some control over the fate of her family, but at the cost of leaving her two children, now aged three and six, behind in Nazi Germany, in the care of their Tante Irma.

If women in Nazi Germany had scant public power, they could still make themselves part of the resistance by silently harboring Jews in their homes, which is what George's mother's aunt, Irma Hasenclever, determined to do when she agreed to care for the two half Jewish children of her sister's daughter. Alice Prym Dumbois, the boys' maternal grandmother, was meek, dominated by the husband who disowned his daughter, and they lived in Berlin. Irma Hasenclever, without a husband, was mistress of the grand Haus Merberich, its vast grounds and its tenant farm, near Düren, some distance away from Berlin, the seat of Nazi power. Tante Irma was vital, a free thinker, a painter and a patron of artists. Later, during the war, she housed artists in the rooms of her mansion, and there were stovepipes from the tin stoves coming out of each window. After the war, she sheltered war orphans in her battle-scarred house, the estate having been fought over as the allies advanced into Germany. Such patronage was to become a family tradition. George's mother would mentor hundreds of dancers in America, teaching them her innovative dance-therapy and dance-notation techniques, and choreographing new works. Her students nicknamed the diminutive firebrand, "the iron butterfly."

The stone and brick mansion, Haus Merberich, was built around an open courtyard, and with its farm, formed something like a small village— a grand house with a domain of tenants and animals. Tante Irma was followed everywhere she went by three or four spotted spaniels, (looking very much like Abby, our first of four multi-colored cockers, which I, as yet unknowing of his family history, brought home for my daughter our first Christmas together. "Don't come in," I met him at the door of our third floor walk-up railroad apartment across from Fort Greene Park, then too dangerous to enter day or night, now a neighborhood dog-walking delight. "I have something to tell you." "You're pregnant!" "No, we have a dog." "Worse," he snapped, but the puppy soon won his heart. We would have cocker spaniels together for the next thirty-five years). In the last apartment we shared, on DeKalb Avenue in Clinton Hill, the same Brooklyn neighborhood we always lived in and loved, George hung a photo of his Tante Irma on the wall across from his side of our big bed alongside two of her paintings, a large sunflower blossom drooping from its weight, and the spire of country church. In the photo, the handsome young Irma, tall and willowy, sits outside on the grass, wearing a loose cardigan over a white blouse and a calf-length wool skirt, her long legs drawn around her. She holds a spotted spaniel puppy from a new litter casually on her lap. The mother dog with another pup suckling stands nearby, looking at her. She pets a large terrier, standing close to her on her other side. She looks out at the camera, an open, intelligent, angular face, with a hint of a smile. Little-boy George adored her. George remembered her loving look all of his life. I could see the slim smile on her face and her twinkling blue eyes whenever Tante Irma looked down on the small, blond cherub looking up, because George wore that same loving look whenever he spoke of his great aunt. From the wall across from our bed, Tante Irma, seated on the lawn with her dogs, watched over George until his death.

Gisela, Irmgard's sister, also lived on Tante Irma's estate with her two teenage daughters, Brigitte and Ina. At some point, perhaps after George's parents left for the United States in 1936, Gisela remarried, to a man named Otto Hoesch who inherited and ran his father's chemical company, Joseph Hoesch Chemicals, still in existence and in the family. This chemical company was immediately commandeered by the Nazis for the war effort. The plant made aluminum alloys used in warplanes. Otto, George's new uncle by marriage, joined the Nazi Party in 1933, as soon as, that is, but no sooner than, Hitler came to power. "A cautious man," his son Henning wrote, describing him to me in a letter, "he was not a Nazi," but he was a card-carrying member of the NSDAP (National Socialist German Workers Party). I received a photocopy of his Nazi Party membership card from the archive in Berlin, along with several letters documenting his Party membership. Thus, George and his brother, Igor, now lived in a blended family of the hunter and the hunted: the Nazi uncle and the two half Jewish boys left behind by their parents. Hoesch, in fact, was a passionate hunter of big game. He kept a preserve in Germany stocked with wild boar and the like and after the war, he hunted in Africa—on his hunting lodge walls were the heads of the big beasts he shot. During the war, at Haus Merberich, when meat was rationed, Herr Otto Hoesch kept his own private locker filled with sausage for his sole consumption. Perhaps, these private extra rations were given to him by his Nazi Party connections. As the owner and proprietor of Hoesch Chemicals, Otto was exempt from military service.

Tante Irma sheltered the two boys. Their two older cousins, Brigitte and Ina, stepdaughters to the Nazi Hoesch, along with their great aunt's many animals, horses, dogs, cows, provided additional comfort and care. George remembered being driven in a black Mercedes Benz through the large iron gates of the factory premises, which were guarded by uniformed Nazi soldiers. Just why the two boys went to their uncle's chemical factory is unclear. But the half Jewish identity of the blond, blue-eyed boys was being kept hidden, and perhaps this trip to the Nazi-commandeered factory was part of this ruse. When he began to be able to remember his early childhood, George remembered the trip through the Nazi guarded gates of the factory with fear.

Perhaps, Otto Hoesch's presence on the estate offered a certain protection to its other residents, as he was a Nazi Party member in good standing. Did he entertain other members of the Nazi Party at the large in-laid marble round table that is now in the large entranceway of his son's large estate in Aix-en-Provence, where he raises organic grapes and makes wine? Hoesch flew the Nazi Party flag from the big house's highest turret, a sign, his son told me, that those who lived below, including their tenant farmers, were loyal to the regime—and should, therefore, be left alone. But the presence of the half Jewish children, hidden there in plain sight, must have added tension. The two boys remembered Haus Merberich as a paradise of sorts, but underneath the opulence and peace of the big estate, there was terror that George began to fully comprehend only at the end of his life. Remembering was the work he was doing as he came closer to death. Five months before he died, George began to write his memoir in earnest. Though he could no longer see what he wrote, his cursive handwriting was clear enough to be transcribed. He was writing many of the stories he told, their details coming clearer over the years since he began being able to recall his early years in Nazi Germany, the memories of which he had repressed until we met, and he found me engaged in Holocaust studies. (George had gastric problems, always, and these grew worse with his cancer treatments and contributed to his death. His troubles with not being able to digest most likely had roots in the early fears he repressed.)

Three-year-old George stood in the courtyard and sang to Tante Irma, leaning out the window above, smiling; she threw coins to him. "My penny for my first performance," he wrote in his diary. His older cousins, Brigitte and Ina, also doted on the little boy; George wrote:

> *Brigitte was the warmest and took naturally to the role of motherly older sister. She and her sister Ina created a significant event of teaching me how to tie my shoelace. I recall exactly where it took place, on the back stairs into the garden on a sunny day. I remember thinking, "even the sun is celebrating," so everyone saw the achievement!*

Gisela and Otto Hoesch had two sons, both born after the war, George's first cousins Henning and Leonhard. They inherited their father's lucrative chemical plant, which benefited from the war effort, and most likely, after the war, from the Marshall Plan. Both, as adults, chose to live outside of Germany. We would meet Henning and Leonhard when George's surviving German family came to see their American cousin act at the English-language theater, improbably called Friends of Italian Opera, in Kreutzberg, in the old communist half of Berlin, when George performed Victor Klemperer in our adaption of the Klemperer war diaries, *I Will Bear Witness*. His German family warmly welcomed their long-absent American relative, and me, his director for the script we adapted together. A year or so later, we were invited to a family reunion to celebrate Leonhard's birthday on his bioorganic farm in Switzerland. There, we saw the small Käthe Kollwitz Pieta on a chest in his hallway, and the Paul Klee displayed alone on an easel in an upstairs room. Leonhard also had acquired the largest collection of Max Beckman prints in the world, currently stored in the Zurich Museum. In Leonhard's ex- wife's home outside of Zurich, we sat on Bauhaus leather and metal, amazingly comfortable, elegant couches and chairs. There were Kollwitz and other fine prints on the walls. On Henning's estate outside Aix-en-Province, with a view of Cezanne's famous mountain, where we were twice guests, a marble bust from ancient Rome sits on top of a low chest, and the large, round, inlaid marble table George remembered from his Tante Irma's estate sits alone in the villa's entranceway. Outside on the grounds, there are old stone walls, fields of grapes, and at various places, one comes across beautiful landscape art, creating meditative places in which to sit and contemplate the light as the sun shifts. Henning collects and trades old master drawings on the world market. Being "a cautious man," guiding his chemical company through the war and the peace, resulted in considerable inherited wealth for the two sons of Nazi-Party member Otto Hoesch.

George and Igor's lives at Haus Merberich were magical, George and Igor both remembered. There are many photos of the two boys to prove it, taken with their parents, and, once their parents had emigrated to the United States, taken, no doubt, to be shared with them, refugees in Pittsfield, Massachusetts, trying to earn their livings as physiotherapists, their successful dance company a memory from a pre-Nazi past. Small George was photographed toddling down to the pasture fence to rub noses with the curious cows, and pet the big workhorses. The boys were doted on by their Tante Irma and their two cousins but the shadow of the Nazi in the house was omnipresent and their parents were inexplicably absent. Once he began to write his past, in his eighties, he remembered scenes in detail:

It was Christmas, near my fourth birthday and I had the mumps. Christmas was unusually elaborate that year. As I was still in bed with a temperature and swollen cheeks, suddenly another, though smaller, Christmas tree appeared by my bed, and soon had some holiday decorations. Anticipation of the perhaps extra special Christmas Eve was growing inside. How extra special would they make this celebration? As one of the most anticipated events in a child's dreams becomes reality, one of my caretakers came to prepare me. She told me the following: 'Tonight, about eleven o'clock or maybe it will be about midnight, you will hear the window above you open. You must not open your eyes. That is the Christmas Angel, coming in with your presents. If you open your eyes and see her, she will disappear, and so will all the gifts.' Of course, my immediate response was, 'there's not going to be any angel, but what if it could be true? I'll just face the wall, keep my eyes closed. That should be enough to fool them in case I do hear the window opening.' Though I didn't believe there would be an Angel I was determined to stay awake even if I kept my eyes closed. It felt like several hours that I stayed awake facing the wall, eyes closed. In complete silence, suddenly I heard the window above me open. Could it be? Was it really happening? I lay perfectly still, now, not moving a muscle. I thought, well, now I can sleep a little. I did immediately. When I woke, several family members were greeting me with holiday wishes. The very first thing I saw was an extended line of German soldiers in various fighting and combat shooting positions, at the end were four of five other figures of Hitler, Goering, Goebbels, Himmler, arms raised in the Nazi salute. Why was I given this, I thought. I never asked or mentioned anything about the toy soldiers.

Despite the mumps, the Nazi soldiers and the absence of his parents, German Christmas Eve retained its magic. Each of the twenty-three years we lived in the big Victorian house we rented in Clinton Hill, George traveled to the Upper East Side to the one German delicatessen he knew still sold the six inch white beeswax candles, illegal to burn in New York. A week before Christmas, he set the candles in their metal holders inherited from his mother and clipped them to straight and strong branches on the tree that stood between the two parlors, adding his mother's old tin ornaments. He spent the next week adjusting, unclipping, clipping again, straightening so each candle would stand erect and burn without igniting the branch above. On Christmas Eve, after a shared dinner, we would gather around: friends, neighbors, my mother, my daughter's father, his girlfriend, his son, visitors from Iraq, Egypt, Macedonia, whoever needed a place to be. George's son and my daughter would circle the tree, lighting each candle, each small flame becoming part of a larger dance of light, amid the green branches making us think we had entered an enchanted forest. We sat in a circle entranced, watching the candles burn (no, there was never a flying spark, but George kept a close eye). We sang carols, and then as candles flickered out, we danced to the folk music of our guests.

By 1938, as war approached and restrictions against Jews increased, the two Bartenieff boys' presence at Haus Merberich must have become more worrying to their parents in the United States and more unsettling to the other inhabitants of the estate. Perhaps, the Nazi-party member-chemical company proprietor was afraid to be found out harboring Jewish children and he wanted them gone, or Tante Irma felt the boys were in growing danger. Probably both. Irmgard Bartenieff returned to Germany alone in the summer of 1938, intending to take her sons back with her to the United States; however, she was unable to leave the country with them. Nor were her sons told their mother was in Germany. She chose not to see her children while she was in the country—afraid of the emotions that would be unleashed since she could not bring them with her to the United States. When George reconnected with his German family in 2002, George's cousin Brigitte gave him letters his mother wrote to Tante Irma from Berlin that proved she was Germany, on her unsuccessful mission to reunite with her children. George had trouble understanding why his mother kept this trip a secret until the end of her life. Perhaps, it was too painful for her to think about; perhaps, she thought there was no point in telling her sons, but he was also extremely moved to learn, two decades after her death, that his mother had intended in 1938, to take her children out of Germany and travel back to America with them. He was told by Brigitte that the boys' "papers were not ready" so their mother was unable to take them with her. In 2003, George inquired about the possibility of reclaiming his German citizenship. He received a letter from the Landesarchiv (State Archive) Berlin that showed there was no record of George's birth. His brother is listed, though his name is misspelled, "Sagor" born in 1929 in Stuttgart. His mother is listed, her maiden name also misspelled, as Doubois, married to "Kan Kogan (Bartenieff), Mikhail" His father's nationality is listed as "stateless," born in "Cherson, Ukrainia," in 1900, and his religion is given as "nonbeliever." There is no record of George. In 1933, his parents must have decided not to register their second son's birth in Berlin. And that there was no official record of George's birth must have been the reason why the boys were unable to emigrate when their mother came to fetch them in 1938. She had to leave her children behind in Nazi Germany for a second time. But the family was well-connected and however it happened, the appropriate "papers" were going to be procured, hopefully before war broke out.

In the meantime, Igor and George were sent away from Haus Merberich, to a progressive school far to the south, in Oberstdorf, the highest point in the Bavarian Alps, where they knew no one, but would be safe. The Rudolf Steiner School was most likely selected by his mother while she was in Germany, as she was a devotee of progressive education, and probably paid for by Tante Irma. Most classes were held outside in the forest, and pagan and Christian holidays were celebrated with communal rituals. The Steiner school was a transformative experience for George. He wrote:

> *I might never have become an actor without Oberstdorf. Oberstdorf ignited in me the world of NATURE, celebrated by RITUALIZED DRAMATIZATION AND MAKE BELIEVE, transferring Nature's Genius through and into dramatization. These rituals opened the world of the playful magic of creating, and wholly honoring the world's regenerative miracle. What gave this year such powerful significance as a formative experience was the constant supreme omnipresence of the spectacular scenery of Mother Nature.*

George was an eco-artist from the start of his life, well aware of the connections between nature and artistic inspiration and the need to relish and respect our magical natural world. In 1992, '93, and '94, at Theater for the New City, he created and produced ecological theater festivals that were focused on reclaiming and sharing Indigenous wisdom. Funded by the Rockefeller Foundation, the eco-theater works were shared with six theaters nationwide. At the first eco-fest, we pulled a large, disemboweled Oldsmobile east along 10th Street chanting a text I wrote. The police tried to stop us and took a few of the performers at the procession's head into custody. We ended in Tompkins Square Park, where we buried the car, with a funeral song for gas-driven automobiles, and planted a tree on top, which was blessed in a ritual led by the late Indigenous American poet John Trudell, and which grows there still. We continued to create and produce eco art. Our 2014 climate-change play, *Extreme Whether*, is about the US government's censorship of climate science. George played Uncle, one of his favorite roles, a John Muir-like environmentalist, living as a steward on the country land of a scientist inspired by the story of James Hansen, who testified before Congress in 1989 that global warming had begun. He was ignored. Hansen is one of the foremost climate scientists in the world, and one of the earliest to sound the alarm. His predictions are most often right; nevertheless, his work was censored under the Obama Administration, and he resigned from the government in 2013, in the same week we presented the first public reading of the play, after which Hanson spoke to our large audience. The reading and Hanson's talk were filmed by MSNBC for supposed inclusion on the Chris Hayes' show, but neither Hanson nor the play ever appeared, another instance of censorship of climate science. Hanson addressed our audience again after the play's opening night. "I hope they can get this play to a broader audience because it makes a lot of valid points and it does it in a more entertaining way than (laughing) the documentaries are just not very interesting so it's hard to reach a wide audience." We took *Extreme Whether* to the UN Climate Conference in Paris in 2015, and performed in French and English as part of ARTCOP, the year the Paris Climate Agreement was signed. The play opened, again, at LaMama in 2018. It had productions in Copenhagen and Oklahoma, too, but it never reached "a large" audience, as say, on Broadway, because, of course, of the censorship of climate science, which exists in the cultural sphere, too.

One day in Oberstdorf in the Bavarian Alps, the children at the Steiner School were made to line up on the road. They were going to watch a parade. The event was seared into his memory:

In May of 1939, the Oberstdorf school received orders to line the students up to stand by the road in front of the school to salute the Heil Hitler greeting as the Brown Shirts paraded into the town. I was right next to the headmaster as the first parade I had ever seen passed by, but the headmaster did not salute or say anything. Why? He stood silent, looking straight in front. Later my nine-year-old brother, Igor, explained the headmaster did not like the Fascists.

George learned from his headmaster how not to salute and became a war protester for the rest of his life. George had been abandoned and hidden, but hidden in plain sight with his brother, surrounded by his cousins and his indulgent great aunt, yet they feared. Otto Hoesch must have feared being found out harboring half Jewish children. Or, perhaps, the women feared Otto Hoesch more. Whatever the truth, the two boys did not return to Haus Merberich.

In summer 1939, George and Igor left the Steiner school and traveled to their grandmother's home in Berlin to get ready to sail on a ship.

George remembers his grandmother warning him to stay far from a certain neighbor, a "bad man" with snarling German Shepard dogs who lived down the road, and he remembers his suitcase was packed with summer things, to look as if he and Igor were simply going on holiday, not emigrating. He was told to break the outstretched Nazi salute arms off of his German toy soldiers if he wanted to take them with him on the boat. Then there was the scene at the dock where but for his Tante Irma's histrionic performance, the two boys would not have been allowed to board the luxury liner, the Europa, on her last voyage across the ocean before war broke out. Again, once he dared to recall it, he found the scene at the dock stuck with him:

> *Tante Irma and Grandmother Alice accompanied us to board the cruise ship, Europa, at Hamburg, August 15th 1939. Tante Irma is the kind of woman you want to make sure is there when you know there's going to be trouble. The Gestapo opened both passports and the Gestapo looked at both passports and said, "Kon Kogan, isn't this a Jewish name?" Never had I ever known Tante Irma to raise her voice or be anything but charming and full of a cordial humor, followed by a family of black and white Spaniels for whom she carried a pocket full of treats. But Tante Irma erupted like a volcano now awakened, a tirade of righteous fury flowed over the Gestapo, "Jews! We have no Jews in our family," she berated the Gestapo. Quickly the black uniforms held out the passports, adding a hasty apology, [Entschuldigung die Sie bitte gnädige Frau.] Two heroines accompanied us up the gangplank and waved Bon Voyage.*

There is a photo once the boys were allowed onto the ship, of the two of them dressed in shorts, sleeveless sweaters, and shirts, looking glum; taller, slender Igor and small George stand next to a stern, hired nanny in white uniform, holding tight to George's shoulder, pulling him close to her skirt, her left arm reaching around Igor's back. They had been saved, but exiled. There was the trip across the ocean, in the care of this nameless nanny, where after-dinner entertainment was the viewing of Nazi antisemitic propaganda films, which gave six-year-old George nightmares. And, then he was reunited with his parents after half of his lifetime apart only to find his father's temper raging. In Pittsfield, Massachusetts, George hid behind the bed while his father hurled shoes and epithets. With his uncontrollable temper, Mikhail Bartenieff bore a certain resemblance to my father and both George and I remembered our childhood terror of and disdain for our fathers' fits. George and Igor debated whether or not to report their father to the authorities for child abuse. Irmgard separated from Mikhail a year or so after the children arrived. She suffered a miscarriage and her husband was absent. She had had enough. "I'm not going to raise these children in Pittsfield, Massachusetts," George remembers her saying. She moved with her sons to New York, where the German émigré community was lively.

Young George was horrified by the hot, humid city, until one day in a gutter outside the Museum of Natural History he saw a slender green stick begin to move. How could a stick come to life? It was a praying mantis, an insect that camouflaged itself by becoming inert, but then the stick began a graceful dance while the boy watched entranced—proof of the possibility of transformation, clear sight of the magic of becoming through movement he would use in his acting. So city-life also held nature's secrets. He began to frequent the Museum of Natural History, and soon, the Metropolitan and the Frick art museums also became after-school haunts. He was a curious, shy child, alone a great deal of the time. Watching a performance of *A Midsummer Night's Dream* with his mother and brother, he turned to her and said, "I want to do that." "Do you now?" his mother looked him in the eye. She immediately enrolled George in Maria Ley Piscator's Children's Acting School, the juvenile wing of Erwin Piscator's Theater Workshop at the New School where Judith Malina, at nineteen, was studying acting and directing. The child George and young Judith appeared together in *Pinocchio* and George played the lead in *The Prince Who Learned Everything out of Books*. His mother never praised him, he used to complain. When he opened on Broadway at age fourteen, she took him to dinner at Howard Johnson's to celebrate and sat across the table, wordless, a thin, tight-lipped smile on her face. George learned to praise others by himself, in reaction to the strict German childrearing practices of his mother, and which his Tante Irama had ignored. Emulating his great aunt, he became a great enthusiast of other people's work. "To praise is the whole thing," he liked to say, quoting Rilke, in a poem I'd lifted and given the poet Robert Blaze in *The Beekeeper's Daughter*.

As George grew more ill, as the side effects increased from the cancer treatments he could not tolerate, and as his immune system continued to weaken, his early memories in Nazi Germany took up more and more space. For much of his life, he had resisted speaking about or even consciously knowing what he lived through as a small boy; now he wrote in his diary, and he wanted to tell people. It was as though the curious, little, blue-eyed blond boy and the angular elder with his luminous gaze were mirror images of one another; both were being cared for and held and each was all alone in the world facing death.

From his earliest life, contradiction, transformation, wonder and terror were mixed. The stuff of art.

What George now knew about himself was the result not just of his serious reflections in his final years of life, but of the trajectory his life took and of the work we did. I was drawn to the traumas I discovered he'd lived. I loved him because of what he had suffered, and for what he had become because of what he'd endured. And, thinking on it now, perhaps this is what love is. We love the hurt parts of the one we love. Love becomes possible when one is engaged not just with one's own pain but finds the pain of the other impossible to ignore, intriguing and noble, needing tender understanding and care. When the pain of the other appears as worthy as yours, even worthier, overall, and therefore deserves to be met, witnessed, and comforted. The pain of the other is to be cherished as it holds the key to who the beloved truly is, why and how the other became; understanding this pain can perhaps help realize more of the beloved's true self and allow the beloved to suffer less. Then, the relationship becomes of equals, two hurt people who wish not to inflict more hurt, but rather to understand the other's and their own, to honor and transcend. We were among the lucky ones who, in the midst of the pandemic, and in the face of a fatal illness, made the decision to grow, to deepen our love and further perfect the vision we shared. And so, we lived with joy for thirty-five years, from the time that we met to the end of George's life. "You and George fit together like two pieces of a puzzle," said a dear friend who knew me before we met and after

George's death. George was not alone when he died. Nor was I ever left alone by myself, until the moment he left this world.

His early life was joy mixed with terror, a terrified joy, joyful terror, and this wide range of emotion, these two clashing forces George was forced to experience very young, were what made his acting unforgettable. He could play two tones, or more, at once, or rather, he could inhabit a huge range of emotion, theme, and dissonance. Opposites. Holding all emotions effortlessly because this is what he knew, life was terrifying but good, and if horribly bad, joy was there, too. In essence, he was always the wondrous, terrified boy housed in the gentle man. He never ceased to marvel at life, even during his most frightful suffering. This wide emotional reach gave him significance on the stage. He was there with a message few people have, signaling from a beyond. Like Artaud's imagined actor "burnt at the stake signaling through the flames," George contained in his flesh the emotional extremes. His fears of having been left, of being, therefore, in his child's head, bad—why else would mother and father abandon him?—and of being dangerous—why else would he have been sent away from Haus Merberich and from the Steiner school?—were met and mitigated by his aunt's, young female cousins', and the spaniels' adoration. By the beauty of the nature around him in which he felt safe, seen by the cows as he saw his reflection in their dark eyes. But danger, incomprehensible to the child, was everywhere. He and his brother were living in the same house with a man who was manufacturing chemicals for a war meant to kill children like him, and growing wealthy from doing so, owing his Nazi masters obeisance. The two half Jewish children were banished from the family home. Yet, at the Steiner school to which they were sent, the transporting nature rituals George was taught provided the five-year-old boy his focus for life. He would become a transformational actor who materialized with his body and voice the possibilities of change and choice. He would contain the two opposites. Not pity and fear, but wonder and terror.

When the new terror of his smoldering cancer hit, hidden in the marrow of his bone, he began to piece together the unspoken traumas of his early life, those that seeped into the boy despite the good care he received on the Düren estate and in the Bavarian forest, and he continued to answer with wonder, to work and live as intensely as he could. From *Us* on, I had often written roles in which he changed form. For our second to final full production, in 2019, *Other Than We*, set in a dystopic future with characters engaged in a utopian plot to doom human cruelty, George would change from a Noam Chomsky-like linguist into an owl, the bird of wisdom, in full view of the audience, in order to watch over the young Newbies engineered by three visionary scientists. Half-animal, half-human, the Newbies are capable of surviving and thriving in the harsh, new, post climate collapse, barely regenerating world but, more important, their minds have been rewired by their creators to connect to their gut-brains so they will be unfailingly careful and kind, taking good care of all that lives, incapable of violence based on fear *and they have language.* Noam titles one of his final books on linguistics, *Why Only Us?* contemplating again his original insight, that human beings, only, among all creatures, come wired with syntax. We each speak an original sentence the first time we talk. Creativity plus syntax, therefore, creativity and language, are linked; we can create stories of origin, tales, nuclear bombs. Why us and no other creatures, Noam asks? And, what, then is our responsibility to the rest of life since we, alone, are able to tell the complex stories of the universe, and with our words invent stories and myths, and, also, compassion as we comprehend and feel ourselves into others' experiences? If followed to its logical conclusion, our possession of tale-telling language, alone among creatures, ought to mean that we become the compassionate seekers, the chroniclers, the singers of the magic of life (as in many traditional cultures). Instead, we use our unique gift to invent cruelties—we are also the only species that murders its own, in vast numbers. Not surprisingly, Noam Chomsky, who built his academic career on his understanding of syntax, has been for so many of us an exemplar of kindness and grace as well as astonishing brilliance. Until his stroke in 2023, Noam personally answered his thousands of emails, sometimes with just a phrase, but always with understanding. We communicated often after Noam's first wife's cancer death about the paradox of what our language-making begets, "In the back of my mind I find it hard to suppress a line from the Analects (of Confucius) defining the exemplary person, presumably the master himself: the one who keeps on trying even though he knows there is no hope," he wrote. We also joked about trivial things like the difference in our equestrian abilities, "Wow, quite a picture. Even galloping horses in the desert? This past summer I had to be led up a mountain on an old nag on a rocky train in the rain and deep mud, traumatic. Down was worse. Never again, to coin a phrase," Noam vowed. We spoke, also, about his grief. "I do occasionally—very occasionally—see some old friends, even for a walk in the woods. But the future is pretty much laid out for me." All of that changed a few years later, when Noam met Valeria Wasserman, his second wife. When I wrote, "That is really super wonderful news." He replied, "Sure is. You'll see why on the fifteenth." We were about to meet at a dinner.

I modeled George's character, the linguist, Opa, on Noam, but his transformation into an owl could only be imagined for and by George. He had started to receive a standard cancer drug, Revlimid, but it drove his white blood cell count down without affecting the cancer. He decided to stop this treatment to be strong enough to rehearse and perform. He was hospitalized overnight between the first and second week, but he did not miss a performance at LaMama ETC in downtown New York. In front of the audience, he changed form, with the help of an ingenious costume designed and made by our costume designer of thirty-five years, Sally Ann Parsons, and her co-designer, Carisa Kelly. Sitting on a stone, wearing large glasses and what seemed to be a cape, an expression of wonder grew on his face; his eyes grew wide, as if he were about to be snatched. From behind, an out-of-sight stagehand popped the head of an owl over his face, with large eye and mouth openings so his amazement was seen as his expression grew more intense. He stood up expectantly, a feathery covering unfurled, covering his front. He opened his arms; the cape he was wearing turned into feathery wings. He was no longer human. He had become an avian creature, all of a sudden, in full view, and we watching in the audience, amazed, could not quite tell how this owl appeared, and with the supple rising and falling of his strong wings, was about to take flight in front of us.

It was magical shape-shifting at which George excelled. I did not give him one single direction; he choreographed every move as he changed from his fragility into the massive strength of the big bird. Even weakened by cancer drugs, at age eighty-seven, he could mutate, emerging from an older intellectual as something other, astonishing the audience, a large, muscular bird. He "flew," as he manipulated his wings. He uttered the whoohoots of the owl. "Watch over us, Opa," the Newbies, who have just gained language, are able to sing, proving their creative intelligence, "with kindness and restraint/with love," and he answers them, losing language himself as his transformation becomes complete: "I will dooo. Whoo. You, you, you. Whoo, Whooo, Whooo." This final shape-change, done on scant budgets and with limited rehearsal time, was, nevertheless, unforgettable. I gave him the challenge to leave human form and become the big bird and he fulfilled it. There was very little he could not accomplish on stage and nothing he would not dare try.

While COVID ran rampant in New York, and the sirens screamed, racing to Brooklyn Hospital at the end of our street, we pledged to one another to refuse to be separated if the worst imaginable thing happened, and one of us needed hospitalization. People were being intubated and dying alone in quarantine, with only over-stretched medical professionals in attendance. We would not let this happen with us. In the evenings, we read aloud; I read to him, rather, as George had macular degeneration and could not read, our shoulders touching. His listening was so acute it felt as if he followed the words on the page with me, and we would stop to discuss a memorable passage in detail. We read great fiction every night, starting, predictably enough, with Albert Camus's *The Plague*, but going on to Thomas Hardy's *Tess of the d'Urbervilles* and *Jude the Obscure*, Ursula Le Guin's *The Dispossessed* and *The Left Hand of Darkness*, Pat Barker's World War I trilogy, Nadine Gordimer's *The Pickup* (George had never read Gordimer and was thrilled by the brilliance of this short, compassionate, timely book, her last). We read *Braiding Sweetgrass*, by the botanist and Citizen of the Potawatomi Nation, Robin Wall Kimmerer, which George loved. We read Rudolf Steiner's mystic book on agriculture with his accurate prediction that the soil is being drained of nutrients. And we slogged through almost all of the Davids' (Graeber and Wengrow) five-hundred-page "hit," *The Dawn of Everything: A New History of Humanity*. George failed to be much impressed. He wanted more vision, not a list of past ways of social organization from which we might choose. But George always wanted more.

We put on masks and rushed out of the house, in furious delight, our fists in the air, learning the chants, to join the first big Black Lives Matter march up Dekalb Avenue, right in front of our co-op building, in the spring of 2020. We were thrilled to be all-of-a-sudden part of a crowd, outside, marching, once again, for what we believed. The protesters were of all ethnicities, races, and ages. (When Barack Obama had been elected, the streets of the neighborhood also filled. We were still in the big house, then; we joined the crowds, and cheered the young people dancing on top of city buses that stopped the traffic on Dekalb Avenue. "I've never before seen Americans happy," said a friend from South America who ran the local convenience store). This time, though, released from lockdown, we were not celebrating; we were enraged by the murder of George Floyd. We continued to protest. George, at eighty-eight, took the knee in the park outside Brooklyn's Borough Hall, his fist raised, in a silent eight-minute-and-forty-eight-second vigil. He had been at the fabled March on Washington in August 1963, with Julian Beck and Judith Malina. He liked to tell how he stepped off the rented school bus at a rest stop. He greeted a Black woman descending the stairs of her bus. She replied, "It *certainly is* a beautiful day." They knew history was being made.

"Ten years is the median survival," his cancer doctor told us, exaggerating the good, as he delivered the bad news. Then, "eighty-seven! You look seventy-seven!" We laughed; ten years from this day George would be ninety-seven. We treated his fatal multiple myeloma diagnosis as a far-off ending. And I promised, many times, not knowing what else I had to give, "You will not be alone." You will not be abandoned again. This pledge was of singular importance to me. I had dutifully left the room, at the nurse's behest, moments before my father died, and regretted it ever since. I had been away doing a play when Julian suffered his fatal hemorrhage in Mount Sinai Hospital. I would remake myself, too, if I could do as I said. And I promised myself George would die at home in my arms. The dogs, too. We had fifteen-old cocker spaniel littermates, then, Cleis and Hermes, whom we both loved. They would die the next fall. Put down in my arms. But we didn't dwell on any of this. We were all alive, despite cancer and age. We would live.

So, he became an owl in front of us, the bird of wisdom. He seemed to take flight. It was my way, too, I suppose, of preparing us both, through the art that we made, for his impending death. This was both unconscious and not. I never said it out loud, though I knew. He would leave his physical form and become ... we knew not when or what. It's called acting, of course, the ability to go beyond who one is, and George was particularly good at changing species and shape, at imagining something else out of this world to be reborn into .... The man weakened by cancer drugs and disease seemed to swoop and rise through a sparkling sky we also saw in our minds' eyes (magical, low-budget lighting by Tony Giovannetti, who lit our plays for thirty-five years). The stronger the imagination, the more convincing the actor. The more the actor sees, so can we; the actor, by seeing in his mind's eye, extends our imaginations. His interior landscape materialized, the inner world of an owl, overcoming the actual physical limitations including his age and his illness, plus the fact that he could not fly. Nevertheless, we saw him grow wings and appear to swoop through the sky. We saw with his eyes; strangely, it felt as if we were inside of him looking out, and taking flight too. This was a magic he worked to his final day on earth. George always seemed to be more vibrant, more alive than the facts of his increasingly limited strength, his loss of hearing and sight. He compensated with the force of his will—vision mixed with desire—presenting a vibrancy that came from within, a power that withstood and could not have come from weakening flesh and muscle, yet did. First, as he transmutes into owl, he looks at the world he is leaving (as a human, that is) with a sorrowful wonder, then he becomes amazed at what is happening, as he grows feathers and wings, and then, he assumes the point of view of the bird, and looks out from the owl's eyes; the human disappears, as he appears to take wing with full power. The audience followed his gaze, saw him transform, watched him seeing into another world. The world beyond, where I suppose he is now, if there is such a place separate from human imagination and wish. I had written his change of form from brilliant thinker to owl as a way, I hoped, of comforting us both, of giving us each the chance to fly free of our fears of his death—how little I knew, then, of death or of grief, how bold in my ignorance I was, and how fearless was he, on stage—and his transformation from man into owl became a transcendent vision. He took the audience with him. We never, he and I, spoke of death, as he prepared to give form to the owl's flight. And I had Noam's age in mind, too, as I crafted the character of Opa in homage to them both, Noam and George, who admired one another, inspired generations, and pursued relentlessly what they believed.

"George was a secular shaman—able to see past the world as it is and through creaturely/species boundaries—here and in other plays George transmogrifies—gender, species so he carries the opening out sense of possibility of your plays—I don't want to take away from the sheer artistry of what he was able to do, but when he comes out from under the wing, he has the penetrating gaze of an owl with eyes that rarely blink, he just stares as his head moves very slowly only from side to side, like an owl—it was an amazing transformation. (That costume was amazing too.)" writes our friend, Ynestra King, who saw him in every play of mine for thirty-five years, and who with her 1980 essay "What Is Ecofeminism?" founded a movement. He never blinked. Owls stare out unblinking, seemingly. Owls blink far less frequently than humans do. So, George made certain he held his eyes open. We never spoke of this choice of his, either. I'm not certain he fully understood what he did.

"Something about this transformation onstage was just magic. Just the thing between a writer and an actor and a costume designer that creates theater. It was as if it couldn't have NOT happened. Surprising and yet inevitable. My heart was following his eyes, and my brain had a moment of how did they do that? A sweep and a shimmer and he was an owl. That was it. Perfect," Christen Clifford remembers.

He had been diagnosed with multiple myeloma in September, after nearly dying of sepsis the previous June. In November, he turned himself into an owl. But truth was, he had slogged through those rehearsals feeling pretty physically miserable, until, that is, he flew at the play's end. The next summer, 2020, with theaters shuttered, we recorded the play for Columbia

University's Earth Institute, on a program hosted by climate journalist Andrew Revkin, who had been partial to our work since he'd seen *Extreme Whether* in 2014. What did George have to say about the play now, writing in his diary as he returned to the script? —misquoting Revkin who, after seeing the play's premiere had tweeted it was "fun and unnerving." George wrote:

> *The more I review* Other Than We *in prep for Andy Revkin's Talk Show Zoom, the more I love the play. "Sweet and eclectic," a tribute to all of Karen's Ecofeminism, especially the last transformation scene which is the kind of poetic theater of some of Ibsen's endings, and creates a perfect heightening of the experience one can only create in the theater reality because we know transformation takes place in nature, where we may actually have witnessed the cocoon become butterfly, the egg become turtle, and so on, and the magic of transformation is a perfect metaphor for the mystery, and in this its representation of the miraculousness of an evolutionary event in the world.*

—

Illness creates its own physical closeness, not the athletic lovemaking of our relative youth. In those early days, we could not wait. We made love in a nook on the stairs of St. Francis of Assisi's monastery, in a swimming pool at midnight at a Tuscan artists' retreat (while others watched from their windows, they told us with smirks in the morning), in my Honda Civic parked at the river downtown, on tables, on chairs, in the middle of a flower-strewn plain in Umbria on a hot summer afternoon, in a prop cage in the theater basement during a rehearsal break. Impetuously, wherever we could. In our last year, sexuality was rarer, but we found our ways, snuggling together, suckling parts of the other's body. Sensuality remained, even ecstatic. I can feel the warmth slowly return to his foot—swollen, bulbous, and blue as I hold and massage it, very gently, so as not to hurt. I am sitting on the floor in front of his chair, working his swollen flesh. His toes and his ankles begin to turn flesh color, and resume recognizable form; no longer do they look like lumps of blue playdough, as my massage restores circulation. Neuropathy is a common effect of chemotherapy, though no one, not a nurse nor a doctor, ever mentioned that to us. Swollen feet that cannot be felt, as if one is standing on stubs. When George met me at Theater for the New City one cold December night the last year of his life, to see Peter Schumann's Bread and Puppet Christmas play, and he arrived without realizing he had no shoe on his right foot, I began massaging his feet in the mornings.

We added a Freudian psychotherapist to work with George, to what we called his healing team. She was recommended by a psychiatrist in London who had become a friend after seeing George perform. George had weekly acupuncture with Nancy, a yoga teacher of mine who had become a gifted healer. Her treatments alleviated George's sometimes terrifyingly labored breathing, perhaps caused by anxiety, and for which his western doctors offered no treatment. His Chinese herbalist MD, Dr. W., lived somewhere in Queens on the down low, made to leave, was the rumor, Sloan Kettering for administering Chinese herbs to cancer patients. Now he met his patients for consultations in diners, but he met George on the telephone. Our Kundalini yoga teacher, Mary, an old friend, gave lessons on Zoom on Friday mornings. We built a holistic team around us. George felt good one sparkling morning in November 2021 and went out by himself to do some marketing; he returned with a bloody nose. He was cheerful. He had tripped on a jutting piece of sidewalk outside Apple Bank on Myrtle Avenue. He'd caught his foot and toppled onto his face. A wonderfully warm Black man had helped him up, he told me delightedly, and his wounds appeared minor. But a week or so later, the long second toe on his left foot became infected. He woke one night in terrible pain. Not knowing what to do, bleary-eyed, pulled out a deep sleep, I gave him a pack of frozen peas to put on the wretched toe. "It's a localized infection and with any luck we can keep it that way," his cancer doctor whispered to me as we sat in a hallway outside the ER, where the infectious disease doctor had also come to assess George. There was talk of amputation, but the toe healed itself, with more antibiotics, of course. Usually, he had a private room, but for this hospital stay, he was in a ward with six beds. We were nearest the communal bathroom and the door. Televisions blared. Once, after a long teaching day, I climbed into bed with George and we both fell asleep. The nurse was horrified. "It's not right." But the infectious disease doctor, who stopped by, thought it was sweet. When George left home in December without one shoe, the other was still in a surgical boot. The toe infection in November 2021, though it resolved itself well, and the missing shoe the next month, were the first times I realized that George might not have long to live. "The awareness will come and go," his doctor, in whom I confided my fears, wrote. Going out without a shoe was also the last time I let George leave the house unaccompanied.

My hands massaging his feet allowed him to begin to feel them, again, as appendages attached. And I, too, as his feeling returned under my touch, could feel him. Bending in gently toward one another. Holding his cold, swollen foot, feeling the warmth return to his toes. Softly bending each one. There was no touch too intimate. Then, we would laugh, too, in joy. Hot flesh bonding us. Relief from the death creeping up from the earth. Icy tentacles turned back, as if we two together had regained power over. Flesh warmed by my hands, blood moving up and down the leg; the foot no longer stiff, unfelt, and blue. The warm toes able to wriggle. We had will and desire, agency. Surely, we'd be let live. Me on the floor, my face bent close to his soft foot, flexible, now, sprung back from the fake rigor mortis of lost feeling and we laughing, delighted by the transformation.

In thirty-five years, a man grows old. Cancerous and old in George's case. His old traumas reemerged to mix with his physical illness. A form of healing occurred as he sickened. Compassion for the hurt and hidden, wondrous child he'd been. He ripened. We spent one memorable night, in February 2022, among many nights we spent in the emergency room. George was out-of-sorts; I did not know what was wrong. By text, his doctor diagnosed acidosis, potentially fatal, caused by the antibiotics, three per day for a year and a half, prescribed by the infectious disease specialist, to ward off another sepsis attack, chief symptom of his weakened immune system, a result of the cancer. "There is no guarantee either way, but he is safer in the hospital," the doctor texted me. I did not think George was going to die and we both dreaded another hospital stay, but we went to the emergency room, again. I followed behind him dutifully as he pushed his IV pole back and forth to the bathroom at the end of a long row of cubbies with cots. "You look a lot better than I thought you would," said his doctor, visiting us in the ER. He would live. Though, like every side effect in the final nine months of his life, this one left him weaker and more depleted. He recovered from each auxiliary illness until he could not, anymore, overcome by will alone the steady weakening of his bodily systems. Persistent diarrhea is one of the side effects of chemotherapy, too. Nothing he took, Revlimid, thalidomide, both with Darzalex, and now Velcade, which is also more toxic than the other drugs, especially to the elderly, caused his cancer numbers to drop very much. He'd gone off the drugs several times in order to have the strength to act. As I walked behind him, to stand next to him at the toilet and fold the paper into the little square packets he instructed me how to make, so he could clean himself, I saw how ghastly thin he'd become, something like a camp survivor in another setting, or cancerous person, no flesh on his lovely bones. His buttocks jutting and raw. His face finely chiseled as an old master's silver point drawing. He looked beautiful, as if he were seeing far away, into another reality altogether, like the line I had given him years before in *The Beekeeper's Daughter*, to comfort the Bosnian victim of rape who was in deep terror, "I saw a luminous light in your eyes, as if you were looking quite far away, into another time and place."

As we looked at death together that night in the ER toilet, we thought: not a worthy adversary, not yet. Never afraid while he lived, or if terrified, comforted by our touch and our breath. Always able to laugh. As I followed behind him back and forth, we took our predicament lightly. Even with his hospital gown flapping loosely around his thin form, wiping a bottom already raw, he never lost his dignity. Did not complain or say a harsh word. In the morning, when someone finally came to move him into a room, I could barely walk behind. I'd been nursing a common yoga injury of my SI joint, but the night, scrunched over his bed on a metal chair, trying to sleep a bit, had left me unable to straighten up. I begged for an aspirin, or ibuprofen to take away the pain, but I wasn't a patient and could not be given anything. "We can't bill your insurance," a hip ER doctor quipped as I, bent in half, limped behind George's gurney. "I'll go slow," the transporter said, and he did. I struggled behind them to a private room and sat in a chair while specialists called by his cancer doctor paraded in and out, with nothing to say. He was better already, on his own, resilient, as he'd always been—a bright light in his eyes.

What I would like to convey is the dignity of the sufferer. And the necessity of the witness. So much better to have suffering acknowledged. Even as he weakened, he never lost the qualities that made him unforgettable on the stage. He wondered at life every minute. Looked with light from within. Delighted. Moved with grace. Amplified every thought with his magnificent, multivalent voice.

George was never present on stage to call attention to himself; he was hidden within the character he'd made. His creation blazingly emerged, a full and captivating presence all its own. He gave of himself to give to another three-dimensional life. This was courageous, generous, and unusual, a self-abnegation of sorts. Like a person giving birth from inside the self to someone else who will become autonomous—a trait most usually associated with women. George would not, therefore, become "a star." A star is always himself impersonating someone else, a star is always there to be seen, first, and does not become another as completely as did George. Nevertheless, for those who saw him perform, his acting remained indelible and cherished in their minds. And in mine. He became the realizer of both of our dreams, as if the active force of my language impregnated him.

After seeing their production of Jack Gelber's *The Connection* in 1960, George wanted to become an actor in The Living Theatre. The Living, always operating on scant budgets and striving for a gritty poetic reality, was also always a mixture of trained actors and amateurs, recovering or current addicts in *The Connection*, for instance, performing alongside seasoned professionals like Warren Finnerty. When Joseph Chaikin, who had performed in the lead role in Judith's production of Bertolt Brecht's *Man is Man*, left the company to form his own Open Theater, George, who had auditioned for the Living many times, was finally called to replace Joe as their next lead. (Joe asked George to join his new company, but George declined. He did not think Joe's new Open Theater would be staging language plays, nor be dedicated to individual character, and he was correct.) George was asked by Julian and Judith to play the lead in *Dog Beneath the Skin*, written in collaboration by the lovers W.H. Auden and Christopher Isherwood. He was very pleased. But just before rehearsals began, a friend of an unknown, first-time playwright, and a former marine, Kenneth Brown, brought Ken's first play, *The Brig*, to Julian. (Ken died of cancer in the winter of 2022, in a Brooklyn VA hospital. George and he remained friends until his death. Ken came to the Christmas Eve parties in our big house.)

"George," it was Julian on the phone, "I have something to tell you. We are not going to do *Dog Beneath the Skin*. We are going to do a new play called *The Brig*. But you can play any number prisoner you choose." Playing "a number" did not sound promising. "This play gave us goose bumps when we read it," Julian explained. "We have to do it." It would give George goose bumps, too. Though he had lost the lead role in the play by Isherwood and Auden, George was thrilled to be able to premiere *The Brig*. Ken Brown had done time in a US Marines prison for some infraction of the harsh rules of conduct and he transcribed in hyper-realism his experience. From the mainly undifferentiated prisoners, known only by their numbers, George chose Prisoner # 6—the only imprisoned Marine who suffers a mental breakdown and runs screaming to impale himself on the fence and has to be carried off. Prisoner # 6 is the only character among the anonymous prisoners and guards in *The Brig* who externalizes his inner life. For The Living, *The Brig* was a chance to experiment with, and fulfill, a uniquely American example of Artaud's theories of theater of cruelty. In fact, a poetic, meditative scene was cut from the play because Judith could not figure out how to stage it. What Judith and Julian determined to do was to put a Marine prison on the stage, in all of its inhumane harshness. A wire-mesh fence surrounded the actors and separated the stage from the audience. There were rows of steel prison bunk beds, and white lines drawn on the floor. Prisoners had to request the guards' permission to cross the white lines. All other talk was forbidden. The hyper-realistic set was designed by the abstract expressionist painter, Julian Beck. One day, Julian left the theater with a Rauschenberg painting the artist had given him. He sold it, for a fraction of what it would someday be worth, in order to pay for the materials for *The Brig* set.

Judith Malina, fierce and tiny, the director, was the only woman involved in *The Brig*. She used the Marines' handbook to establish and maintain a fierce rehearsal discipline. Actors were punished by physical activities, push-ups, running in place, and by fines, for the slightest infraction of rehearsal rules, for arriving late or for speaking out of turn. They were made to conform or to suffer. Rehearsals were intended to teach by experience the soul-deadening reality of becoming subject to arbitrary power. George got a broken rib from a punch to the gut by an untrained actor. Many of the performers quit in despair, but George become more committed. He was thirty years old, recently married to Crystal Field, and, again, putting experimental work in the avant-garde over and above any commercial acting job.

George kept a "*Brig* Log" in which he wrote about the moment in the play when he had "to act"—to break free of the enforced routine and freak out. He wanted to arrive at his character's mental disintegration naturally, internally, intentionally, without it being perceived or looking false, as if predetermined. Judith, he writes, did not always know how to help actors mine their feelings:

> *The production is progressing but I have to be constantly aware of Judith's technique of giving "results" in her directions (the Erwin Piscator method with plenty of all the fanciest theories quoted), I am slowly putting my inner life together, slowly feeling it, seeing it, but it ain't easy, since in this play the reality doesn't allow the character to reveal himself except in one moment in the whole play; everything has to lead to that moment.*

While other actors quit, George understood as well as Judith and Julian the importance *The Brig* would have for the theater at large, with its riveting, monotonous, terrible cruelty revealing the greater tragedy of increasing militarization and incarceration; he committed himself more deeply to the avant-garde theater he would nurture and create for the rest of his life:

> *I believe in this play more and more. In fact, I'm getting some of that old enthusiasm back, that I had in those first days, just after I had read the script, because now, at last, I am in the realm and*

experience of performing—I feel and hear this play even while I am concentrating on the down-to-earth business of "doing my task" in the scene—or scenes. This play is a great something, a real trailblazer. The fantastic thing about this play is that the author was given an actual reality in life from which he lifted all the actions that make up the story of this play and he came up with a highly expressionistic work This is very rare, very rare: that such heightened expressionism exists in any life that we could come up against, but of course, we in the 20th century, have known many variations of this life. This play is a poem; a very cruel, long-lasting poem; reality has been taken unto a poetic plane, because intensity, tension, music and rhythm, are all wedded into this grueling experience!!!

As you can see, I think this is great work and I love it and I am deeply proud to be associated with bringing it to life. It is my fervent wish that we can last for at least three months. As usual, they don't have a penny and are getting deeper and deeper in debt. They, of all people, deserve to be subsidized, but of course, because they are dissenters, and they are real dissenters, and not phony ones, or successful dissenters, who give generous lip service to ideas; because they make very limited compromises and they're in front of radical movements, such as the Women's World Strike for Peace, they will never get a subsidy—anyway, meanwhile, back at the grindstone ...

—

After George's death, Hugh Burlington, another performer who, like many people in the Living Theatre, was not a trained actor, and is now working at Federal Express, wrote to me about the production of more than half a century before, and George's role in it, still vivid:

George and I were in prison together. We were maggots in The Brig. *For two hours we were humiliated and beaten by sadistic guards. Many actors dropped out during the rehearsal period. Many others after the play opened. Not George. He persevered through hundreds of performances. His character (#6) broke down crying and screaming, "Let me out of here." He charged the chain-link fence and tried to climb out of the cage. The guards dragged his clawing hands off the chain-link and put him in a straightjacket. Weeping pathetically, he was carried away by medics. His performance helped move the US Congress to launch an investigation into brutality in the Marine Corps' brig system. Few actors impact the world the way George did. Thank you, George! I will never forget you!*

Few actors in the American theater commit their considerable talents as fully as George did to addressing injustice while acting brilliantly.

Peter Schumann, creator of the Bread and Puppet Theater, first saw George perform on a flatbed truck in Central Park at an anti-Vietnam war arts festival where George also first saw Peter's puppets, gigantic and small, being maneuvered in slow motion across the Great Lawn. (Where I first saw them, too, the impression unforgettable of great theater-puppet art; I wrote about Peter's work in my first book.) George and Crystal were performing an abridged history of the Vietnam War, acting generals, state department officials, presidents, grunts, victims simply by changing their hats. Peter was impressed by this comic economy and George thrilled to Peter's so-expressive papier-mâché puppets. George and Peter became lifelong friends. They collaborated on the fierce antiwar play *Woyzeck* by the German playwright and revolutionary, Georg Buchner. It was a favorite play of both. George was the only actor. Acting with life-size puppets manipulated by puppeteers, George played the hapless soldier whose life is ruined by the army and who stabs his common law wife to death when he finds her in bed with the Drum Major. In the final scene, George as Woyzeck is about to be hanged. As the curtain falls, he kneels on a box, a noose around his neck, completely deserted by humankind. Even in the scratchy, ill-lit video, the humanity with which he endows his hapless character is intensely moving. As always, on stage, George gave full attention and respect to Peter's out-sized puppets, loving his puppet wife. The master puppeteer and the actor collaborated, again, on a play they created together, *Diagonal Man*, which toured Europe after its New York premiere. Michael Romanyshyn, one of the puppeteers, now proprietor of a Vermont maple syrup farm, tells the story:

> *In Bielska Biala at a puppet festival, we discovered what the show was really about. This was during martial law in 1983 after the Solidarity movement had been crushed and the head of the government, General Wojciech Jaruzelski, was trying to thwart a Soviet invasion. Food was scarce and it was a tense and uncertain time. The theater was packed and from the moment the performance began we knew something was very different.*
>
> *The audience responded to George's lines and embraced him as if he was them, neither up nor down, caught between two superpowers. Diagonal Man said: "He wants Bread not Death AND Fire Without Smoke" And at the moment in the show when he recited the lines from the ballad in Polish: "On his way to the sun, he lives like a dog. Does he live like a dog on his way to the sun?" The audience stood up and all together yelled YES! It was a unifying cry of joyful distress. The acknowledgment of collective fatigue with a tinge of optimism. At the end of the show, George was mobbed. People crowded around onstage, hugging him with tears in their eyes. It was a wild and moving scene we'll never forget. He was Everyone and only George.*

"Go for it," yelled an unseen voice in the dark, as if from on high, from across the street when we kissed for the first time. We had stopped beneath a single, bare light hung with a wire shade in the archway of a public garage, and, lit from above, turned to one another. "Go for it," the voice yelled, again, and we kissed. It was after a performance of *Us*, which had already been slammed in the mainstream press, as, of course, had *The Brig* when it first opened. Audiences didn't care and they kept coming—which would happen to us so many times with our plays. What had the person across the street seen in our urgency, our pain, our desire, our need? I imagine all was clear as if written in white exhaust across the night sky: it's *this* or nothing ever lasting, it's now or never, what you've wanted and lacked, what you desired and feared you'd didn't deserve. We would not have kissed that night had we not known this was a pledge to unwind two complicated and frequently miserable personal lives, to disentangle from a past that clung like sludge to our insides, that had turned me meek, stoop-shouldered and guilty, like a schoolmarm, and indeed, I was adjunct teaching so many classes I would soon get walking pneumonia, and that had prematurely wrinkled his face, so he appeared, then, tortoise-like, to be peering out from a prehistoric past in which he'd been crushed—when he was off-stage, that is. We would not have stopped on the dark street, in the chill New York mist, underneath a bare lightbulb unless to be spied by the angel who flew by and called out "go for it" so we knew we'd been blessed from on high, though neither of us believed such a preposterous thought, neither believed in anything … but the love we desired so much. If we hadn't stopped, if we'd walked on, oblivious to the fact of being watched, seen, blessed, then all of what I tell would never have existed. Our lives would have continued separate, desperate and pinched. But we'd given ourselves already in the rehearsal room as I watched him become and transform. And he had given to me, as he used my words to do what he wanted to do on the stage, shape-change. Language to which he gave physical form was his medium. We weren't any more young.

His acting in *Us* was a revelation. I had never seen such physical acting in a poetic play and I suspect few people had. When he won his Village Voice Obie award, and he said about his performance in *Us* that "there are some plays that get a rise out of an actor," a laugh went up from the crowd because everyone knew by then we had cast our lot. Transformation was our desire and goal, in our personal lives, in the theater, and for the violent and unjust world in which we lived. In this, we were kin to Judith and Julian, and to Joe Chaikin, Jack Gelber, Peter Schumann, our colleagues and friends. Though all of our aesthetics were vastly different. George wanted mainly to do new plays. Joe, when he turned from devising work himself, would gravitate to the classics to direct and act, but also new plays by his friends Adrienne Kennedy and Sam Shepard. Like George, he would do Beckett; like Judith and Julian, *Antigone*. In truth, each of us loved the large passions, the poetry of a theater with high stakes. We each felt that if we could give form in our different ways to those moments in which transformation occurs as a living, observable thing, then social and individual change would be possible, and would be witnessed as possible by the audience. People would not be condemned to repeat the violent legacies of their past, but might grow, blossom, sink deeper roots. Trauma might become undone, peace appear, and the natural world would be honored and loved. We were idealists. Opposed to the Vietnam War and to all the wars and invasions to come. We did not view our artistic work as separate from the values we held in our lives. We did not work for hire. Each of us wanted nothing less than nonviolent social change. We were pacifists and we put our bodies on the line. We broke the law in civil disobedience actions for what we believed (Thoreau-like, also as rebels in the Romantic tradition). And we each went to jail sometimes. We all thought our work was to show metamorphosis onstage and that the transformational experiences might, through the actors' bodies and voice, enter the audience's flesh and bone. Breathing together, the word materialized. The World as One. That possibility glimpsed.

There are two moments still vivid from the play *Us*, of which there is no photographic record. George became a stallion in front of the audience. Dressed, again, only in that clingy underwear, he stepped into the role, his back arching like the rippled neck of the big horse, his muscles taut beneath his skin like a hot-blooded, highly bred animal, his feet pawing the earth. There were lines that accompanied his physical transformation. The female character, Hannah remembers the childhood scene (which happened to me as a young teenager at the stable where I rode). She watches the frantic mating of stallion and mare. Around the ring, the men from the stable also gather to watch the mating, making crude sexual comments. No one notices the girl, barely tall enough to peer over the ring wall. The lines were not his, but the image was his to create as she spoke; and he gave the emotion, the raw animal sex, to the audience, while the woman actor, playing her young-girl self, describes the mating to us, and feels for the stallion, spent, standing alone in the ring. As a teenage girl, I had been given a quarter horse stallion to exercise, King Hand III, and had run through the woods on him. Girls were not supposed to ride a stallion; we were too weak to pull him up if he took the bit in his mouth. And he threw me like this once, galloping across two roads to dump me in the stable yard, but more often than not, the supple mass of horse between my legs was evidence of my power. In the play, Hannah bridles the horse whose sexual prowess startles her, and she rides him bareback into the night. "I sing into his ears because he cannot. Because he runs for me as I sing." While George in his flesh showed this bond, his feet like hooves, barely touching the floor, their galloping.

George, playing Michel's mother, stepped into glittery, silver platform high heels, and, then, with the big shoes on, he stepped through the tunnel of a slinky silver jersey dress, which he pulled up over his suddenly feminine form, one hip jutting out. He put on the clear plastic mask and the poufed yellow hair of his "mother" who sat in front of her mirror, arching a shoulder, turning this way and that for the best view of herself, as a narcissistic woman does.

"Don't tell me that, because I don't want to hear it," he/she (the child's memory of his mother) says. "I don't want to hear it because it is not true. It is not true because it could not possibly have happened. Because it could not possibly have happened it is not true and I don't want to hear it ..."

The speech turns suddenly seductive. She asks her son what he thinks of her hair, asks him to admire her, and she praises him, catching him in her narcissist's web. At the end, she bursts out in anger, denying what her youngest son told her about his older brother, Andre,

"Did not sodomize you over and over again ... He did not say he'd kill you if you told. Don't tell me this because I don't want to hear it. I don't want to hear it because it is not true. It is not true because it could not possibly have happened it is not true and I don't want to hear it. Do you want to kill me? Do you want me dead?"

She (George in his female mask and dress) swings away from the mirror to stare hard at the audience.

How did the same actor hold both the larger-than-life, self-involved mother and the stunned, frightened boy, seeking comfort that was not to be, in one body, one voice. Why, when looking at the actor in outlandish drag, could we also see and feel for the hurt child? Because he, George, empathized with both—the woman terrified of the truth that would bring her imagined world, in which she is beautiful above all, cascading down, and the frightened child trying to speak up to save his life. The woman pushing the ugly truth away, transforming it into the stories we tell precisely so we might never know, and the boy, with the truth stuck in his throat, showing the terror he hopes someone sees in his eyes.

It was a trick George perfected all his life, to step into someone else, human or animal, in front of the audience, and take us instantaneously deep into that private other life. With his shape-changing body and voice, he was able to reveal how we might become another in an instant, or more truly ourselves, or change to reveal the sentient life of an animal. This is transformational acting which the American avant-garde of the sixties and seventies pioneered. And transformational acting is the artistic proof of the political belief that we can change, systems and selves, and become other than we are, and, as important, feel increased empathy for one another. No wonder people remember for years George as he was on stage, in one role or another of the hundreds he played with such compassion. Our work together would return him to acting full-time in my plays, but also at regional theaters, and at The Public Theater, on Broadway in *Fiddler on the Roof* and briefly in Al Pacino's *Richard III*, (someone gave Pacino a bouquet of flowers, Pacino turned and gave them to George, "these should be yours." Pacino had always admired George.) Off-Broadway George played Morrie, in the revival of *Tuesdays with Morrie*, and he won a Best Actor award when the production transferred to Philadelphia. He was in Steve Martin's comic *The Underpants* at Long Warf in Connecticut, and at Hartford Stage. He worked with our friends Olympia Dukakis and her husband, Louie Zorich in a Chekhov marathon. But George loved the new poetic-political play most—that was our bond, and my luck.

In a 2015 interview for the Lower East Side Oral History Project conducted by performance artist Penny Arcade in our living room, George spoke of his fascination with the plays I wrote, while I was in my home office, at work:

> *My whole life until I have to say until I met this person who is present in this house, until I met this person, I was looking for a theater that answers all the things that I want to do in the theater, which is to be able to act in another dimension, to create something where you don't know quite what's going on but it's transcending something, and a lot of that has to do with language.*

As if he swallowed the words and they worked their magic by transforming him from the inside out, he became inhabited, first, and then he materialized a character who was not him. He drank in the words of the playwrights he loved and found his character as a lover finds their beloved. He became an admirer, a cherisher of all his character was.

From 1987 until his death, he premiered ten new plays of mine and one we created together from the Holocaust diaries of Victor Klemperer, most of which had multiple productions in New York and Europe and toured. In the final years of his life, his last stage acting, he would perform major roles in two new plays I wrote and directed, which our small theater company, Theater Three Collaborative, co-produced, *Other Than We*, at LaMama and *Blue Valiant* with Farm Arts Collective. Shortly after the vaccines, just as lockdown was lifted, in 2021, we staged *Blue Valiant*, outside at Farm Arts Collective in Pennsylvania, and filmed it for release on YouTube where it remains to be viewed. "These last two plays," George wrote in his diary, "are a new level for the personal and creative in Karen's work. This is also why I want very much to realize performance of *Blue Valiant*, which is (an) even more daring departure in Karen's style." He was in a race against time, he well understood. George would also record the speech of the Talking Fish in my short play, *Troy Too*, which he performed posthumously on tape eight months after his death, at HERE Performing Arts Space in Soho, in May 2023. Then he "acted" with our friend Lydia Koniordou, one of Greece's foremost classical actors, also a television star and a former Minister of Culture. Lydia and George had always talked about acting together. They met when Lydia staged my adaptation of Christa Wolf's novella *Kassandra*, for the Tisch School of the Arts. After his death, Lydia, as Hecuba in *Troy Too* would react to each nuance in George's voice as the Fish.

George was embodied, he was attentive, he listened onstage; one remembers most "the silence he conjured between thoughts," says Penny Arcade. A silence as if to let us in, to think/feel with him. A silent attention that gave the other actors on stage room to be. He made exquisite specific choices, which he could do because he had been so thoroughly trained, also as a dancer by his parents, early on, and his malleable body and resonant voice were at his command until the very end of his life. "The minute he opened his mouth, the entire audience was spell-bound and hushed," Kathleen Chalfant says. She shared the stage in his last live performance. *Blue Valiant* was one of the first pieces of live theater performed in the country, if not the first, immediately after the lockdown orders were lifted. We were racing against cancer, dealing with a pandemic, so that George and Kathy could act together, again.

Between the ages of twelve and seventeen, I became a somewhat accomplished equestrian. Good enough, that is, to be given wealthy people's purebred horses to exercise: a gray Welsh pony with flaxen mane and a tail that swept the ground I named Moxie, so high stepping and beautiful he stopped traffic when I rode him on the trail next to the road; the chestnut quarter horse stallion King Hand III; a skittish, liver-colored cutting horse called Spider Web; a tall, flashy, and ill-tempered strawberry roan Saddlebred, Candy Kid, whom I rode often when he was a school horse and whom I fiercely loved. After he was sold, I was allowed by the new owner to exercise him. I'd gone to the horses for comfort, to escape the violence in the house and my own uncomfortable teenage years. One had to be calm around or on top of a thousand-pound animal, but more than that, the horses looked at me with deep, feeling eyes. I felt seen. I was comforted by their breath, their animal smells, by leaning against their warm necks. During those years, I spent every hour I could in the barn, mucking out stalls, currying, saddling, wiping down. I hung onto the wise words of the dark-skinned men from the Caribbean who were called stable boys, especially a man named Martel, who became my source of wisdom about horses and life. My best horse friend, Joanie, a natural rider if ever there was one, whose seat was so deep and hands so light she seemed indistinguishable from the horse, died from an illegal abortion. At the Catholic funeral her sister, who must have arranged for the procedure, was hysterical with guilt—though no one spoke about any of this, official cause of death was appendicitis. I saw foals born and watched horses die, saw a horse shot who had broken his leg, and watched the stallion and mare mate. I was thrown many times. I stopped riding as my father grew more gravely ill, and I went to college. But all that I'd learned in the barn, how to *be* around forces much larger than I, how to communicate by a shift of one's weight, the pressure of knees, the twitch of a little finger on the reigns, the cluck of a tongue with a powerful animal, how to be as if one with a nonhuman life, felt, and feels, essential. I hadn't sat a horse since childhood until I went to Egypt, for the Cairo Experimental Theater Festival, in 1998 and '99, and in the early mornings rode Arabians in the Sahara desert. I loved it, thrilled that my body remembered. George, who was head of the judging panel the second year, insisted on coming with me once. He gamely flapped along on his forgiving horse, and returned to his role as judge, "Dr. George" everyone called him, with a flaming red bottom and on wobbly legs. Then, in 2017, on a whim, I booked several hacks on English thoroughbreds during an academic conference in Surrey, British horse country, where I was launching an anthology of four of my plays. I had never ridden thoroughbred hunters before. They are big. At tea with Kathy Chalfant, I mentioned I was going to go riding in England and might break my neck. "Not a bad way to go," she laughed. I agreed. She told me that her family had owned seven hunter-jumpers that her children rode and showed. She loved horses. I hadn't known. "I'll write you a play," I said. We laughed, but I did.

Blue Valiant is the one play during his life I did not write with George clearly in mind—Don Leadly and Elmer Holsdorf were in my head, the two men who had owned the stable where I rode, both crusty and wise, very different one from the other as Don was rough and uneducated, a hillbilly, really, who used to put his feet, with their manure-caked boots, up on the office desk, lean far back in the chair and pick his teeth, and Elmer a homosexual, gentleman stable owner and recognized saddle horse show rider who was partnered with my riding teacher, Gavin Beglin, on whom I had a teenage crush; knowing he lived with a man, he was, for me, a wise father figure. "She has those eyes and she knows how to use them," Gavin said to my father one day about my dark eyes, so like my father's deep flashing ones, when he picked me up at the stable. My father was furious at Gavin's sexual remark, innocent though it was. What my father didn't know was that the deep red scabbed line across my neck came from accident on a horse I did not dare tell my parents about. We'd been riding through the woods, Gavin in the lead, when a vine somehow caught me around the neck, my horse walked on, and I was left hanging. I never told them about the multiple times I was thrown, afraid they would make me stop riding. On my first time up on a horse, twenty-year old Ranger, every child's first ride, Holsdorf had seen me in the ring and called out: "That's good on Ranger." I was hooked. Sam was my compilation of every wise horseman from my childhood. I had no actor in mind for the role. I did not think George would like the part and it was smaller by far than Kathy's long role, Hannah Doyle, the bereft wealthy woman who decides to buy the untamable horse. But George felt for the man, Sam, so unlike him, and Kathy, of course, wanted to act again with him. I understood later, after George died, that I had also written the play as a meditation on grief, prefiguring a future life I did not yet know. If I'd fully understood, then, what I was writing, I would have recoiled. Hannah Doyle, Sam Brown, and Maya Zelaya, a refugee child from Honduras separated from her father at the border during the first Trump years, as well as the horse, Blue Valiant, we come to find out, have each lost the people closest to them. Sam is mourning his wife. Hannah, her daughter, dead from opioids. Maya mourns the loss of her family and her country, an immigrant child alone in a strange land. The horse mourns "his Sally," the girl who raised him from a foal, after the old mare died giving birth, the girl who, while experimenting with drugs, falls and breaks her neck while misguiding him over a jump at a horse show. When the horse stands, stock still, next to her body refusing to move, bending his neck toward her lifeless frame, he is brutally beaten by Sally's distraught father. The loss of Sally and the beating turn the horse wild. The drugged horse is dumped at Sam's barn with $5000 in cash. He's untamable now, racing around Sam's pasture, jumping the fence, threatening those who stop their cars on the roadside to admire the astonishing beauty of the blue roan. Each character begins the play alone, and each, including, of course, the horse, is unable to articulate the full reality of their pain. Grief exists beyond language, inexplicable, un-relatable. The horse, magnificent, dangerous, and enraged, becomes the metaphor for grief, untamable. When people asked me in the months after George died whether or not I was angry, I would yell back them, "of course not," but grief makes us so furious we cannot even admit our rage to ourselves. In the play, the characters are drawn together by each one's deepening awareness of their unspeakable loss, and by their fascination with the magnificent horse.

Sam Brown, his final character, seemed nothing like George, except that George would endow him with a compassionate gaze that was not consciously in my script, but that George found there. George could not sit a horse, but like Sam sitting overlooking his pasture, George, so close to death, also stared into a vastness. Sam believes in the wisdom in the flesh of the big animals he loves. Observation, deep looking. Words, too, like riddles, the thing and its opposite. Maya, a Spanish speaker, the immigrant child, takes refuge in the horse's stall. A new family, of sorts, forms at Sam's barn, each learning the language of the other. Sam works stealth reins as a sort of *deus ex machina*, undetected, yes, like a demigod. Sam's oracular role in the play was not clear to me until George began, in rehearsals, to embody him.

I wrote *Blue Valiant* quickly. I'd done all the research years before when I was a kid hanging out at the stable; the memories bubbled up, now, many of which I shared by text with George's doctor. We often texted back and forth about things other than George's health. He liked my horse tales and I liked remembering and sharing with him. But the big problem we faced was however do you put a horse onstage? I didn't want to use a puppet. This had been spectacularly done and at great expense in *Warhorse*, and by men wearing masks in psychological drama *Equus*, two British imports. But I wasn't certain, other than through the characters' words, how to visualize the animal. The play sat with the question unanswered. I decided to throw George a fancy eighty-seventh birthday party in a downtown restaurant with a performance space, in late January of 2020—just before the pandemic began. Though several people stay home sick with what seems like a flu, many of our friends are there. My twin brother, John, and George's son,

Alex, give the birthday toasts. Kathy Chalfant performs a section of Eliot's *Four Quartets*. George does several of his favorite speeches: Victor Klemperer, and Uncle's pond speech from *Extreme Whether*. Downtown doyenne and the evening's M.C., Penny Arcade, riffs about George's storied career, producing and mentoring artists like her. Stephen Said sings. George retakes the mic and entertains the crowd with a long, impromptu, comic monologue about his life in the theater. Though *Blue Valiant* is written and everyone likes it, we still have no idea how to stage the play. Arthur Rosen, the composer of incidental music for our work over the years, approaches Kathy at the party. Kathy asks Arthur, "What if he were to create the horse's voice—and play the horse on a piano?" Arthur believes he posed the question to her. I didn't overhear so I do not know who had the idea first. Nevertheless, we jump at the thought. Piano as horse, brilliant. We decide at once to begin workshop rehearsals, to see, if with piano-voice, the horse might interact with the other characters. A reading of *Blue Valiant* is scheduled for April 6, 2020, at New York Theater Workshop; there is always the chance they might also produce the play once they have heard it read. But as the novel coronavirus spreads, the theaters shut down. The reading is canceled.

March 14, 2020, one day after the official lockdown begins, we violate the national quarantine in order to sneak in one horse rehearsal in Kathy's living room, where there is a piano. We need to hear if music-as-horse will be convincing, if strong chords, fists slamming on wood, feet galloping on piano pedals as if hooves across fields, might give voice to the wounded equine's inner life. George is wildly enthusiastic. He gives the composer strong notes. We try moments again. Yes, we anoint the piano as the horse. We will not see one another in person again for over a year. We find the composer an empty studio with a piano (he only has a keyboard at home) in deserted, dusty Manhattan in which to work. We go there once, driving with the composer through the deserted city. George has just been released from hospital for something or other. He is using a cane for the first time. He's weak but attentive and he gives the composer more good notes. George is so much better at directing music than I. George, in league with Arthur, the composer, is co-creating the horse. We do a Zoom reading of the play, without music, in May 2020, with a moneyed producer. Everyone, including the so-called producer, is thrilled. (The producer finks out, but we continue our work.) We are racing to bring *Blue Valiant* to the stage while George's strength holds. But all the theaters are closed. Our costume designer, Sally Ann Parsons, knows Tannis Kowalski, who runs Farm Arts Collective on her organic vegetable and flower farm just over the New York Catskills border in Pennsylvania, a place many New Yorkers fled to in the pandemic. Tannis offers us a co-production, outside, over Memorial Day weekend. We will reopen her theater to live audiences. Nina Kamberos, publisher of Laertes Books, and of my recent plays, offers additional funds for our production. As one of my other functions, aside from producing, directing, and writing, I have to take a five-hour training to become the COVID compliance officer in order to rehearse with the two Equity members, Kathy and George. The cancer doctor writes a letter to Actor's Equity asserting our rehearsal room, with its five windows and open door to a garden has better ventilation than his hospital. Nevertheless, Equity, which demands a certain air filter, declines our request. We lie and tell them we are rehearsing outdoors. The doctor is following the progress of the production closely.

In April of 2021, we meet to rehearse in the Brooklyn studio; we all are recently vaccinated and boosted. We are again in a rehearsal room where George and Kathy work fast and deep with delight, two consummate actors egging each other on, *and* the horse finds voice through Arthur at the piano.

Blue Valiant will be our last play. Though George and I both know this, we never say it aloud. We are going to film the production in the hope it can be widely seen. There is a producer who promises to present the production to Audible (nothing will come of this, but nevertheless, we have the performance on film). We stop for a drink and a snack outside after rehearsals, as we'd often done over the years. The cancer doctor calls. George has missed his chemo appointment. He's off treatment for rehearsals, I tell the doctor. George is too weak to walk home and we have to wait for the bus. Chemo-brain makes it impossible for him to remember all his lines, no matter how many times we go over them. He knows all his longer speeches; it is Sam's repartee with Kathy's character Hannah he can't keep straight in his head—quick, short and idiosyncratic. We go over his lines at home every morning. Kathy, who has several very long speeches, and Henry Chalfant are doing the same thing at the same time. "This is beautiful," Henry says, reading George's part as I am reading Kathy's for George. We joke, Henry—filmmaker, artist, photographer—and I could act the play together. Kathy and George can watch. A week before we open for our two outdoor performances only, we bring in an Equity stage-manager and Millie Ortiz, a lovely young actor who will play Maya, the refugee child. Our design and film crew come to a final run-through in the rehearsal studio. They are all steamed. George will need earphones we decide at the very last studio rehearsal. The stage manager will stand behind the audience and behind the four-person film crew, and read the lines into George's, and sometimes, too, into Kathy's ears. Pacino used earphones in order to be prompted in *Richard III*, George knows because he was the production. Usually, this sort of thing takes technical rehearsals, as there is lag time between hearing the words and saying them, but we have had no rehearsal time. No matter, there will be a dress rehearsal at the farm. We arrive at Farm Arts Collective in Pennsylvania, where we are to perform outside. It is a brilliant, clear, warm late-May day. That night, working like a well-oiled machine, our team, including the horse photographer Ellen Lynch, whom I found on Facebook and have not met until now and whose beautiful, huge images of horses we will use once the sun has set, manages to focus the projections, and the lights are hung on poles as construction work is completed on the raised stage. George is ecstatic. He likes nothing better than to see artists working together, everyone doing whatever is needed without thought of job description or hierarchy. We each help move, place, and wire things, solve problems. We are all so happy. We are "back" in a theater again, outside of the greenhouse over which a large white drape, for the screen, has been hung, on an organic vegetable farm. I have our two aging cocker spaniels, Cleis and Hermes, on leash as I watch and give my thoughts. "These are beautiful," Henry says., as the horse projections are seen for the first time. He is one of the five-person film crew. Ellen makes a crucial edit while the projector is being placed—our horse is gelded in full view. We will have all day tomorrow to rehearse.

The next day, the temperature drops into the forties and the rain starts. Our dress rehearsal is rained out. We have had minimal rehearsals, and now we lose this. We try to run lines in the greenhouse, but the rain pounds so hard on the plastic roof we cannot hear anyone speak. We give up. It pours all the next day; we will be rained out, but Tannis tells us she has uncommon good weather luck and not to give up. The rain stops exactly at 6 pm. It's freezing for May, but the sun has come out. We have just enough time to dry the stage, hang a few horse blankets as masking, and set some bales of hay. The lighting and projections have yet to be seen as they will only become visible for the first time once the sun goes down, roughly at the perfect time in the play for the horse's large images to appear on the white drop hung from the greenhouse roof. There has been no rehearsal with the earphones, and yet, they work so well, or, rather, George and Kathy do so well, the stage manager, too, that the audience cannot tell when they are being prompted on the spot. The first performance is beautiful. We are ecstatic. The audience comes with blankets and they huddle against the cold, but no one leaves, and they love our play. We have it on film, with four different cameras, too. I cannot imagine a second performance can be as good. Usually, there is a drop off right after the tension of opening night. The second night performance is often the worst. George's doctor texts to see how it has gone. I answer, "brilliant." We are so happy. It pours rain all night and all the next day. It's even colder and wetter than the day before. It is still raining as we drive to the theater, just in case. But again the rain stops, just in time to mop the stage. We get in a second performance as if by magic. It is very cold. The audience comes dressed in layers, with blankets, but is in a celebratory mood; they've heard the play is good and they want to see a live performance after months of the lonely pandemic. George is on stage in the biting cold for the entire play. I leave him there rather than have him laboriously climb up and down slippery steps. Sitting in full view, overlooking his world, overhearing Hannah's long monologues and scenes with the child who appears, Sam Brown takes on the resonance of the creator of all of this. The one who, with stillness and penetrating gaze, nurtures and prods. Kathy calls the performances "our miracle."

George sits stock still on a metal chair, in thirty-nine-degree, unseasonably frigid May weather between downpours with an all-seeing gaze, though he is legally blind and I never am quite sure what he sees, surveying the world Sam has made at his stable, and the community that forms from these hurt people, the hurt horse. Sam Brown, George's final creation, becomes omnipotent as night falls and the stage lights cast him in their glow, his look showing a way we might go if we dare give of ourselves as thoroughly as the old actor does dare. Frail, yes, but his voice rich and full, he makes careful decisions to maximize his force. The final performance of a play after a long run is quite often the best, actors are no longer bound by constraint, they try what they've been longing to do but were frightened of. And this second performance of a new, never-before-staged play, is the last live performance of this actor's long life. He creates a rare and consequential presence, a horseman who nurtures. We have it on video, on YouTube to this day where it can be seen: *Blue Valiant*. George's lastness, the final moments he moved and spoke on stage with consummate force. Two performances on two consecutive nights in the bitter cold, going from stormy sunset to dark. We did not speak of it like this. We knew, of course. Everyone understood George would not be onstage in all likelihood ever again. He, of course, would have thought the same. But we never said so out loud. So, the two performances were nearly mystic, the hardships, the play's brief fulfillment, as if he had to encompass all the knowledge gained from a long run, from his long life, in fact, starting as a boy, and there was no overacting, nothing but strict attention paid so that the two other actors might thrive. Frail, cold, some lines coming to him through earphones, yet in complete command of his skills, making choices at every moment, as generous as he'd always been, his pauses, his intonations. He did not falter or halt. The final performance of a life carefully wrought.

Not only could we not repeat; we would never again ... there was no future ahead. We never said this. We had our fifteen-year-old spaniels in tow. George, despite my warning, opened the door to the top floor bedroom where we were staying. My girl dog ran out and immediately tumbled down a long, curved, hard stairway, ending in a heap in the kitchen. As she fell, I said to myself, "whatever happens, don't yell." The feisty old girl jumped up, seemingly unscathed. Good that it all went so well, amid the weather crisis. Crisis is inevitably part of the opening of any play. George and I thrived on it. The others in the company and the film crew had celebratory drinks in the hotel bar. George was too weak. We didn't care. We climbed into bed in the big Victorian house where we stayed, that belonged to Lee Nagrin who founded Theater Three with us in 1995. Snuggling with our old dogs.

His deep attention to others on stage drove every actor deeper into themselves and made them feel safe enough to take emotional risks. The final performance of his life was strange enough to be a fitting end to his strange stage-life, in the freezing cold, outside on a farm before seventy-five people, captured on film. Yes, "George made everyone a better actor," as Kathy said.

"In theater, where everything is some sort of a lie and a convention, from a cardboard tree to a wooden rifle, George delivered truth. The words he uttered, the gestures he made, the mimics he performed, they all created completely believable characters whom audiences fully trusted," film director Arsen Ostojic writes. "He was a great actor because he was a great man." He was a great man because he gave himself to wonder and combated terror, and though the two remained unalterably mixed through his life, the result was intoxicating. George exuded joy. He was happy to see you, happy to be. He was invariably kind. And uniquely present. He was singularly unafraid to become.

"Showing is a kind of loving," he would croon to me often. He was speaking of the most intimate sharing in which we indulged, but equally of giving of the self wantonly in the theater space. He liked to tell of the time when he was naked on stage, and the fire marshals came to inspect the theater space, and he greeted them hastily wrapped in a black plastic garbage bag. He would splay himself open, emotionally, his body and voice. He never stopped going deeper, as he committed himself to favorite characters over the years. He worked slowly, methodically. As his sight dulled, he would sit waiting for meetings or his many doctors' appointments, going over his favorite speeches. He had a repertoire he had memorized over the years, Hamlet's soliloquies; or Faust, learned from his mother in the German; Victor Klemperer; or from my plays *Extreme Whether* and *The Beekeeper's Daughter*; favorite long speeches by the environmentalist Uncle and the poet Robert Blaze. He would come home beaming to tell me, "I'm getting better!" or "I finally understood that line," after performing in his mind. He loved his last character, Sam Brown, the crusty old horse trainer, nothing at all like George, rough, ungrammatical. But George was attracted to the felt wisdom in the man's unlettered ways, how he conjured the horse's violent past from his behavior, and to the poetry in his simple words. "Nature is God," George frequently said. If his last role was nothing like him, in my mind, he so loved the wily horseman, standing or seated in his chair for the entire play, that he made him oracular—as if watching over the pasture, the animals and people, since time began.

Because of the deep quality of his listening, the attention he paid, other actors became deeper, more attentive, more nuanced, too. They began to embody their characters more fully. Their egos receded. They gave themselves more completely. They became more like George. This was true whether they were already accomplished actors, like Kathleen Chalfant, or young and relatively inexperienced, like the actors we often worked with on our limited budgets. Everyone became better when acting with George. By his example, his carefully chosen words of instruction, he turned our actors into a cohesive company with every play. George, who loved to mentor, delighted in telling the story of Harold Clurman, his first director at age fourteen. In 1971, Clurman was the theater critic for *The Nation* and George invited him to opening night of newly formed Theater for the City. Clurman made a mistake and came a night early in his fedora, a coat with a cape, his silver tipped cane, and a young woman on his arm. Inside the theater, he found George up on a ladder, painting the ceiling, his face and clothing paint-smattered, exhausted. George was mortified, "Harold, I'm so sorry, it's tomorrow, the opening …" Clurman waved him away, "Look," he yelled in his stentorian voice, "What The Young People Are Doing!!! Making Theater!"

In the theater and literary history of the western world, I know of no relationship similar to ours, in which a younger, lesser-known, very often critically-reviled woman playwright is accepted as the equal partner of an older, established male actor and producer, and returns him, through leading roles she writes, to his full excellence on the stage, all the while he devotes himself to the development of and to producing each one of her new works. And they live together in harmony for thirty-five years. Our friends Judith Malina and Julian Beck had something similar, but George and I were physically in love; we remained wedded to poetry and character, and to the poetic play, crafted and well-acted, a commitment Judith and Julian abandoned for collective creations. If I would not have been able to become without him, it is also true that he needed me. We inspired one another, perhaps like William Godwin and Mary Wollstonecraft or, more so, Percy Bysshe and Mary Wollstonecraft-Godwin Shelley, Wollstonecraft's second child, both those couples married so briefly. Visions intertwined, work done separately or together, impossible to conceive without the other. Long, rambling, interesting talks day and night. Romanticism: reverence for nature, materializing through language social possibilities beyond the strictures of an ever-industrializing, hierarchical, increasingly violent world, the necessity of physical closeness, of bodies intertwined in love, Mutual Eros, in order to fully conceive mutual artistic vision. The impossibility of separating the flesh from the word. In our plays, we sought to transgress the boundaries between the social world as it is and what we might become, to explore the permeable boundary between what exists and all that can be imagined in the mind's eye. We sought to show nature as alive, divine, and shape-changing. To incorporate nonhuman sentient wisdom through animal presence. To defy convention. Exult in change. Practice, on the stage, as in life, nonviolence. Be outrageous for the fun of it. Instigate delight. In these ways, our project aligns with the Romantics. Our plays in production stood against both the violent state and interpersonal violence. We dramatized resistance. We dramatized nurture and love. We went in service to all that hasn't happened yet, but yet could happen still, if we dare transform and materialize our desires.

I am speaking, obviously, of our intentions which we sought to fulfill in our productions, of how we spoke to each other, and to others, about our work and of what we believed. And we spoke to one another constantly, at all times of day and night. Ours was a conversation that lasted thirty-five years. We loved most to wake at 4 a.m. and talk until 6, to fall back into sleep, dream a bit, get up and get to work. We wanted ongoing relationships with other artists, and we worked with many of the same people again and again, most notably lighting and sometime set designer Tony Giovannetti, costume designer Sally Ann Parsons, and photographer Beatriz Schiller. All had roots in the avant-garde. With the performance artist Lee Nagrin, we founded Theater Three Collaborative. We worked with Ruth Maleczech and Vanessa Redgrave in a piece called "Collateral Damage," at LaMama, during Gulf War I. We worked with Najla Said, Edward Said's daughter, for four years in multiple readings and two productions in London and New York of my antiwar play *Prophecy*. Najla, who was evacuated from Lebanon during that conflict, played three parts I crafted especially for her, inspired by the emails she sent from her family's home while Beirut was being bombed. Kathleen Chalfant played the female lead in *Prophecy*. George and she were husband and wife in a long, complex, sometimes quite humorous marriage. Najla played the woman for whom Kathy is betrayed, the Palestinian-Lebanese mother of Allan's out-of-wedlock daughter, a part also played by Najla. We worked with Christen Clifford for decades in three productions of *The Beekeeper's Daughter* and five of *Another Life*, and with Di Zhu, who is now co-producer at Theater '86, in *Another Life, Extreme Whether* and the fourth production of *The Beekeeper's Daughter* in 2016.

I had sworn off the theater after I felt we botched the third production of *The Beekeeper's Daughter*, on Theater Row. I wasn't wrong. It had taken us several years to raise the money. Then we miscast badly and I gave the play to a Croatian director who was far too harsh with it, rather than direct it myself. Though successful in two previous productions, the play failed, now. I was suffering, when a voice spoke in my head: "Why not do something nice for George." I'd just read a glowing page one review in the Sunday Book section of the *New York Times* of *I Will Bear Witness*, volume one of Victor Klemperer's just-translated Holocaust diaries. "Would you like to make a one-person play out of this?" Our neighbor happened to be from Germany and worked in publishing. She knew the German publisher's phone number. George was on the phone with him the next day. In the publisher's Berlin office at the same time, there happened to be a New York theater producer who knew George's acting. We received the English language dramatic rights to the two books immediately. Perhaps the publisher thought we were bluffing. It was an unlikely task, adapting two, five-hundred-page personal diaries, filled with hundreds of characters, for one man. Volume two had not yet been translated when we began years of work. As always, if we'd known what we were letting ourselves in for, we might have stopped to consider, or perhaps not. Turning the diaries of Victor Klemperer into two dramatic one-person plays would become the defining point of the last third of George's life. It would take us three years to create two texts, one from 1933 to '39; the other of the war years, and the deportation of the Jews, ending shortly after the firebombing of Dresden and defeat of the Nazi government. This work would demand virtuoso acting and allow George, finally, to connect to his earliest memories in Nazi Germany. He wished to perform the assimilated German Jewish professor in the "VK," as he called it, because Victor Klemperer, too, experienced the life-saving reality of "good Germans." Klemperer's wife, Eva, like George's German Tante Irma, had stuck by him. Jewish men who remained married to non-Jewish women were among the last scheduled for deportation.

Not knowing how to begin, but captivated by the diary, we met filmmaker Margarethe von Trotta at a luncheon at BAM, after a showing of her documentary film about Rosa Luxemburg and asked her about process. "Read the book five times or more," she advised, then select. We each had our own two volumes of the thousand-page diaries that we read and reread. We would not change or write one new word, but we would edit and re-edit mercilessly. We would cut within sentences and string phrases together from different paragraphs on different pages, in order to create a dramatic thrust. Each volume was crisscrossed, underlined, and heavily marked. We began, separately, to trace out a story. We compared. We argued fiercely, as we always did. We each loved sections we had to exclude. We hung on until we had to let go, of, for instance, the entire comic story of Klemperer learning to drive at age sixty in Nazi Germany, and the petty cruelty of the forced euthanasia of Muschel, their cat. We were trying to extract a drama from a man's personal, hidden, illegal diary. If his pages had been discovered, Klemperer would have been sent to a concentration camp immediately, yet he kept writing. His urgency to leave a record drove the drama we made from the fine English translation by Martin Chalmers. Klemperer had a novelist's eye for character. In a few sentences, he sketched an unforgettable person, and George made it his business to get to know them by physically assuming their posture and voice, not mimicking, never losing sight of the fact that this was the character as Klemper saw them, becoming, that is, Klemperer in the act of seeing. After George performed at the Holocaust Museum in Washington D.C., a librarian took him to their film archive to view films made by the Nazis to show how "well" they were treating Jews. He wrote:

> *I really felt I knew this person, (it was Frau Pick, a major character in our play). I mean if I had met her on the street, I would have recognized her. This person comes out of the factory and has to change from her clogs to her shoes. I said, I know this person. And sure enough, they showed her luggage with her name painted on it for deportation to a death camp, and it was her.*

—

In the fall of 2000, we staged workshops on two consecutive nights for an invited audience of Part I (1936-42) and Part II (1942-45) of our dramatic version of the Klemperer diaries at HB Studios in the West Village where George taught. He was still holding a script. Our friend Olympia Dukakis was in the audience. Olympia was strikingly, wonderfully honest, prone to obscenities if disappointed or disturbed but, when moved, she gave elaborate praise. Olympia, too, was a much-loved teacher and with her husband Louie, she ran theaters. She came barreling down the steps of the theater to greet George on stage. She raved her delight. She thought the work important, marvelous, his acting superb. I quoted Olympia's fervent words in faxes I sent, there were only fax machines, then, to virtually every producer I knew in New York. Within the day, we heard back from Classic Stage, well-established and respected, on 13th Street; they wanted to produce *I Will Bear Witness*, the 42-45, years, that February.

The creation of *I Will Bear Witness*, for which George won an Obie award in New York for his acting and which he toured to Washington D.C., London, Berlin, through Germany and Austria, including to Dresden, where Klemperer lived and taught, became George's sustained confrontation with his buried past as a hidden child in Nazi Germany, and with the terror he bore, which had gone up to this time, he was nearly sixty years old, unacknowledged by himself. His performance of the Klemperer diaries in Berlin reunited him with his Germany family, including his two first cousins, the sons of the Nazi chemical plant owner, Otto Hoesch, who traveled from Switzerland and France to see him perform in the Kreuzberg neighborhood of Berlin, at the English-language theater improbably called, Friends of Italian Opera. There, too, was the elderly cousin Brigitte who had cared for George as a child on the estate of their Tante Irma. There were younger cousins he'd never met. Almost to the entire, large, German family, in fact, most living outside Germany. In the final months of his life, George wrote:

> *The moment I finished reading the* Times Book Review *of Victor Klemperer's* I Will Bear Witness, *I was tantalized and captivated; somehow, I sensed an enormous challenge, this was what I had been looking for, a dangerous but a familiar cultural ordeal of hiding in full view, protected by others at the very last moment. It took us a year-and-a-half just to edit the first volume. What I could not anticipate— was the way or ways these daily details of Victor Klemperer's reality would affect me. Victor had to make his own yellow star to wear at all times, even on his waistcoat when taking out the garbage. Three times during the period we were rehearsing for the first public reading, I had to stop and go to bed for several days."*

George, too, made his own Jewish stars, and he sewed them onto his coat jacket and vest before every performance. He had buried his early fears deep. Now the Klemperer diaries demanded he reconnect. As we worked on and reworked our edit, trying to turn a man's hidden diary into a stage play, George felt the strain of both the material and his own life. He took to the bed in our downstairs bedroom, but we continued to create a text even as he was too weak to sit up. He lay on his side, a pillow under his head, as we argued and worked. Klemperer's trauma reignited his own buried terrors, sapping his strength, yet there was no way out but through.

While George struggled with his hidden past, I wrote of my struggles to direct the production which would open at Classic Stage Company on 13th Street in New York, in February of 2001, in the midst of a heavy snowstorm, the farthest uptown that a play of mine ever got: "how, not to interfere, to make the transfer from rehearsal hall to theater into a new precision, while retaining the spiritual aspect—the feeling that it is almost impossible to be witnessing *this* yet, here we are, and here he is, and he is in it and outside it at the same time." George was ravaged by entering Klemperer's life, yet both actor and author are, somehow, by some somber strength of spirit, which is also particularly German and what both Klemperer and George loved about being German, able to record and bear witness to the unbearable, in meticulous detail, with grace and dignity. Each was also accompanied by a woman, an artist-wife. Klemperer's Eva was a composer in her own right, and a constant presence throughout. "It is important he not try to suddenly 'act' nor I to 'direct,'" I wrote. "Purity is what we want, what we are after." In the end, George achieved the feat of becoming Victor Klemperer, and materializing through Klemperer's body, heart and mind, with the most subtle changes in posture, voice, gesture, the fifty-two other characters we selected and whom the diarist drew sharply from precise observation, who stepped out of the actor in an instant to make themselves seen. Without miming, without mimicking, without indicating, without "acting", without changing costume, George found how these people could speak as if we had access to Klemperer's mind, where their images lodged, as they appeared to him. Each brief, haunting, as if in a dream, materialization of each doomed Jew Klemperer knew was unique, understated, and immensely moving. At once a memorialization and a vision of life. In Klemperer's city of Dresden, where George performed at the same university where Klemperer taught before the war, and to which he returned during de-Nazification, then in the East of the divided country, a man who been a student of the real Victor Klemperer burst into George's dressing room before the show. "How are you going to perform him," he shouted at George. But after the show, "you were completely him. You had his voice," the man said.

At the same time we rehearsed, and as George regained his strength, he took the initiative to learn the Tao of sex, as if a reward for me, how not, that is to ejaculate prematurely, or even ejaculate at all, so that, he brought me into a new presence in the act of love which is so far from the masochistic-ecstatic letting go of old (when whoever the partner was, climaxed, that is), but which is full of thrill—the thrill of how long can I maintain my presence, my thereness, my awareness of being loved and loving, I wrote in my diary. In all ways, we were revived by the challenge of crafting *I Will Bear Witness*.

"Yesterday, after a long time 'positioning' himself correctly within the letters section of the Klemperer, G. says, 'Maybe by going through this, I will come out free of the past,'" I wrote in my director's notes.

Klemperer is made to deliver letters announcing deportation the next morning, a certain death sentence, to eight of his fellow occupants of the Jewish ghetto in Dresden. Made to deliver these letters by the Jewish officials, who for special favors and rations, run the ghetto for the Nazis. Klemperer, the mandated angel of death, tasks himself with becoming the witness for the condemned. He meticulously describes, in his detailed novelist's way, exactly what he says to each person and what they say, if they can speak, and how they look as they hear the news that they have been selected for a death march. In a brief paragraph he devotes to each one, Klemperer paints an indelible portrait of each of the damned, a vivid memorial to the soon-to-be disappeared:

> *Even more pitiful was Frau Bitterwolf in Struvestrasse. Again a shabby house; I was vainly studying the list of names in the entrance hall when a blond, snub-nosed young woman with a pretty, well-looked-after little girl, perhaps four years old appeared. Did a Frau Bitterwolf live here? She was Frau Bitterwolf. I had to give her an unpleasant message. She read the letter, several times said quite helplessly: 'What is to become of the child?', then signed silently with a pencil. Meanwhile the child pressed up against me, held out her teddy bear and, radiantly cheerful, declared: 'My teddy, my teddy, look!' The woman then went silently up the stairs with the child. Immediately afterwards I heard her weeping loudly. The weeping did not stop.*

By bearing witness even as he performs his terrible task, he defies the Nazi need to dehumanize and disappear these eight Jews. By witnessing he defies genocide, whose point is to leave no witness alive. We staged his letter delivery along the downstage edge, as close to the audience as we could get. George held eight white envelopes. After he delivers the news—do they scream, do they cry, or stoically walk away, he tells us in a few detailed words—he drops a white envelope. Each death notice letter falls to the stage like a small coffin, hardly making a sound, yet seeming to hit with a thud. The last time this person was seen and understood. Eight times, the same staging repeated itself with eight different, carefully observed reactions, which are the last recorded memories of each life. It is not easy to bear witness to such a task as this, and the actor's body bore the increasing stress, with the subtlest of movements. He looked into each face before his mind's eye, he let us see what Klemperer saw, he recorded each reaction, and dropped each letter like a guillotine blade.

And then: "Now Klemperer is an island, surrounded by death," George says to me. And he writes: "for me personally, this is the hardest thing to say, 'Kätchen Sara, etc. I count them all among the dead.'" We stop yesterday, not knowing how to say this line. I say, "it needs space around it, silence. It is his memorial to his friends, all he can allow himself, a somber listing of their names."

George could give, and nowhere did he give more of himself, or dredge up more of his past than to do this one-person play, which in many ways gave him his own story back with the compassion he learned to feel for Klemperer and his myriad characters. If there can be such a thing as a Holocaust play with a "happy ending," this one has it, and it is difficult not to believe that Klemperer's insistence on recording in his illegal diary his daily humiliations and fears and painting his portraits of his friends, contributes to his survival. As if words matter. Klemperer escapes deportation because the day before the death march order would have been delivered to him as one of the few remaining Jews, the Allies firebombed the civilian city of Dresden. A war crime that freed those who survived, including both Klemperer and his wife, Eva. George was particularly proud of the feat of staging the firebombing of Dresden by himself. I had objected. I did not think he could do it, but he insisted.

Even as he describes the horror of the bombs and the fires in Klemperer's words, he is running through them, dodging flames, throwing himself into a ditch. It was an improbable acting feat of the sort George loved. I am certain this is the only time the firebombing of Dresden has been put on the stage—certainly, by just one man. At one performance, three women survivors of the firebombing sat in the first row, complimenting him afterwards on the veracity of his performance. "That is exactly how it was," one said. George, trained by his father as a dancer, choreographed his movements himself.

Klemperer and Eva grab a few things, when the air raid is heard. He has his diary pages in his briefcase, and he runs outside. "At that moment a big explosion nearby. I knelt, pressing myself up against the wall, close to the courtyard door. When I looked, *Eva had disappeared.*" Now he is truly alone, facing the flames.

George moved as he spoke, with great precision. Klemperer runs, hides, dodges, jumps, is struck by debris, "something hard and glowing hot struck the right side of my face. I put my hand up, it was covered in blood. I felt for my eye, it was still there." The actor's movements become faster, his voice more exhausted, but, still, he never stumbles over lines even as he jumps into a bomb crater and falls to the ground. Though separated in the firestorm, both Eva and Victor survive. Miraculously, he finds Eva unhurt, on the terrace of the ruined city. "We greeted one another warmly," Klemperer writes and George says, with Germanic understatement. Reunited with his wife, Klemperer rips off his yellow stars and he throws them away (George tore with one sharp stroke each star he sewed each night onto his costume, preferring to do this task himself to ready himself for performance). He and his wife walk and hitchhike into Russian occupied territory. There they find temporary refuge in the home of an acquaintance, and Klemperer writes what we called his "Angel Speech," a poetic hymn to life and love everlasting, riddled with wry improbable insight. My favorite piece of writing in the entire diary. George delivered the speech in his white shirt and vest. His arms spread out like angel's wings as he spoke.

> *18th March: Sunday morning, downstairs just after seven. Brief morning reflection arisen from great love. In fact, the main point, after all, is that for forty years we have so much loved one another and do love one another, in fact, I am not at all sure that all this is going to come to an end. For certain, nothingness—the loss of individual consciousness, and that is the true nothingness—is altogether probable, and anything else highly improbable. But have we not continually experienced, since 1914 and even more since 1933 and with ever greater frequency in recent weeks, the most utterly improbable, the most monstrously fantastic things? Has not what was formerly completely unimaginable to us become commonplace and a matter of course? If I have lived through the persecutions in Dresden, if I have lived through the 13th of February and these weeks as a refugee—why should I not just as well live (or rather die) to find the two of us somewhere, Eva and I, with angel wings or in some other droll form? It's not only the word "impossible" that has gone out of circulation; "unimaginable" also has no validity anymore.*

Then George turned and walked upstage to a small wooden door that had been present on stage but unopened the entire time. With this exit, Klemperer and Eva return to their beloved home in the outskirts of Dresden which, also, improbably, remained intact (and he to his university professorship in what was now East Germany and to writing a widely read book, *The Language of the Third Reich*, a primer on totalitarian regimes.) George left the stage, and the Nazi terror, through that small door up center. The ochre-painted door has moved with us from house to house and is in what was our last shared apartment. It stands behind the metal statue of Nijinsky dancing that was on the first landing of the wide staircase of Haus Merberich in Düren where George was a hidden child. When he visited his Tante Irma after the war, she said with her wry smile, "If you like it, you shall have it," and she sent it to him in New York.

The day before we opened in Berlin, George was interviewed by a journalist who asked, "What is it like coming back to the city in which you were born after all these years?" "Oh, it's nothing, it's fine, no problem at all," George, waved her question away cavalierly, whereupon he immediately lost his voice (which never had happened to him before) and he was almost unable to perform his premiere but for a savvy doctor who treated his condition with grave seriousness and prescribed Ricola in his pockets so he could slyly suck on them during the show. The city of Berlin gave George, as a returning German-Jew forced from his home, a mansion to stay in designed by Hitler's favorite architect, Albert Speer. Huge, square, and concrete, the guesthouse was in Grunewald, the still posh suburb that had been home to the artists of the German film industry, rather like Beverly Hills. Grunewald was also where, from the local train station, the herds of the rounded-up Jews of Berlin were regularly transported to the death camps. One could almost see, still hovering in the air, these lines of people, their shoulders hunched, wearing layers under their drab winter coats, standing quietly dejected, waiting to board the trains. Trains to the death camps ran on the same tracks, interspersed with German freight and commuter trains, so completely "normalized" was this genocide. The guesthouse was empty of guests but for us. There were housekeepers, but we never saw them and caught only glimpses of their white uniforms as they disappeared down the long halls. Our rooms were straightened, bed made, and elaborate breakfasts of cheeses, sausages, bread, jams, freshly squeezed orange juice, and coffee, far more than we two could eat, were mysteriously laid out for us each morning by these ghostly servants. When I had to catch a very early flight back to New York after the first week of George's performances, I got dressed, ate, and slipped back into bed for an instant in my coat, my arms around sleeping George to whisper goodbye. He fantasized that I was his mother singing a song in his ear, the same song she sang the morning she had come into his bed on his great aunt's estate to bid her three-year-old good-bye before she left him there and fled with her Jewish husband through Cuba to America. He had not remembered this song before.

If art can heal and wound, or, perhaps rather profoundly shake up, as it can and must, *I Will Bear Witness* became the defining life-artistic-event that allowed George to confront his buried past, the traumas inflicted and carried until then, unattended, in his flesh. Creating and performing this work breathed into him a new depth, both as an actor who is able to profoundly embrace his character(s), enter and materialize them, and as a man who began to understand himself, his own bouts of terror as a small child that lived in his gut. He was sixty-seven when we completed the one-man play, and had twenty-two more years to work and live.

In 2017, shortly after the inauguration of Donald Trump, when we were all reeling from having a right-wing fanatic as our new president, Christen Clifford suggested George and I put together a short version of the early diaries of Victor Klemperer for performances in living rooms. George jumped at the chance. He and I re-edited our script of volume one of the diaries, 1933-41, into a thirty-five-minute version. It began:

> *For something like three weeks now the depression of the reactionary government. I am not writing a history of the times here. But I shall nevertheless record my embitterment, greater than I would have imagined I was still capable of feeling.*

And ended:

> *But the danger is so great and so omnipresent that it makes a fatalist of me. This manuscript is my duty and my last fulfillment. I shall go on writing. That is my heroism. I will bear witness, precise witness!*

George sat at a table or desk in various living rooms and lofts in Manhattan, Brooklyn, and Queens. He spoke as Klemperer recorded his thoughts. Then, there was discussion of those times and our own. People shared stories of family histories and spoke of their present fears. "The Living Room Klemperers" were performed free, a gift in troubled times. Everyone needed to share. "We spoke quietly because the windows were open," is one of Klemperer's lines and there was a similar feeling of newfound fear among New Yorkers shocked by the election results. We had no idea how to survive the presidency of Donald Trump. (As I write this, his second term has recently begun; yesterday, he called himself "King".) George felt a new urgency returning to the character of Victor Klemperer after more than a decade. He loved the intimacy of the living room performances; being so close to his audience, he could easily share the man's inner thoughts, which felt, often, very much like their own, without raising his voice. It was not just changing the world that George sought; he wished to show the art of it—the quiet courage and commitment, the persistence it takes. Klemperer and his secret diaries were the perfect vehicles. From the very start of Hitler's rise to power, keeping such a diary, if discovered, would have led to imprisonment or worse, being hung (there was a gallows in the yard of the Dresden police station) and Klemperer understood the risks. George also wanted to document that there were Germans, then, and Americans, now, who were afraid yet determined to do what they could to stay decent and kind. Whether it was another potato, or an offered handshake, or the offer to hide the diary pages, neither Klemperer nor his diary would have survived without the aid of decent, anti-Nazi Germans, who put their own well-being at risk. George's Klemperer performances were his way of giving thanks to his Tante Irma and to the headmaster at the Steiner school, the people who kept him and his brother alive and showed the little boy George that individual actions make a difference. That if we do not act well in troubled times, it hardly matters what we do when times are good. George felt it both a personal artistic delight and an intimate public service to share Klemperer's early shock at the Nazi regime with Americans reeling from Trump's election, in the intimacy of private homes, without any financial transaction, as if speaking truth were already against the law, yet necessary then and now. We did not even pass a hat. "The Living Room" were a gift. Klemperer writes:

> *The dominant feeling is that the reign of terror can hardly last long, but that its fall will bury us. I for my part will never again have faith in Germany. In fact, I feel shame more than fear, shame for Germany. I have truly always felt a German. I have always imagined; the twentieth century and Mitteleuropa was different from the fourteenth century and Romania. Mistake.*

George spoke carefully, considering his words, in a low voice, as if afraid of being overheard, or as if he voiced the fears in the minds of his attentive audience. We scheduled twenty or more living room venues. Our audiences were small, but the work stuck.

Prophecy, in 2006, was my first big play since *The Beekeeper's Daughter*, 1995. In-between had come our years of work on the Klemperer. Then came the attacks of September 11, 2001, and soon enough the invasion of Iraq. *Prophecy* is both a memory play informed by my years as a young anti-Vietnam War activist and a play about the moral injury of a young Iraq-war veteran. George played the unfaithful husband, Alan, head of a human rights organization, to Kathleen Chalfant's Sarah, actor and acting teacher They were a delightful team—touching and deep, their marital squabbles recognizably amusing. Najla Said had been visiting family in Lebanon in the summer of 2006 when Israel invaded. She remembers, "My Post Traumatic Stress Disorder (that up to that point I didn't even believe really existed) jolted me into a heightened state of awareness and fervor, and I began sending long email missives to everyone on my contacts list, one of whom was Karen." I was in Macedonia on a writing retreat, staying in Stalin-era cabins built for Soviet workers around its one lake. I walked on the beach in the early mornings and wrote. I created three characters for Najla: Hala, a Palestinian Lebanese human rights worker; Mariam, her daughter from her affair with Alan, furious at her absent Jewish father and at the atrocities committed during the war in Lebanon; and Miranda, the Puerto Rican girlfriend of the deeply troubled Iraq veteran. "Somehow, she had taken everything I had said and expressed and created three different women for me to play ... that contained an essential truth that Karen had found inside of me ... Moreover, the story of *Prophecy* is also the story of the healing power of theater," Najla wrote in her afterword to the published play. We did six or more readings of *Prophecy* in New York, and one at the Kennedy Center, all of them full with extremely appreciative audiences. Sometimes, Maria Tucci (a friend of Jack Gelber's who had been in his *The Cuban Thing*) read Sarah and sometimes Kathy. We were hoping an established theater would take the play on and fund its production. Finally, we received an opportunity for a co-production in London, with an English cast, and Najla who came to London with us. We opened *Prophecy* in 2008, at the same small, now defunct, New End Theater where we had played

I Will Bear Witness. I cashed in my NYU pension to pay our part of the joint production. We received excellent reviews and high praise from many, including Vanessa Redgrave and David Hare, and my favorite comment of all time from Corin Redgrave, who came down the aisle with his wife Kika Markham, on opening night, saying loudly, "Harold must see this!" But Harold (Pinter) as Kika gently reminded Corin "was poorly" and he would die soon, and Corin was losing his memory. Back home in New York, we still searched for a producer. "It's brilliant," the artistic director of the Public Theater, Oscar Eustis, said to me with tears in his eyes after a reading. "It's too risky," he explained to George and me in a closed-door meeting several weeks later. "I couldn't have done *Stuff Happens*, now." Finally, New York Theater Workshop offered to rent us their small theater. To fund *Prophecy*, George went in person to every peace organization in New York and he sold them large blocks of tickets. Luminaries from the nonviolent activist world, Noam Chomsky, Chris Hedges, David Swanson, Laura Flanders, agreed to do talkbacks. There was a buzz about the play.

Noam Chomsky and I renewed our acquaintance while George and I struggled to produce *Prophecy* in New York. We had not seen one another since our never aired CBS interview on the lawn at MIT in 1973. Now, Noam was to give the 2007 annual lecture in honor of his friend Edward Said at Columbia University and Najla was acting in my play, in three roles written for her. George and I were coming up the aisle of the crowded theater searching for seats; Noam was making his way down to the podium to speak. He smiled warmly at me. "He recognizes you," George said. Noam never went to the theater but two years later, when he was barely going out again after the death of his wife, he agreed to speak with the audience after a performance of *Prophecy*. We moved from our small ninety-nine seat theater to the larger theater next door so we might accommodate everyone who had bought a ticket for our production on any night, and others who wished to be present at a rare public appearance by Noam in New York. Uncharacteristically, he let his emotions show. He was "glad" we changed locations, he said, because he was "so moved" by the play, he was afraid he "would not be able to speak coherently in the same space." My memory play had evoked in him "all the memories of all the wars of my life." Later, more formally, he wrote, "The play is a remarkable contribution and I hope it will reach many people." That same night, the *New York Times* critic Charles Isherwood was in the audience, distant relative of Christopher, whose play *Dog Beneath the Skin*, was jettisoned by the Living Theatre in favor of *The Brig*. The next morning, there was a long, scathing, not to mention demeaning, review of my play in the *Times*. "Good actors acting badly in a bad play," is the first sentence and it remains seared into my brain though I stopped reading after that. What happened to Julian with his *Sleep* play, now happened to me with a play I dearly loved. Different critic, decades later. Same newspaper. And the review spelled the death of any future production for the antiwar memory play. When I came home from walking our dogs, I saw the paper lying on our doorstep and picked it up, but the entire arts section was missing. George had already read the review, hidden it, and replaced the paper on the front step. He greeted me "acting" as if nothing had happened. We ignored the review as well as we could. Our audiences were full for the rest of the run and the word on the street was good. I bought chocolates for the cast that night. Chris Hedges wrote about *Prophecy* in his 2010 book *The Death of the Middle Class:* "It is only when artists control their own work, as Malpede did with *Prophecy*, that great, socially relevant theater can be sustained." We "sustained" *Prophecy* over five years, with a half a dozen fine readings before full, appreciative audiences, and two small productions in London and New York.

In 2016, when George had his first sepsis attack, we had no idea what happened when he began to come apart on the Midtown city street, shaking uncontrollably. "The nearest hospital," I said to the cab driver, as his condition worsened; we had been heading downtown toward Brooklyn. When we arrived at Bellevue's emergency entrance, I jumped out of the car and screamed, "My husband has just had a stroke." Although, in the cab, George had been able to remember his heart doctor's name, not I. "That's not a stroke," the attendant said as George was loaded onto a stretcher, and this calmed me. Bellevue, the City's public trauma hospital, is an interesting, humbling place—like Brooklyn Hospital down our street, its doctors have a commitment to medical care for all. Inmates from the notoriously cruel Riker's Island detention center are brought to Bellevue for medical treatment, and armed guards sit outside their rooms. George's mother worked there treating polio sufferers in the 1940s. George was dressed and ready to be released after a two-day stay, when a doctor came into our room and told us we should not go. The blood tests just back from the lab showed sepsis, an infection in his blood that could kill him if we went home. "If his fever spikes, again, by the time you get to another hospital, there may not be antibiotics strong enough to treat him, and he will die." George got undressed and got back into the hospital bed. We would be no wiser about what was the cause of his blood infection when he was released from Bellevue Hospital several weeks later, without explanation, and with no follow-up treatment, and no recommendations for future care. We knew it was sepsis. "These things happen," the resident said. "We don't know why," and discharged him. His second sepsis attack was relatively mild. I was out of town visiting my daughter and her new baby, but I could tell as I left, George was out of sorts. When I phoned him from Texas, he was clearly ill. His son took him to Lenox Hill Hospital while I flew back. By the time I arrived at the hospital, his heart doctor was in charge and George had been moved to the heart patient floor for monitoring of his atrial fibrillation; the sepsis, if that is what it was, had been forgotten. His third sepsis attack was clearly serious, but I was sitting next to him at breakfast when he began to shake. "Let's go to Methodist," I said, because it was close by in Park Slope. He was very, very ill for several weeks. Shopping at the Park Slope Food Coop, I met two friends and told them about the recurring sepsis. "It's his immune system," they both said. When he was finally released, we demanded further tests. The infectious disease doctor read the results. "Go see Dr. ____," he said, "it's probably nothing but he is our new hematologist."

Cancer doctors rarely witness the effects of their treatments. Even ours, who was empathic, who genuinely liked and admired us, as we did him, who came to our plays, rarely saw, nor seemed to understand, most probably, he blocked out, the extent of the suffering George endured. The doctors order the chemicals by computer and sometimes come around to watch the infusion begin, then they are gone. For reasons I could not understand, George's doctor refused to admit or address his frequent breathing problems. He would not give us oxygen at home, saying the insurance would not pay for it. In October of 2020, just a year and a month after cancer treatment began, George's breathing became so labored, I knew we needed other intervention. I phoned Nancy Allen, my former yoga teacher who had become an acupuncturist and made an appointment. When we arrived at her office door after a long, terrifying walk down the hall which George could hardly negotiate, George's breathing was so tortured we thought he might die. She considered calling 911, but instead we managed to get him up onto her table; with a few needles to his chest, his breathing began to stabilize. Nancy would treat George weekly until he died. When he was too weak to go to her, she made house calls. Also, because Nancy actually looked closely at George's body, which cancer doctors seldom do, she was able to point out sores on his legs that might be infected. I sent his doctor photos and, on a Saturday, he ordered antibiotics. Antibiotics were the treatment for everything, again, with no understanding shared with us about what they would likely do to George's digestion. He refused to take the probiotics I bought for him, not wanting to ingest another pill. Nancy took George's ailments seriously and treated him with careful touch. She introduced us to the Chinese herbalist MD, Dr. W., who prepared his daily doses of herbs, changing them every month to, as he said, "outwit the cancer." The three of us, Nancy, the herbalist, and I, had a suspicious view of biomedical treatments, far more suspicious than George. We supported him in all his medical decisions, but also urged him, as his side effects worsened, to consider going off treatment.

So, our life together the final two years of his life became a struggle to do our work, to stay happy—surprisingly easy, actually; we were happy together, always—and to endure what was a slow slide, so slow we could often convince ourselves, in lockdown for much of this time, that it was not happening. Sometimes we wept together at night, then, found a way to restore our calm. I would read to him because language healed him. I would stroke his belly. We would laugh. The last time we experienced genital love in the last year of his life was also one of the fullest experiences we ever had, a last radiance, a gift. He came into the bedroom naked with an erection. I was already in bed, naked, as I always sleep. I was not expecting to see him like this. He stood at the bedside, which is the perfect height for him to slip himself into me as I put my legs around his neck. He hoisted my hips from underneath like a much younger man, like someone who was well again. Every touch between us was an act of love. We sat together on the couch leaning into the other's shoulder while I read Hardy, Gordimer, Camus, the words from my mouth to his ears, an intimacy perfect in and of itself; our talks about what we had read a deepening. He slipped himself into me standing at the bedside, slipped himself deeper it suddenly felt than ever before, and I opened myself wider and deeper than I had ever been. He began to thrust, and I opened more, letting him in to an innermost core. I made the sounds of great pleasure; he, too, standing there thrusting. I looked as we dove deeper still, he inside me, me holding him in a circle of hips, legs, feet linked behind his head, my butt off the bed, urging him in, rising and letting go, rising to meet him again, both of us making sounds of effortful delight and as I looked up I saw the cancer doctor entering George from behind, as George moved his hips inside the circle of my legs thrown around his neck and drove himself deeper still into my open self. And I had such pleasure, we two together rising, falling, moaning with joy, with the mirage of the doctor hovering and thrusting behind George. I was shocked at myself, that I'd imagined the doctor at this moment penetrating George from behind. It was a threesome in which we were engaged. Yes, I wanted the doctor to keep George alive. Grief, the threat of grief was all I knew then, driving me wild. I imagined the doctor could save him; I imagined the doctor thrusting himself into George from behind. Grief is a species of madness. Worse for the depth of our love.

Cancer treatment is brutal and over-treatment is almost inevitable so long as suffering mixed with hope appears to promise a longer life. The Chinese herbalist had been emailing for weeks, "they are killing him." But he had nothing to offer but his herbs, he was associated with no hospital, and George was afraid to trust him solely. In late winter of 2022, Nancy, our acupuncturist, began urging George stop cancer treatment, as his body was clearly now too weak to tolerate the cancer drugs, but with a caveat: she was concerned his cancer doctor would refuse to monitor him if George refused more injections and wished to make certain he would. George was easing himself toward saying "no;" he had stopped treatment of his free will to perform *Blue Valiant* the previous spring. Then, it had been an easy decision for him. He needed all his strength and concentration. Acting well trumped longer life in his mind. George would stop or take treatments as he wished. But now, in spring of 2022, I asked that the celebration of his life and career scheduled to take place at LaMama, in January, on his ninetieth birthday, be moved to October. I feared he would not live through the next winter. He wanted to perform Uncle's long speech about nature and death, one his favorites, "In those days nature intervened in all our words, we painted with our tongues … we would exit as we'd come, simply, unremarked upon," and the angel speech of Victor Klemperer.

For George, ordinary events, even mishaps, were often wondrous. His eyes would light up. He had a particular tone of voice, excited, intimate, as if what he related was in strictest confidence, but he just had to say it aloud, to make a story out of what had happened to him, give it place, no longer a random occurrence but changed into a tale told, remembered, remarked upon, shared. Feeling unusually good one morning, he left for a walk, to do some marketing. When he returned sooner than I expected, his face bloody, he waved away my concern. Yes, he had fallen on a patch of rutted sidewalk right outside the Apple Bank, but he'd been lifted upright immediately by a particularly kind and comforting, strong, Black man. He spoke in that excited whisper that might have carried to the last row of a theater, so perfectly placed was his voice. No broken bones, just a bloodied nose. He'd been saved by human kindness. Did I not understand how lucky he was? That a toe later became infected was not yet part of the story. On another journey the last spring of his life, he went alone with Patrick, his chosen driver, who is also a journalist originally from Congo who treated George as an elder with great respect, to the Lighthouse to consider computer programs for people with limited sight that might allow him to edit his journals. "I was left alone for a long time in a large hall with huge white pillars," he told me, "And, then, the strangest thing: I felt I was back on the ship coming to America." Who left him there, while he waited for someone to escort him downstairs to the car, and for how long didn't matter. He'd been transported back in time. For the young, sensitive child in care of a nanny he barely knew on a German luxury liner in the middle of the

Atlantic, going toward a new country, to parents he had not seen in three years, the journey must have been wondrous and terrifying at once, those opposites that defined his life and gave shape to his talent. Now, here he was, left alone in a large, white-pillared space, staring out into emptiness, as if lost on a vast Expressionist stage set that externalized his terrors. Didn't I understand how amazing his experience was? Ever the precocious child making meanings to live by. All of life seemed to fill him with joy, the old man alone locked in a white-pillared hall become the small boy on deck of the big ship, holding tight to a post, looking out at the vast blue. The little boy inhabited the old man and unlike for most of us, that little boy was still intact. He had been neither silenced nor quashed. He still jumped up and down, pointed and screamed, "look, look." He was still discovering everything for the first time. He was embraced and held by the man he'd become. This, too, is what gave George's acting such force. Watching him act, we also experienced what he shared as if it were new, the wonder of the first time and the last, the epiphany, was what he gave.

George was going to die within the year. We both thought so, though we did not say this aloud. Increasingly, as his body grew weak, it seemed he was living in two worlds at once, the years of his tiny boyhood in Nazi Germany, with the cows and their warm noses, his great aunt's humor and kindness, the nature mysteries of the Steiner School, and the many terrors, unnamed to the child, menacing wherever he went, and, this year, 2022, the year of that was going to be the final year of his life. His sight was dim and his visions were increasingly hallucinogenic and so when he told me of the large hall with the huge pillars in which he'd been left, alone, by someone unknown, and taken out, again, also, by someone unknown and led down to the waiting car, I felt his experience might not have happened at all; it might have been a sort of waking dream that he had, or a vision. His excitement when he told me made it seem an initiation—into an afterworld of some sort. He was readying himself, perhaps, drawing on all that he knew that he was, and though he complained, sometimes, he was afraid of death, he had not been afraid in the large, white room; rather, if he had been there at all, he'd been enthralled. He'd seen something he could not explain—both like the boy on the German ship, sailing into a new life of he knew not what and the elderly man looking beyond his life. He told me in the excited voice of a person relating a mystery that the non-initiate cannot grasp.

If Barbara Deming danced toward her death, wide-eyed, expectant, naked, creating a lesbian feminist ritual surround, and Julian Beck faced his premature death by denying death existed, George remained the storyteller he had always been. Only the character he wished most to inhabit at the end of his life was his own self, the wide-eyed, exuberant boy who sensed the violence to come because he lived with and escaped the Nazi menace. In his last months, he entered, reentered and fully embraced, recognized and understood this childhood self. He materialized the boy-child through vivid memories he recalled and told to me, to close friends, to his acupuncturist, his doctor, and his psychotherapist and to his friend from London, the psychiatrist, Dr. David Bell, with whom he had zoom conversations every week. He wished us all to see, understand and take-in this child-self as he wished to make vividly alive every character he embodied on-stage. He found and relayed empathy for his child-self, the one who he was and from whom he grew into the generous artist so thrilled by the quirkiness of the natural world and her creatures and so appalled by the violence of humans. Perhaps this full embrace he extended to himself at last is why, though he feared death and spoke openly of his fears, he will appear to die unafraid.

Our first crisis was November's toe infection, the result of that fall on the rutted sidewalk. Then came our realization he could not anymore feel his feet, and the addition of a psychotherapist to augment what I called our healing circle, and my frequent foot massages. In February, the acidosis hit. He developed shingles, also a common side-effect of the drugs he was on, and because he refused to take one more pill, lack of the medicine prescribed to prevent it. The constant constipation George suffered from the cancer drugs, and his weakening digestive system gave him two hernias, the larger of which was particularly painful. A heating pad sometimes helped. He sometimes wore a truss, which he found extremely uncomfortable. He caught COVID in April, 2022, the result of our foolhardy decision to pretend all was normal and take a visiting friend out to dinner at a very good nearby restaurant. He had to take a reduced dosage of Paxlovid, which had just then become available, because Paxlovid is hard on the kidneys and George's were failing, no doubt, the Paxlovid worsened his overall condition even if it might have kept him from more serious COVID. Too many side effects, too much weakness. I lost a front tooth, broken off at the root, as I regularly do lose teeth under stress. When I came home after hours being drilled on in the dentist's chair, George yelled at me for spending so much money on a tooth, and I wept. We were on edge, but we were not yet speaking of death. George was still going in for regular cancer infusions, and he continued to write his journal.

The first weekend in June, I texted his doctor that George was not "well enough for treatment."

"Bring him in Monday, I'll check him out." George's doctor cleared him for treatment, with a cursory pat of his hernia. And he scheduled a scan of his intestines and colon in the coming week. We were scheduled to meet with the hernia surgeon also in a week or so.

During these nights, he was often in pain. We were reading out-loud Diane di Prima's *Recollections of My Life as a Woman*. Her complete commitment to the downtown bohemian scene, her work publishing and supporting others, brought George great cheer and made him forget his pain, his fear. He delighted in di Prima's life, so like his own. He revived on her words. Sat up, determined to get back to work. Language was his best medicine. He was coming down with a cold. I read him a short remembrance I'd written about our much loved, late spaniel Cleis and her improbable life; falling through the ice, surviving a pit bull attack, her conversation with a black bear. George loved what I wrote; he had been telling me for years, "If you want to be a success, write about the dogs." His cold seemed cured.

During the days, George was intent on his writing. His last written memory was also his first. He shared the passage with me, which he seldom did, and asked me for notes:

> Crib—white metal bar—bare, empty room ... alone ... no one comes. Cry. Yell. No one comes: Pull myself by white bars to standing ... rocking crib forward, moving crib towards door ...

crying ... yelling ... rocking crib over, rolling of crib. Finds glass, knocks glass over, starts to put pieces in mouth. Chew. Swallow. Door opens. Brigitte sees George, smiling chewing pieces of glass. Brigitte calls for help, quickly gathers up glass remains. Tells help to get mashed potatoes and put it down George's throat. George is now happy, everybody pushing mashed potatoes into mouth. "Just keep swallowing. Here, here, take more, that's it, keep eating it all." How George was happy. They were all taking care of him, three little mothers were fussing.

We lived a mirror image to his primal memory our final spring; one of our last erotic adventures and perhaps our night of the broken glass triggered the earlier memory of the glass he broke in rage as a toddler because he wrote about it soon after. I woke abruptly from a deep sleep. Where was he? He was not in our bed next to me. I got up in a haze and wandered down the hall to his private bathroom. I found him, seated on the toilet, naked, surrounded by shards of broken glass, twinkling in the night light. Bright red blood bubbled on his right big toe, shimmering like a faceted jewel, where a sharp shard of glass had punctured his flesh. He was alone in a sea of glass. He couldn't get up or he might further injure himself. Pieces of glass covered the floor. He was marooned in this shiny, treacherous sea. I bent down. I was also naked, my breasts that once had stood upright, now hanging limp, my small waist, larger hips, the wrinkles in my skin, my legs unshaven, my thinning pubic hair once thick. "You are so beautiful," he said, as I bent, each orifice exposed, to clean the blood from his toe, carefully inspecting the wound, in case a piece of glass was stuck. "You are so beautiful," he whispered, again. "You are so beautiful," I said. Squatting exposed next to him. He was vulnerable and wounded, shimmering in his sea of glass. We continued sexual contact almost until the end, if it was just my tongue on his penis, his hand inside me, simple gestures, that pleasured us. But I remember this moment with him seated on the toilet surrounded by glass, his blood bubbling, as a consummation. The Night of Broken Glass, Kristallnacht; his Huguenot mother had had the sense to flee Germany before it occurred, leaving her terrified children behind. From her Berlin apartment window, she watched a friend be arrested, dragged out from the building next to theirs. She knew it was time to go. The jam jar glass shattered on the floor, large, jagged shards, and the baby George in his crib, breaking and eating glass, in order to be comforted. "You are so beautiful," he said, as I knelt amid the shards, and I thought to myself, "no one will ever say these words to me, again." "You are so beautiful," he said. This terrible pleasure, both of us naked surrounded by broken glass. Almost injured. A shard had punctured his skin. I looked at his beautiful red blood shimmering on his toe, and heard his voice, resonant and full of love, "you are so beautiful," he kept saying to me, for the last time, and the last time, again. Now, everything was to be for the last time. "You are so beautiful," never again. "You are so beautiful," he said. I would not let him see me weep. The last time. The last time again. So beautiful now. You are. With a soft tissue, I stanched the blood on his toe. A gesture as sacred to me, now in my mind, as any I have ever made. Like putting a child to the breast for the first time. Kneeling naked, my legs splayed in front of him, open and unprotected as one is in love. "You are so beautiful," I wrote the sound of his voice in my head. The last time. With tenderness kneeling amid the shards of glass. "You are so beautiful," we each said. He had not yet written the paragraph about the little boy alone, his rage at having been left, his unbearable fury, smashing the glass and trying to eat it, to swallow rage down and injure himself. We were not angry now. We did not say, but we knew, this was the last time; it would now always be the last time. The last time. So beautiful. Now. Never again. How beautiful you are. How like a small child he was. "Baby George," I sometimes playfully called him. His penis dangling into the toilet bowl. Stuck, rooted before me in a sea of glass. His vulnerability was mine to love, mine his. I carefully washed his toe with soap on a tissue, and slowly pulled his toes apart to inspect them for hidden hurts. I found none. How open with one another we had become. I picked up the pieces of glass I could see, swept the floor. We were always breaking glasses, he and I, wine glasses fell from our hands at the sink, they cracked as if by magic as we filled them at the table. They broke when we made a toast. The beauty of it all. The terrible beauty of blood and glass. "You are so beautiful," he crooned. The last time. Almost our final erotic act, across a floor of glass, I squatted at his side, careful not to injure myself and ministered to his wound. "You are so beautiful," he said, as I knelt before him to clean his toe. His wounds and mine, all that we carried, all that we'd given one another over the years, shared with each other, spread out before us on that floor, shattered, as our life was, the dangers and the delights, broken and sparkling there. I took his hand. We walked back to our bed. We crawled in, for the bed is high and you need to pull yourself up.

The beauty of our sorrow. The joy and terror intermixed through his whole life. His naked beauty in my eyes, mine in his. Perhaps it sounds strange to say this, but our life in those months, from the time that I knew he was dying, seemed blessed by a deepening of love, which was as close as I could come to acceptance. We were going to go wherever was needed, together, without animosity or any sense we had not lived well as we could, done what we wished, aided and abetted one another in all our desires, each of our follies. We were going to finish as we'd begun: radiant, amazed.

We went dutifully, stupidly, to his treatment, on Wednesday, June 8. "He is too sick," I had said to the doctor who cleared him for treatment despite my misgivings. I lived with him. The doctor did not. We should have known to stay home. As the nurse approached with the shot, we both cried out, "no, not this week." The Darzalex shot was given, now, only once a month; we had both forgotten this was the week. "The order is in the computer," she said and drove the needle deep into his stomach, pressing and rotating its sharp point to better distribute its contents. We were under doctor's orders, but the doctor, of course, was not there to see. By the time George got to the elevator bank, he was in such pain he was unable to walk. I left him leaning against a wall and went to look for a hospital wheelchair. It did not occur to me to ask anyone for help, and no one came to help us. I wheeled him downstairs, outside, and he managed to get into a cab. Each bump on the Brooklyn roads created a new spasm of pain. When we got home, I ran inside to get my desk chair to use as a makeshift wheelchair. The porter at our coop, Edgar, a good friend—"George always looked at me with respect"—not a young man, saw us struggling in the parking lot and took on the task of wheeling George in the rickety desk chair over the ruts in the asphalt to the ramp. George moaned in pain with each bump. Edgar helped George onto the living room couch. He was soon on the floor, I lying next to him. Helpless and terrified, he writhed.

I wrote a play about the United States torture program, *Another Life*, about people who inflict pain on others in order to get results, most of which are verifiably false, because to make the pain stop people will say anything, "yes, I was." "yes, I did," "yes," "yes," "yes" only let me live pain free for a minute or more, when in reality they had been sold to the US troops for bounty, and know nothing, nothing at all of what they confess to know. Pain is another country. The more the victim writhes, the less human they appear to be, the harder to identify with that. The one in pain, even when lying next to him on the floor as I was now, inhabits another place, unreachable, by language, by touch. What used to be words, capable of description, at least that, where does it hurt, there, here, how does it hurt, they always ask on a scale of one to ten, words are now sounds, moans, groans. Language, George's love, gone.

Abbas Noori Abbood was in three productions of my anti-torture play, *Another Life*. Eubulliant and charming in real life, and on the stage, his acting grew better and better because he was acting with George. The two formed a bond. Abbas spoke two thirds of a long story I took from *One Thousand and One Nights* in Arabic, while with movement acting it out, adding an extra beauty to my bitterly ironic, surreal play. Abbas played the Egyptian cab driver, Abdul. The character was based on the true story of a New York cab driver of Middle Eastern descent who did a good deed during the attacks of September 11, bringing a victim to their home, and was erroneously labeled a "terrorist" and incarcerated. In the play, he becomes the indentured servant to Handel, the oligarch George played, CEO of Deepwater, who becomes a billionaire supplying mercenaries and interrogators to black site torture centers. In real life, Abbas, living in Baghdad, cheered alongside his father their liberation from the dictator Saddam, until, that is, the American tanks rolled into the city and he understood this was an occupying force. Coming home from university one night, Abbas was caught in a crossfire between the Americans and the Iraqi insurgency. Abbas did a deranged dance of terror across our living room, as he narrated the scene. He was a body spasmodically dodging bullets, trying to get home. Cancer is like being caught in lethal crossfire between two competing armies, the disease marching in and the toxic cancer medications to blockade it. Hunkering down and fighting it out.

In bed at night for two weeks, George was unable to sleep, but lay awake, eyes blank staring at the ceiling, going over and over the terror of his early years. The cancer sufferer is the abandoned child, there is no safe harbor from the pain of having been left, dropped from the community of the healthy, those who can count on life. He tried, overcome by the urge, to relieve his bowels, time after time, using MiraLAX and Chinese herbs with properties to combat constipation, to no result. He would go to the toilet and come out a defeated man, the urge gone, the pain remained. And this went on and on. Because constipation is a side effect of his cancer drugs, it was hard, at first, to understand that his bowel was blocked.

"Why me," the cancer doctor suggested George might ask at our second meeting, the one in which he had biopsy results. "Why me" was a question George had not thought to ask, and never asked. But the body in pain screams the question out, wracked and writhing, moaning, unable to find the slightest relief, the pain mounting hourly, without remit. Why him, asks the witness to the sufferer, sitting on the floor next to the couch. No amount of fussing, raising pillows, finding coverlets, wiping the sweating brow, whispering love, alleviates the pain of, in this case, an undiagnosed blocked bowel. We did not know the cause, the source. My twin brother and his wife were on their way to Europe and stopped for the night. George, ever the charming host, walked himself to the table. He could not eat. But with every muscle he could muster, he acted "health," he was charming and funny for a bit. Then he went back to bed. I phoned the doctor. Neither of us knew what was wrong, and the doctor agreed, this time, we should not go through the emergency room. He will try to get us a bed. George will need a scan. Perhaps, he says, the cancer has grown tumors. Nancy volunteers to come to the house for a second acupuncture treatment of the week. She works slowly, gently, with concentration, trying to affect the constipation, to get his bowels to move. She says if there were an obstruction, he would be in constant pain at the spot. She thinks, therefore, his bowels are not blocked, but she later does more research on hernias and discovers there might not be a constant pain at the site of the blockage. As her treatment proceeds, George begins to throw up, but he cannot vomit the insides of his gut, only bile coating little bits of food, slimy pea-sized pieces. On Thursday, he lies comatose, sleeping finally, after many sleepless nights, eyes half-open, as in death, his mouth hanging loose. At night, I lie next to him, waiting for his breath to stop. We cry a bit. We pledge our love, the only comfort we have. On Friday morning, the hospital calls. They have a bed. He can be admitted directly, not after waiting hours in the emergency room.

Pain departs as completely as it comes, sometimes. So it is, at last, after nearly two excruciating weeks, when the hernia surgeon's assistant manipulates the hernia, thus unblocking his intestines, allowing him to begin eliminating a week's worth, or more, of waste from his body. I take a photo of the toilet bowl full of black liquid and text it to our doctor, as proof. The cancer doctor has not been there in the middle of the night, for the wretched retching, the eyes open staring at the ceiling, blank with terror.

Now, out of pain, bowels unblocked he lies in his hospital bed, alert, speaking as he does so often about his early life in Nazi Germany.

In hospital on Saturday, after the good news that there are no cancerous tumors in the stomach, he complains his heart is racing. He is getting potassium because his level is low. "Low or high," says the articulate nurse, Lisa, is the same result, "lethal arrhythmia." "You don't want that," she adds after a pause, but because his hearing aids aren't in, I have to yell the words "lethal arrhythmia" loud enough for him to hear. George, out of terrific pain, also has no interest in anything to eat.

Our doctor arrives, with a new resident in tow. My brother is there sitting in the chair at George's head, and I in the corner chair where I've been found permanently these days. The doctor tries, without success, as he has a quiet voice, to make himself heard. "Your scan is pretty uninteresting," he says. "What?" He repeats the bad joke again. Would it be "interesting" and to whom, the cancer doctor only, of course, if the scan revealed tumors in the gut … then what could be done? "You have kidney failure" is another remark casually dropped.

The doctor arrives with his resident the next morning. "Well, you did it again," he says, "you got well." George will be discharged. My brother and his wife leave for their European vacation. George's son Alex picks us up. George wants to go out to lunch. The day is bright. We go to a Japanese restaurant in the neighborhood. We sit outside and eat, making small talk. One of George's favorite things to do is to go out to lunch. How we met.

It takes three days before we are back in the hospital.

At dinner, George barely eats. He has a quarter of a glass of white wine, a third of a vegetable pie, half a sweet potato with butter. It's Wednesday night. He has been losing energy all day. In the morning, we sat outside in the sun. After dinner, I read a few more pages by Diane Di Prima. We tumble into bed at 9:25 and I am immediately asleep. At 11 pm, I wake because George is retching on the toilet in the bathroom we call "mine" as opposed to "his" down the hall. I phone the doctor: "he is retching on the toilet." "You have to go to the emergency room." "I thought so." I tell George and help him dress. We have just purchased a wheelchair, but I've not yet attached the footrests. No matter. I call a car. The driver is quiet, concerned and helpful. We drive, barely speaking, to the hospital entrance.

There are perhaps fifteen people ahead of us. Intolerable. I tell the admitting person at the desk she has to let us jump the line. She does. We get inside but are consigned to wait, again, in the hall for the mandatory echocardiogram. Finally, we are let into the crowded emergency room and are assigned cubby thirty-seven.

At last, at perhaps 3 am, a young doctor appears. "I will give him morphine for pain." He has had stomach X-rays, but that is all. George drops off to sleep, mercifully. I keep asking, for hours, it seems—but time has long since lost meaning, it is eternity here—for help, for knowledge. Did they take blood? What has been done, exactly? On a cot in the same cubby, an Orthodox man and his wife await a prescription to treat his urinary tract infection, the doctor buzzes in and out, to attend him. We are without medical attention. As they leave, the wife wishes me "good luck." Do we need "luck," I wonder to myself. Are things that bad? Her husband's urinary infection is "nothing" compared to us. Closer to morning, a seriously injured young Black man is wheeled into the other half of our cubby, with much attention. A blood transfusion is begun, and shortly after, explaining that he is very sick, and there will be many people attending, they move George to cubby thirteen, near the doctor's station. Where we remain until 4 pm the next day. With nothing being done. As the morphine wears off, George's pain intensifies. Two young residents visit and suggest discharge. The cancer doctor, who has visited us in the emergency room so often over the years, is out of town. He is speaking at one of his "conferences" that resumed as soon as the COVID lockdown ended.

Then, in late afternoon, his cancer doctor texts, "I just talked with surgery. Hernia is stuck and not reducible. When did he last take Xarelto?" "Last night about 9 p.m." A surprisingly tall and portly Asian man dressed in unusual red surgical scrubs is suddenly attending to George. He is going to put a tube down his nose to drain his stomach liquids. George resists. He is frightened. He cries out. He flails on the cot trying to protect himself. I take his hands in mine. I have to hold his hands down on his distended stomach so he can't fight back, saying he mustn't resist, saying words of love. The big doctor in red pushes the tube into his nose, and threads it down his esophagus. I have become his accomplice. George is being done to, helpless. I am in shock. I text to his doctor: "General anesthesia. Surgery today. You know this; I am just trying to take it in. I would not say 'no' but I am speaking with George. What are the chances?" "Taking it in?" his doctor questions. He does not seem to understand how helpless we feel. "Yes. That he has to have surgery today with general anesthesia. This happened in an hour. Until the hernia doctor's team came, they were talking about discharging him. Then suddenly it was the tube down the throat, which he fought but then grew brave, and the surgery and the general anesthesia. He is taking all this in," I am precise as I can be. "It's a load," his doctor texts back, "but there is no choice in the opinion of surgeon." "Yes, I realize," I text, but I am in shock. His bowel is blocked. Without intervention, he will die a gruesome death, poisoned from the inside. His bowel blocked, unblocked, has been blocked, now, for several days. It is 6:15 in the evening. George is in the care of the hernia surgery team. World class, I'm told. After a night and a day in which nothing happened while George lay suffering everything has suddenly become efficient. The large Asian assistant even puts his hand on my back and asks, "how are you doing?" The first time anyone in the hospital ever inquired about my feelings. I have no idea how I answered him. I was in shock.

Once the tube is in place, George is moved to a private room on the sixth floor. The tube down his nose spills brown liquid into the jar on the wall. I am sitting close to his bed; my leg and bare foot are stretched out toward him on the mattress. George grabs tight to my foot. His doctor arrives, back in town. George's son, whom I've called, stands at the end of the bed looking down. George does not let go of my foot. This might be our last embrace; nevertheless, we are smiling, yakking. Our mood is strangely exuberant. As if he is about to go on stage and we've gathered here in his dressing room, not into the operating theater to repair an impacted intestine that would kill him. Alex and I follow his gurney to the surgery prep. The surgeon appears, large, dark, and handsome underneath his mask. "I can do this in a half hour," he tells me. Confident, as world-renowned surgeons are. Inspiring confidence in us. I lightly kiss George. I go back to room to wait. I gobble a bagel with lox; I haven't eaten all day. I call a friend. True to his word, the surgeon phones me before the hour is up. Success. The bowel was impacted but not decayed. The hernia has been repaired. I phone his cancer doctor, on my way down to see George briefly in recovery. My voice breaks. I hear his doctor's voice break too. We had both been terrified.

A few days later, all is well. The cancer doctor arrives to see George in recovery, where every organ is being monitored. His every extremity is wired to machines. The doctor stands at his bed. George impulsively grabs both his hands, "I have to thank you ..." He is effusive. I can see the doctor's discomfort, but I don't dwell on it. George launches into a vivid description of the surgical team, their expertise, how they danced in unison around him, fulfilling the surgeon's orders, "all speaking Chinese. It was just like a performance. Thrilling." "Were you awake?" his doctor asks, incredulous at the joyful description. "The last thing I remember is the surgeon, orchestrating everyone, saying, 'I can do this,'" George describes the scene as if from an opening night, or a good tech rehearsal: competent people doing their work, in rhythm. The doctor is charmed. George's enthusiasm for the expert dance of the surgical team is infectious. The cancer doctor says, "well save his number because you have another one." (He has a smaller hernia on the other side, but they had not dared operate on two; it is likely this would have to happen again but George and I do not think about that right now. He is alive and out of pain.)

Saturday afternoon. I am scrunched on the window ledge next to his bed in the recovery unit. George is feeling good, though he is still attached to monitors everywhere: ankles, arms, heart. But we are in a good mood. Outside the sun shines. It is June. The trees are in leaf. On a website called Pawrade, I find a liver and white, beautifully marked six-week-old cocker spaniel puppy, very cute, and "look(!)" I cry out, "He is named Percy!"— Percy Bysshe Shelley II is the name I had chosen for our new spaniel. I had been ordering and canceling orders for a spaniel pup all spring. First for a springer, then for a cocker. George was too ill, I thought. Now, it is summer. He is recovering. Now, I tell George that our former spaniels, Cleis and Hermes, surely sent this little puppy to us, from that cloud where all good dogs go, and they had him named Percy. "So Kahwren will shurely know," I mimic how Hermes spoke in my ear. He's a beauty, I can tell. I, a mutt, am a snob about animals. As I liked the horses I rode, so with my dogs, beautiful conformation and well bred. Dogs need a job, I think but I don't say. When I return to teaching in the fall, this little dog will stay home with George. "I'd better pay for the puppy, now, before someone else does. Okay?" "Okay," says George, "but you'll have to do all the work." I agree, joyously. With a few clicks, it is done. Percy, our fourth spaniel pup, will be delivered straight to our door in three weeks. Madness or sanity? Like George's Tante Irma, like Virginia Woolf and Elizabeth Barrett Browning, haven't we always had spaniels. Three months after Abby died and we buried her with a basket of her blue balls underneath the red rose bush in our, then, backyard, I ordered littermates Hermes and Cleis from a breeder in South Carolina—the first purchase I had ever made on the internet. Hermes, a blue merle, is the only dog whose voice I have heard distinctly in my head. He spoke loud and clear, with a spaniel accent. "Kahwren" he called me. Together we wrote a short play, "Hermes in the Anthropocene: a Dogologue," staged at three or four colleges and published on-line. But Hermes was George's dog, invariably charming and kind. Cleis, named after Sappho's daughter, was my girl, blue-eyed, light brown and white, she had been abused at the breeders by a springer spaniel and came to us traumatized. "Don't you see, she is not a dog at all, but an angel, sent here to get you through this," the breeder, a devout Christian wrote me. The spaniels made certain I was outside in all sorts of weather. When I hit a block, I would walk the dog or the dogs until the sentence I needed appeared in my head, or the right turn of event for the scene I was stuck on. The gods, but I just did, again, when I go to type dogs, it comes out gods more often than not, the dogs slept at my feet, under my desk. I cried so often and so hard in the days before we called the vet to come euthanize Cleis and Hermes—now I know I was crying not just for them, but for the end of the life they shared with us. I held Clee and felt her heart stop. Hermes, too, while George sat on a chair next to us. We followed their bodies the vet pulled in a little wagon out to the vet's car. She loaded them into her trunk for cremation. We took ourselves to lunch, told dog stories and drank—a wake of sorts. We have now been dogless for over a year. With George in and out of hospital, it is easier not to have a dog. Percy is paid for by American Express. He will arrive in three weeks, but for now it still seems unreal.

The doctor appears. He has been riding his bike in the park and affirms it is a beautiful day outside. George can be released on Monday. There has been another terrible mass shooting, this time of many children, in Uvalde, Texas. This latest collective nightmare has registered with us, but barely. As the doctor circled the long meadow on his bike, he tells us he fantasized shooting into the crowd, rather amazed at himself. "I think many people are having the same fantasy," I reply sourly, rather amazed at him myself.

We go out to dinner, just we two, as we have done every year on my birthday, June 29. We eat outside at a restaurant nearby where we often go. George is in a wheelchair. But we are gay. As we finish our meal, a man emerges from the restaurant and sidles right up to our table. He stands too close to me; looming over, he looks down at me and says, in a voice I find sinister, "I watched you eat that whole fish." I had had the branzino and though I'd put a few choice pieces on top of George's crab pasta, it was so; I had, in fact, eaten most of the fish. So, he watched me eat a whole fish … ravenous. What else might I eat, with gusto, if given the chance? I'm speechless, somewhat terrified, also furious. In the way that such mini-assaults leave one jangled with emotion, inarticulate, afraid often to answer back. George doesn't hear what he says. I do not repeat the remark. What gives him the right, by what laws is he granted permission to comment on my eating of fish, but women are always under such scrutiny. We are always being told. Our appetites condemned. We are always watched. We are always, even now, at my age, potential sexual victims: we deserve it because of the lusty way we devour an entire fish. In full view. At a restaurant table. Now, with the recent overturning of Roe, one can feel the sexual menace in the air. We've been returned to our "proper role." Fish eating becomes provocative. I ought to eat gruel. She was asking for it, after all. Our appetites are to be condemned, policed. And, I think, too, it is because George is obviously so weak, confined to a wheelchair, that this man feels he can sidle up to me and say what he says with a leer.

—

On July 6, a Wednesday, George has an appointment with the head of urology. He is to remove the catheter that George has been using since the surgery. When I get out of the shower, I find George, dressed with hat on at 7 am, sitting in his wheelchair already waiting by the door. I want to cry, but don't dare. The appointment is at 8:45, and close by. George waits patiently. Patrick, the driver-journalist with whom we've become friends, picks us up in an hour. With his usual courtesy, he greets George warmly, and helps him into the car, stashing the wheelchair in the back. The urologist wants to leave the catheter in (a huge disappointment) and put George on Flomax for a week. I phone the cancer doctor, and he and the cancer doctor discuss. The urologist, I realize too late, finds this a hostile move on my part, but he agrees to abide by George's doctor. He says he will take the catheter out and see if George can pee. The office is freezing, though outside it is very hot. They stick us in a corner next to an out-of-use desk, with a flimsy curtain between George's chair and another, which is likewise occupied by a man with a urinal; the nurse hands a plastic urinal to George and leaves us there. George pees on himself. I find a bathroom, and I walk George the few steps down the hall, so he can have privacy, and perhaps empty his bladder. He seems numbed; he's passive and sad. I stand outside guarding the door; someone stops to yell at me. Didn't I see the room is marked "staff"? Now, with George on the other side of the door, I do start to cry. I actually hadn't seen the sign—what if I had? It's too late now. George's urine flow is not very strong, but the urologist leaves the catheter out and he lets us go. "Make another appointment for October," the angry urologist dismisses us. The thought flashes through my mind: George will be dead by October, and the urologist knows this. Patrick doesn't answer his phone, nor can I find another cab; there is construction outside and the noise of jackhammers is loud. It's very hot, but we decide to walk; rather, we decide I will push George up Clinton Hill in his chair. We stop for lunch at a Middle Eastern restaurant on Lafayette Avenue. He eats lentil soup, hummus, baba ganoush, pita bread, and drinks two glasses of iced mint tea. We are suddenly happy. The ghastly scenes at the cruel urologist vanish. So does George's passivity. We talk and laugh. It is like so many lunches we've had. Like the first, when I suddenly asked how he felt. Now, I don't ask; I know. But we push death away and are merry. It is often like this in the last weeks. Normal life materializes all of a sudden, the kind that goes on and on, uninterrupted, especially on long summer days. George becomes lively and funny. We look at one another with those looks of deep love people remark upon more and more, that seem singular, somehow. Someone or other would say, then and after he died, that they had never seen two people look at each other with such deep love. To us, our mutual gaze seemed regular but as we approached his death, we took to looking deeper and deeper, as if to stare straight at the source that makes one one and not any other, and our love seemed released at these moments, to dance between us in the air, in the space between souls, and this is what others sometimes saw, our love dancing there. As if love were rare. So we ate and we talked and we looked. I have not a memory of the words we spoke. I remember the food and the heat, our laughter that releases us from the humiliations we had just suffered, from his pee on his pants, my tears, the urologist's cruel dismissal, and we clung to one another with our gaze.

From here on, the hill home becomes steeper. The cheap wheelchair we bought in a rush keeps getting its wheels stuck on the tree roots that rupture the sidewalks every twenty feet. I am helpless. It's boiling hot, plus I am wearing platform sandals. We are still blocks from home. We are invisible to the white people passing by. They see in us their mortality from which they shy. Black people see our suffering, akin to their own; they see George is about to meet the same mysterious force who has sheltered them, who has embraced all the loved ones they've lost. From "out of the blue," Black women descend like ministering angels, clucking over George, laying their blessings on as if we all were in church together, and we are so much needing to be blessed.

The first time the wheelchair is stuck in a rut, a single Black woman sweeps in from somewhere and helps me get him over the hump, in the next block, two Black women appear, lifting wheels, fussing over us; the third time, three Black women with three small Black children arrive as if by miracle—they maneuver the increasingly rickety vehicle. Am I making this up or did their skin shine, like angels bathed in eternal light. Black people, perhaps most especially Black women, do not shy from others' suffering. Black women have grown wise from heavy blows. Here, I am simply quoting James Baldwin when I say the suffering of Black people has made human our inhuman nation. I know from my experience in the neighborhood where we've lived for thirty-five years, Baldwin is correct. We are blessed to live here; even if now gentrified, enough of the old spirit remains. This is the center of the Black Democratic party. No one wins an election who does not have support of the churchwomen from Ebenezer Baptist, on our corner. The Attorney General of New York, Tish James, is a neighbor. From here, Hakeem Jeffries was launched to power. In this neighborhood, walking dogs or not, taking children to school, we say "good morning" to people we know and do not know, a chorus of greetings starts our days. On the hot street trying hard to get home this afternoon, we are cared for and blessed by neighbors who seemed to me, then, angels. Because I could not have gotten George home by myself. Because they must have been watching out for us.

Our new puppy, Percy, arrives by puppy transport from the Midwest at 3 am the next morning. I meet the young transporter on the street. He puts a trembling, terrified fur ball into my arms. By the time we get to the apartment door, the pup has relaxed between my breasts. We are bonded for life. I put Percy on the bed to meet George; he snuggles and licks. Soon after, when I try to put puppy Percy into the dog crate I've dutifully bought, he screeches in terror, throws himself against the bars. I haven't the heart to stuff him in, not after his long, terrifying trip from Indiana, not after being wrenched from his litter. I bring him to our bed, where he stays his first night. He paper trains himself inside his playpen over the following days. He is adorable and chill. He insists on snuggling close to George, licking his face. He lies at George's feet, if George is up, pen in hand, sitting at the table, writing his diary and looking out at the trees.

Percy arrives on July 7. On July 11, late in the night, George falls to his knees on his way from the toilet. He and I manage to maneuver him into a chair. We have to call 911 to help him back to bed. No, we do not wish to go to the ER. They take his vitals and leave. Kind as always, the EMS people are. "For God sakes, woman," he yells at me two days later, completely out of character. Wednesday, July 13, and he is back in the ER, a catheter has to be put back in. He has developed a urinary tract infection. There will be more antibiotics.

I have to buy a phone charger. I've left mine at home in the rush to get to the hospital. Coming back, the security guard stops me for no reason; I'm wearing my yellow "ER Visitor" sticker plastered against my black sweater. "My husband is in the ER." "You can't go there." "I have to go there." I walk past the guard. I'm met at the door to the ER by another large security guard. "Caucasian wearing a black sweater," he says into his phone. I want to laugh, yes, I happen to fit the description, but they cannot mean me, whatever for. "I've got her." He grabs my arm. "You went past security. You don't obey our rules." I do my song and dance, husband, old, ill, I must, I need to, etc. etc. But no. He marches me back to the front desk, holding tight to my arm, and stands me in front of the hall guard who sits on a high stool behind a small desk, like Gabriel at the gates, before whom I must grovel in the front of people. "I'm so sorry, etc., etc., my husband blah, blah. You have to, please, please. Please let me go. Forgive me. I am so very sorry." "You see when you obey the rules, we let you go," the large guard sneers down at me. I am free. It is an exercise in the futility of power over others, the stupidity, the flaunting of authority, the cruelty, pomposity, idiocy, uselessness … endemic in the "criminal justice system" just not usually felt by the Caucasian woman in a black sweater. But perhaps my vulnerability is clear to them. They are not going to let me "get away with it" anymore. After all. Though they don't know this, my name is "Karen," a pejorative nickname for white women.

George is admitted to hospital, again. The catheter goes in and comes out, and goes in, with increasing pain each time. He stays for nearly a week. When Peter Schumann, whose wife, Elke, died the summer before, hears how ill George is, he phones me to speak to him. I leave the room but can hear George's laughter from the hall, and his wondrous voice. The two friends since the 1960s are reminiscing. One morning I throw up and cannot go to the hospital. I ask his doctor for news. He tells George, "your wife wants to hear how you are." George begins to recite the first lines of Uncle's speech that he loves, that he hopes to perform again at the LaMama celebration of his life on October 20. He is line-perfect on the video I am sent: "So, we shall surround our pond with rosemary, thyme, and eglantine, partridge pea and blue-eyes grass …" but his resonant voice has cracked. I am walking the puppy outside when the tape arrives on my phone. I listen, trying to be glad, but I'm horrified. George speaks in a raspy whisper. Did the doctor not know? I am losing him. Piece by piece. He can no longer walk by himself. I will never again hear that magnificent voice. A voice that held every feeling in the world. His voice is gone. That for years sang my words. Peter calls back a few days later. "He's not who he was," I warn him. "Never mind. Put him on." They laugh and joke again. Again, I listen from the hospital hall. George is still who he was, even though his resonant voice has cracked. So few people address the ill, not even their close friends, boisterous and unafraid as Peter did—as if nothing could come between George and him, certainly not imminent death.

He will come home to die. We have requested palliative and hospice care. We will have neither. The palliative care doctor, a portly blond woman in a white coat with an unfortunate German name, Goering, does nothing but read us the list of the non-resuscitate options. His doctor has "sent his regrets," he is too busy to attend. Why had I thought of this as some sort of inverse graduation, from hospital where he'd spent so much time, to hospice, home to die, and why had I thought his cancer doctor's attendance mandatory? I thought his heart doctor and the infectious disease specialist would also come to say their good-byes. The odd trio that treated him together for several years. George and I used to joke that they were a Gilbert and Sullivan chorus. One portly and tall, (Dilmanian, the Albanian, we called him) one short and with a sort of sideways walk, impish (the cancer doctor), and one inbetween, the youngest, an infectious disease specialist with a name that rhymes with sepsis. They had danced in and out of his hospital rooms for three years. Smiled and clucked, made small talk, sometimes about politics, sometimes about books. Wouldn't they come now, now that George was so sick that they had nothing to offer, nothing, that is, but themselves. Doctors, I realized, are not good at dealing with death. They are in retreat. Nothing they know can have the effect they wish, pushing back death. To each question about various means of resuscitation, George, who is sitting up next to me, gaunt in his hospital gown, which is open at the back, answers "no" in his cracked voice: he does not want this or that extraordinary measure. So-called palliative care specialist Dr. Goering checks the boxes off. She and her team of residents look at us pityingly. "How long have you been married?" she asks. They cluck in sympathy. I want to throw something at them. But she abruptly leaves with her team. She is done. She never gives us the Do Not Resuscitate order she has filled out in our presence, nor does she offer a word of counsel. Her job is not palliative care, I dimly realize, it is purely administrative; she is there to transfer us officially from the hospital's liability to that of hospice. Now, hospice can bill Medicare (though we will never benefit from any hospice care).

My daughter arrives the same day with her two small sons, six and three, to say goodbye to George. We come home from the hospital by ambulance. Carrie Sophia helps the two women ambulance drivers hoist George in a sheet from the stretcher onto our bed. Her children, his stepgrandchildren, stand on the mattress at his side. The pup snuggles in. George takes his stepdaughter's head in his hands. He beams. He has always adored her. "I *am so happy to see you, Carrie*," he croons. "No one," she responds, "has ever been so glad to see me in my life." They were always a team, his stepdaughter and he—in the midst of her worst teenage rebellion, he always said, "Don't worry about her; she has a great gyroscope." He was right.

If George is going to live, he has to get up. At least to sit, if not walk a few steps. Hospice has no one to send. No nurse, no physical therapist. No advice to give, not even over the phone. I hire private health aides for the weekend; it will cost $3000 but I cannot care for George by myself and my child has gone home with her children, back to work. A woman arrives. We help George into a chair. I wheel him to the table where he writes, where we eat, so he can look out at the trees he loves. The pup sits at his feet. I give him a protein drink with a straw. For an instant, all is well. He has to use the commode. I wheel him back to the bedroom. The aide and I get him up from the wheelchair and set him down again on the commode. He has a bowel movement and, in the next instant, what looks like a mini-stroke. He faints, for an instant. He comes to immediately, but is very weak. We manage to get him into bed. "He needs the emergency room," the terrified aide says. "Call 911." I phone his doctor, first, who, again, is out of town, at one of the "conferences" he goes to on the weekends, and who says to me, "if you're ready for it, you can leave him in bed." Ready for it? I brought him home so we might have weeks, a month or more. He would get up. Walk, even with a walker, recover some strength. We would play with our pup. Friends would come. I am not ready "for it", nor, I hope, is he. At the same time, I see.

Hospice would be able to rehydrate George in our home, if we call them, but they do not do so on the weekend. It is Saturday. The aide and our neighbors who have just come by to visit urge me to take George to the emergency room instead. I am in shock, but I am not ready for "it"; neither is George. I call 911. The EMS young people could start an infusion now, at home, but they can only do so if they are then going to take us to the closest emergency room, and they can *only* take us to Brooklyn Hospital at the end of our street if I put the medical directive Do Not Resuscitate Order into their hands. But I do not know what became of it. Dr. Goering never gave it to us. (Medical directives we filled out when we made our wills, six years before, are stashed in his mother's roll top desk drawer, but I have forgotten this, of course.) We cannot leave without the missing DNR paper. Through all this, George is lying silent in the bed, listening. He does not speak while we debate his fate as if it is no concern of his. Yet he must be listening. Is it that he can no longer talk? But I don't have time to think about this. We need to get him to the hospital, now. I grow slightly hysterical. It is my fault I cannot remember what happened to the DNR order. Finally, the young, invariably kind EMS people realize that the hospice that has provided us no service must actually have his medical orders, or they would not have taken him as a patient. Goering must have faxed the order to them. EMS is correct, and the young man calls hospice and, yes, they will fax the DNR order, which they do indeed have to Brooklyn Hospital down the street, the nearest emergency room. The same public hospital where Anthony Fauci was born. We've been there before, once when George was in arrhythmia; they'd stopped and restarted George's heart. We had just that night opened *Another Life* in a festival uptown. We'd gone out to celebrate with my mother who had come to see the work, and George had ordered some vodka and rum fancy concoction and become quite drunk, as neither of us had had very much sleep for several weeks, racing to stage the play in which he had a huge part. Once I'd gone with a case of influenza just to make certain it was not pneumonia. We arrive at the Emergency entrance by ambulance. A huge sign on the wall reads, "No Visitors Allowed." A large guard sits at the door. I walk past him, alongside the stretcher carrying George. The guard does not stop me. He sees the crisis we're in. I'm Caucasian, in a thin red sweater this time, escorting my dying husband. Inside the freezing ER, George is wheeled to a curtained cubby. Three nice young doctors, two female and one male, start the IV, shoving the rehydration fluids in as fast as they can. I am communicating with George's doctor by text. He is out of town, in Philadelphia, at another of the frequent what he calls "conferences" he attends. I fancy he presents his research papers. I don't know yet what he actually does. I give George half a tuna fish sandwich, ever-present inpatient refrigerators. We have eaten many of these densely packed mayonnaise and tuna, tasteless concoctions during the years of his long chemotherapy infusion sessions. He chews, as if hungry, but later I find the masticated bits on the edge of his cot. He had taken them out his mouth. He is no longer able to swallow food.

"I feel I am losing sense and language," George suddenly says, the first words he's spoken since he passed out, and his voice sounds restored when he speaks, as if shocked by awareness into full resonance again. So I do hear his full voice one final time, saying words that hurt so much. He is losing himself, leaving me. With his usual fine sensibility, he knows exactly what is happening. "I am losing sense and language," he said. I lay myself over him. Kiss his face and chest. I can think of nothing to say. He has been so precise. "Sense and language, language and sense." I cannot contradict. I walk some feet from his bed and I start to sob. Holding myself tight. Crying hard. I am freezing. He is losing "sense and language." He knows best the state he is in. The words sting. The air conditioner is blasting. I have only a light summer sweater over a seersucker jumpsuit. I cry harder, perhaps, than I ever have, standing alone, away from his cot in an empty part of the emergency room. I am so unstrung, I cannot comfort him. I am losing my heart. I stand shaking and sobbing by myself while he lies all alone. Someone approaches me from behind and drops a heated sheet over my shoulders. Warmed, I calm. I go back to his bed. He is lying in his own excrement, again. Much of my time the last ten days of his life will be spent cleaning his bottom, as gently as possible. There are no aides. I search for pads, towels, wipes. The doctors have given him as much liquid as they can. We have been here for four or five hours. The ambulance has been called. We are waiting to go home, again, for the last time, we both know. "Sense and language," his words repeat in my mind. Losing language and sense, sense and language, losing them. Language, what he loved most.

While we are gone, our neighbors, Mariah and Henry, clean and straighten the house. They do the laundry. Now I cannot find anything, but house is clean and neat. They have taken George's expensive heart medication for family members of theirs, and his expensive eye drops, too, but I don't care. Henry had been going with George out to lunch once a week during the spring. They've become friends. The hired aide has been dismissed. George is put back into our bed by the ambulance drivers. I am alone with my love. He has been silent. He is no longer able to speak. I lie down on our bed, next to him. On Monday morning, I manage to take the puppy to the vet. His son, Alex, stays with him. "Dogs need a job," the vet says. Alex will come after work and stay the nights with us from now on.

People begin to come to our home to say their goodbyes: our dear friends, Jan and Winston. Jan, a wonderful writer who counseled George and listened deeply to his stories. Kathy, who starred with George in *Blue Valiant*, and Henry, who put together the crew that filmed it. Sally Ann, our costume designer. Our old friend Lydia, a great actor, once under the short-lived, progressive Tsipras government, the Cultural Minister of Greece, calls from her home in Athens. We haven't spoken in years. She had "a feeling," she tells me. I put the phone to his ear so she can speak with George. They had always wanted to act together. Bread and Puppet puppeteers call from Vermont and sing to George over the phone. Dara, his student, who wrote a play about Edward Hopper under his tutelage, brings a scented candle I will burn the last night of his life. Another Lydia, playwright and novelist, happens to be in New York from her home in Germany. Stefanie, who runs a nonprofit in Bed-Stuy, whom we met years before at a yoga studio and for whom George once directed *A Midsummer Night's Dream*, free, with her Paul Robeson High School students. Beatriz and her husband, Johan; she has been the photographer for all of our plays and has taken hundreds of photos of George in many roles. Michal comes several days in a row. She is producing the *Coffeehouse Chronicles* at LaMama, where he'd hoped to perform Uncle's speech one last time. Now that event will become his public memorial. JoAnne calls from Nova Scotia; she directed George in many plays for Mabou Mines and at the Public Theater. Clove, Lee Breuer and Ruth Maleczech's daughter, calls from California. Paula Singer, a very old friend, has lost her husband the month before. She is here in New York from Boulder; we walk in the park together while Alex is with George. His oncologist makes a surprise house call. He gives George some protein drink through a straw. He swabs his mouth, as he had done during the sepsis attack a year a-half before; now he shows me how to do this every few hours. He and I share a chaste hug by the bed. We are losing him. The oncologist, not hospice, sends me a Fed Ex package of mouth swabs. The next day while George lies dying in our big bed, a visiting nurse I have never before seen appears at the door, to "take his vitals." She is appalled when she sees where he lies, in our large, carved, wooden bed. I have to have a hospital bed delivered immediately and put in the living room of our apartment where George is to be moved. When I refuse, she begins to harangue. I must have a hospital bed. Why? Because, this is the way it is done. She has no other reason but her voice rises, because, because. Finally, beaten down I say, "Okay." She begins to call in the order. I know we haven't long. Immediately, I change my mind. "No." She begins to shout at me again, but this time she leaves in a self-righteous huff. When I promised he would not be alone, I also meant he would not be put in a strange and uncomfortable bed where I cannot lie next to him and hold his hand. A bed he would need to be hoisted into. He hated hospital beds with their uncomfortable mattresses. He is to die where we loved, made comfortable with pillows.

These last days become strangely joyous. We are in a heightened state, staring down death as he lies in his own bed, surrounded by close friends. George can see and hear; he can open his arms wide as if to embrace those who have come. He follows all that is said. His eyes sparkle and he shares in our laughter. We tell many stories. I sit on the big bed next to him. Others stand or sit in chairs at his side. He is propped up on pillows, beaming. We are reliving *Blue Valiant*'s production, with Kathy, Henry, and Sally Ann, those freezing, stormy days, just over a year ago now, outside on the farm. George's last live performance. We are laughing at our own audacity, our refusal to give up. George relished the insane difficulty of live theater. He loved performing outside. The driving rain on the greenhouse roof, which made it impossible to hear the lines. Our lost dress rehearsal. Yet the projections, the lights, the staging worked well. We never thought we could do it, but the rain stopped just in time, twice in two days. The second performance even better than the first. We made the film, which is stunning. (Many people have watched it on YouTube.) Kathy calls it "our miracle"; meanwhile, she has broken her arm on a vacation in Italy. She fell out of a hammock. They have come home early and are with us now. She had a torn meniscus while we rehearsed the play and was often in terrific pain. She was putting off surgery, which, eventually, she did not need in order to perform. Today, her arm is in a black sling, held against her white summer dress. She acted a similar arm injury in the play, and had worn that same sling, then, as a costume piece. She presumed to know the horse too well so he rammed her. He taught her that we approach the aggrieved with care. The hurt are prone to lash out. "The moment you said your first line, the audience was held in a trance," Kathy, smiling, gesturing with her good arm toward the imagined crowd, reminds George. She had a long entrance through the audience. She felt their attention and what a fine way to enter a play, through a rapt audience the other actor has prepared for you. Or, why people loved to be on stage with George, his generous attention, his intensity. He is graciously dying. As he lived. He is present to hear from many who gather around the big bed or who phone how he is loved. Everyone has memories to share. What fun we had and against what odds. In community, creating.

All these final five days, we are up most of the night, George and I, talking, I talking to and with him, though he is mainly silent, but for sounds, and odd words. He is alert. He takes everything in. I tell him he is being "called back," an expression I've learned from Black friends. I tell him he will "join the ancestors," which I myself, an unbeliever, do not believe, and neither I think, an unbeliever like me, does he. We talk. I talk to him about our work. He is always most alert when we speak of the work we've done together. Whenever I speak about art or nature, he brightens.

On the morning of July 27, I write: He is still alive, odd what comfort that brings. The beautiful, resonant voice is gone, but the flesh remains. He is ever more so slightly alert at odd moments. I finish my shoddy version of a sponge bath. I give up thoughts of changing his shirt, and I clean his bottom, again, I hope, without rolling him over, which I cannot do alone. I was so tired all last night that I could not sleep. Every muscle and sinew ached with fatigue, too tired to rest; it was an odd sensation. Finally, I slept for several hours. We woke at sixish.

On the morning of July 28, I write: A quiet night, sometimes I thought, our last. We hold hands. I rub his belly. I weep. Sometimes, sleep. He breathes, heavily or lightly, refuses the offered oxygen, pulling the hose from his nose. He is, again, most engaged when I begin a riff on our work together. How important it is not to know exactly what you are doing. How in the space between the knowing and not knowing, the magic happens. How little I have ever known about anything I've ever done. Then, he reaches for and takes my hand. Now, once, again, we know nothing. We are on the brink.

On Friday night, July 29, after everyone has gone, Alex is asleep on the couch and George and I are alone. He manages to whisper to me, "I'm afraid." George is an animist, and so, I suppose, am I. If we believe in anything, we believe in the sanctity of the living world. His time in the Steiner school in the midst of the Nazi horror taught him to find comfort in the Bavarian forest, where many of their classes took place, seated at the base of a tall tree on the loam of the earth. When he was still able to walk to the top of Fort Greene Park, he would spontaneously throw his arms around a particularly grand old elm on the pinnacle, planted by Olmsted in this park initiated by Walt Whitman, and meld his body into its trunk, until he looked quite like a sprite emerging. He would murmur words of endearment to the tree. At the end of his life, when he could no longer act, nor walk that far, he spent hours writing in his diary, at the table in our first floor apartment where, if he looked through the geraniums on the window sill and above the cars in the parking lot, he could see a stand of trees. He delighted in this view, scant though it was. His macular degeneration meant he could not see the words he wrote in his diary in his cursive script; nevertheless, he continued to write:

> *The number one proof of God—it is The Tree. The kindest, most loving of all creatures on earth is the tree. Trees of all kinds, both large and small give everything to support all other life, as home, as food, both fruit and its own body while alive and in decay. As shade from the heat of the sun. As hiding for creatures that can climb, burrow into its body, in death and decay it creates new soil. As home for birds, for insects, squirrels, ants, bears, and Homo sapiens. How does one creature give life to all?*

Wheelchair-bound the last weeks of his life, he would make me stop to admire how a particular tree behind a building on the corner of the campus of Pratt Institute reached around the brick wall. "See," he would say, "how it reaches toward the light." When I pass it now, I stop. I fancy I can see

George's form inside its trunk; his arms are those branches reaching up. George's tree, I tell Percy, the pup.

When, on the night of July 29, his last full night alive, he managed to whisper to me, "I'm afraid," I knew we should speak of nature, or I, to him, saying many of the things we always said about the beauty of the eternal life force to which he is about to return. The glory of the natural world whose future we fear for from climate change and war—what will happen to the spirits of all our departed should humans continue to destroy earth's ecosystems? I speak to George, on and off, for hours the night through, lying next to him, holding his hand—but this is a dialogue, truly. I am repeating sentiments we share, as he lies unmoving in our bed, his eyes still sparkling, somehow. The life force is eternal, I say—do I believe that myself? But we both do, I know, this is why we fight so hard for the health of the natural world. "Of life only there is no end," I say, quoting Shaw. My own terrors to come I do not yet know. He is dying, I understand. But he lies alive, now, next to me. We are still in the midst of a conversation that began years before when we met doing a play and I asked him how he felt, and our life is not over yet. I am not alone. Never have our moments together been more precious than now. Never was our communication deeper. You will go back into life, I tell him, and the spirit that is you that, too, will manifest in a thousand ways, my darling.

So, we stay up talking all night—as we often did whenever a crisis in life or work occurred, talking things through till the light dawned, then grabbing an hour of sleep. I always relished our nighttime talks, but none more than this, when now I dare speak for us both. His words issuing through my voice. I am trying to feel what he might say if he could. He says nothing more. I say everything I can think to say about death, from a pantheistic place. You will become a part of all life. I promise, again, and as I have said for several years, you will not be alone. I love him, I tell him. I say he will be out of pain. How happy we've been. How divinely happy he made me. I say these things over and over. I have no words of wisdom. I do not believe in Heaven. I do not believe he will "wait for me there till I come." I do not believe we will ever see one another again. But I believe his spirit will live even if fractured into a million pieces in wind and wave. And his spirit will live inside of me and in so many he touched with his joyous grace. Softly,

I speak into his ear, touching his flesh, kissing his face, resting my head against his chest.

As morning comes, George squeezes my hand, which has been in his all night; with the strength he has left, he says, "that was good." His last words.

I hover around his bed all the next day. Or sit on the bed with him. Michal arrives; I take the puppy out for short walks. George is calm. We are waiting for a nurse, who is a friend of a friend, but her tire blows out on the George Washington Bridge; she never arrives. Lydia is there for a while. Alex has gone to work. When I am alone with George in the late afternoon, I pick up one of his legs. It is completely limp. All week, his legs had been rigid and straight. I know he is dying now; he is dying from his feet up. I text his doctor so. His doctor has been reading Keats with his wife. He sends me the college paper she has written on "Ode to a Nightingale" and suggests I might find solace in the poem's well-known final phrase: "Was it a vision, or a waking dream?/ Fled is that music:—Do I wake or sleep?" I am not consoled but I am reminded to read aloud to George this last night as we did so often during the pandemic. The Romantics.

I read a few more of Keats's poems to George. I read "Ode on a Grecian Urn," of course.

> *Beauty is truth, truth beauty,—that is all/ Ye know on earth, and all ye need to know.*

It is night, now. I turn to Percy Bysshe Shelley, our puppy's namesake, and a poet we love very much. I read him "Ozymandias," harsh though it is,

> *Round the decay*
> *Of that colossal Wreck, boundless and bare*
> *The lone and level sands stretch far away.*

And then I read George's favorite poem, Judith and Julian's favorite, too, "Ode to the West Wind." The last words he hears.

> *Drive my dead thoughts over the universe*
> *Like withered leaves to quicken a new birth!*
> *And, by the incantation of this verse,*

Scatter, as from an unextinguished hearth
Ashes and sparks, my words among mankind!
Be through my lips to unawakened Earth

The trumpet of a prophecy! O Wind,
If Winter comes, can Spring be far behind?

I lay myself close to him, my hand on his heart. I listen to each breath, as his breathing grows shallow. His heartbeats come farther apart. "Agonizing," his doctor texts me. But I don't yet feel so. He is here, now. There is no place I would rather be. He is still alive under my touch. Perhaps, he still hears the poets' beautiful words.

I feel his heart begin to slow under my touch. I wait for his heart to stop. I wait. Each heartbeat keeps us as together as we ever were. I wait. There is no answering beat of his heart. He dies in my arms, as I'd promised. It is 2:08 in the morning. I cry for a long while, covering his still body with my heaving one, holding him. "He is gone," I text his doctor. I won't hear back from him until late the next morning. "What had to happen, happened," he writes. "You made it softer and more humane."

To be completely truthful, I was holding George, drifting in and out of sleep, after I'd read, but I was awake as his heart slowed, awake with him until he took his last breath. Shortly before, I had swabbed his mouth and given him a bit of pain medication, as he seemed to be in some distress. Before and after, he was peaceful. Alex is asleep in the living room. Percy demands to be lifted up through the night and he licks and kisses George's mouth, snuggling with him, gently. George looks beautiful, ruddy in complexion as his heart slows and stops. I had my hand on his heart for a great part of the night and that wounded muscle beat with enormous will, like the bell in a clock tower, so it felt, for as long as it could. When his heart stops, I lay myself over his body and I cry, and cry. I cry my heart out, his chest wet with tears. Alex hears me and he comes in to sit with us. When I have wept myself still, I leave the room, so Alex can have some time alone. I send an email death announcement to a circle of friends: "Good night sweet prince. And flights of angels sing thee to thy rest."

George's last words he spoke in the early morning of his last day play in my mind, "that was good." He had never hurt me once, well once or twice, for an instant, until we talked it out, the same with me, of course. I could not remember an unkind word either one of us had said, though, of course, there had to have been some. Nor a crisis of health or career, nor a personal hurt, we had not shared. Giving and taking comfort as we could. "That was good." Had he meant our final talk the night through, when I tried to comfort him with my secular, animistic words about death, and promised him, again, he would not be alone? Did he mean the theater work we had done, his long career, the characters he inhabited so wonderfully on Broadway, off and off-off, on tour, in the street theater, the plays I wrote, we produced together and in which he starred? "That was good." Did he mean the parties we gave, our children and friends, his granddaughter, his step grandsons, our four cocker spaniels, our intimate meals, the novels we'd read during lockdown, the protests we'd gone to, the Peace Salons we hosted in our home, the huge Living Theatre Seders we held for which I boiled and peeled 100 eggs, and the Christmas Eves in the big house, the tree lit by candles, the house by the lake we'd had for a few years, until we sold it for airfare, to take the anti-torture play to London, our laughter, the long hours in the ER and hospital we shared? Did he mean the night of the broken glass on our bathroom floor, or his memories of his boyhood in Nazi Germany, Tante Irma's love and the big family estate, the cows whose noses he'd kissed, all the early memories that came flooding back once he was sick and the sense he made of them, now? Did he mean all that he'd given to the many artists he'd helped by producing their work at the theater he co-founded? Did he mean his entire eighty-nine-and-a-half years on this earth? Did he mean the living world, the trees in Fort Greene Park he spontaneously hugged? "That was good," he said to me in the early morning of July 29th. The last words he spoke. I felt his final heartbeat. George died in my arms at 2:08 in the early morning of July 30. Like the creator he was: "That was good," he said, and it was.

—

In September, I scatter George's ashes with friends:

In a pine wood on the Bread and Puppet land, the trees fifty feet tall or more, straight black bark, green needles branching out far above our heads is the memorial grove. What you think you cannot do alone, put your hands into the ashes of the one you loved, his earthly remains, they are gritty with burnt bone, if you do not know, becomes possible, even sacral, in community. There is a line of Yeats, a signature line, so-to-speak, I have always loved. "Think where (wo)man's glory most begins and ends/And say my glory was I had such friends." Yeats, too, made a theater with those he admired and loved. The Bread and Puppet Theater, sixty years on is going strong. Our Theater Three Collaborative is being laid to rest this day as we leave George's ashes here in a grove where many of our artist-friends are also commemorated with small memorial houses or other structures. To the right lies the grave of Elka Schumann, a small mound of earth, already growing things. Her body is here because the land is hers; the remains of her friends are memories only. Judith Malina has a small edifice down the slope. She introduced George and me when she directed my play *Us* in which he starred, for which he won an Obie. Grace Paley is to the right. My friend and George's, who anointed our early relationship with her words, 'I am so glad you two are together," at a protest march against the Gulf War I. There are many others including Bob Nichols, Grace's husband, who wrote the early street theater plays in which George performed.

We are, for the moment, the survivors, Peter and I. He is holding his trumpets, with which he led the Bread and Puppet brass and percussion band as we walked and danced from the farm down the slope to this pine grove. "I found Lady Gregory at eighty on her knees, planting trees," Yeats writes. On her estate at Coole Park is a large oak in which the Abbey artists carved their names, visible still. "That inquiring man, John Singe," wrote Yeats, "who dying took the living world for text."

"Nature intervened in all our words. We walked with beauty inside and out …" I wrote in one of George's favorite speeches as Uncle from *Extreme Whether*, a speech he was rehearsing in his final weeks of life hoping to perform it once again at LaMama's Coffee House in his honor, now his memorial service.

With me are Ynestra King, my friend of forty years, a founder of ecofeminism, Michal Gamily, who is producing George's memorial, Patrick Mintu, a journalist from Congo who became our trusted friend and driver in the final year of George's life and George's son Alex. All will speak. Alex will read from George's diary about playing *Diagonal Man* to rapturous response in Poland, caught in martial law. Michael Romanshyn and Howie Cantor were also in Peter's production of *Diagonal Man*, in which George played the sloping fellow, feet on the earth, straining toward freedom that very freedom the Polish audience was straining toward. The banner from that play, done in the 80s, marks his memorial mound.

"Bring something to nail to a tree," Peter had said on the phone. I have George's Irish cap, which he wore as Uncle and again as Sam Brown in *Blue Valiant* and which he wore on many trips to doctors, hospitals and back, and many walks, shorter and shorter they became, around our neighborhood. George loved trees. He wrote about them, delighted in them, often hugged them spontaneously.

Underneath the hat, surrounding the tree's tall trunk are tubs of wildflowers, gathered by the puppeteers too young by half a century to have known George when he rehearsed *Woyzech*, *Othello* and *Diagonal Man* with Peter on the farm, before I knew George. I have a photo of George as Uncle, holding the same hat, dressed in the deerskin robe designed and made in the shop of Sally Ann Parsons, our costume designer for thirty-five years, which also lay atop his coffin at his funeral service, outside on a glorious, hot day at Greenwood Cemetery. Now it hangs on the wall in my Clinton Hill apartment, next to the large Plexiglas panels of the tree branches in full leaf that set the stage for *Extreme Whether* at LaMama.

These are the strands of our community, intertwined over decades, with roots far back in theaters like Yeats' poetic Abbey, or Brecht and Piscator's epic ventures. Theaters meant quite simply to show the way, or, rather, to show images of another way. Theaters made from ideas, the particularity of their creators' talents, puppets or poetic texts, in every case visions of lives fulfilled, a world at peace, equality, community, nature honored, verdant and alive.

I did not believe I could put my hands into his ashes. That flesh I so much loved to touch. I have brought the African wooden bowl I bought on Myrtle Avenue and painted green, decorated with gold leaf. It was Sniffley the frog's urn in *Extreme Whether*. George carried it for his young friend, the bereaved Annie, set it on the ground for her funeral song, "Sniffley was/ And the world was, too/The most decent frog/The most beautiful place/We knew …" Now, I dip a brass scoop into the box full of ashes and I fill the urn with them. Put on the lid and set the wooden bowl on the ground, under the hat, next to his photo against the tree.

There are ashes to be scattered, their grit on our fingers, and memories to be shared. Peter tells of his first sight of George and Crystal Field, atop a flatbed truck in Central Park, telling the story of the Vietnam War, its generals, soldiers, victims, simply by changing hats. It was George as clown he first encountered, also a vital aspect of this poetic actor, and he was enchanted, as George was excited by Peter's puppets, huge and tiny, in the Sheep Meadow. They became friends that many illegal wars ago, a friendship that remained and deepened in the final weeks of George's life when Peter phoned him the hospital and they talked and laughed and George felt seen and restored. Again, Peter called. George less able to respond this time, "that doesn't matter, put him on the phone," and they laughed together a final time. At the end of that phone call, Peter and I planned for this day. George knew his ashes would be scattered here and he approved.

What he did not know in life was the full beauty of this place, nor how many others of his friends' memories he would be near. What he could not guess was the sublime beauty of this late summer Vermont day. Michal, Nesta, Patrick, Alex, and I stand at the tree while the light fades, and changes on the photo of George, until he glows, then dims.

No, I did not think I could do it. Could not have done it by myself. Only in community, only held by the energies, the memories, the presence of these friends could I have done this thing. Put my hand into the ashes of my love and scattered those that did not fit into the urn to the wind. One by one people come to do the same, a handful of ashes, words, and thrown, the ground beneath the tree now has grey circles of the ash that did not blow in the scant wind.

Nothing is possible without community. The Bread and Puppet is the perfect example. We are welcomed, entertained with a new, short, beautiful and biting play, fed and housed by the puppeteers and Peter still scattering his visions far and wide. Parts of the company are in Istanbul, others on tour, others here on the farm making "before the Apocalypse" pop-up plays for parking lots.

Peter is at the outdoor kitchen, in the white chef's apron another of his close collaborators Genevieve, also memorialized right next to George, also a cancer victim, had given him. "The last I have," he says. He is making latkes with fresh applesauce for our communal dinner after the ceremony. Those of us who have stayed late at the tree return hungry for drink, food, comradeship, including my cocker pup, Percy Bysshe Shelley II, who came to us in the last weeks of George's life, and who binds me to life, now. He, too, is ravenous for Peter's latkes and begs with excellent success.

"We are next," Peter says to me as I stand beside him in the outdoor kitchen. As impossible for each of us to have imagined life without our partners in art and love, as impossible for us to imagine our own ends, made more desirable by deaths of our beloveds, and yet we cling to life. Peter calls it a "half-life" and I, newly widowed, agree, or a nonlife, I might say, as I leave behind the life I've known, making theater with the man now dead. To these moments, when out of the rubble of modern life, its constant disasters with other, greater disasters yet to come, we cling, only because around us are our friends, eating latkes, drinking wine, laughing, building a bonfire as the cool sets in. To the pup who snuggled with George the final days of his life, now crunching latkes, licking his lips, asking for more. We are always asking for more.

Nothing is possible without community. This day on the Bread and Puppet farm with generations intertwined, new friends and old, allows the most sacral of acts I could not have done by myself alone. I could not have sent my lover's ashes to the wind, the earth, nor nailed his hat to a tree. I could not have. So much I could not have done without George, without the community we built around our work, so much I could not have imagined alone became manifest together. Nothing is possible without love, of the work, of one another. Everyone, alive and dead, in this grove together thought the same, that we must, against all odds, against the awful commerce, the madness for money and destruction that dominates and crushes all that lives, create. Visions of life through communal acts. That we must make work and share it, like ashes scattered to the wind, as useless, perhaps, impossible that any lasting structure might result. Nothing but ash, nothing but love, insubstantial things, have we to give, to offer, to give of ourselves and finally give ourselves running through the fingers of others to the earth. Nothing but our visions, in words or puppets, with actors, with music, with joy.

That we have lived this way. That I lived this way with George. That George and Peter, over sixty years, worked together and apart to tell the same story, the story of the earth, our rightful place on earth, our pledge not to destroy, not to grasp, nor hate, but to create.

Chapter Three:
There Is No God of Grief

The Greek word for grief is *thlipsi*, but there is no god of grief in Greek mythology. We know grief through the mourners: Orpheus, who births music from his sorrow; Demeter, who smites the world with famine in her rage; and there is Pentheus (*pathos*), whose mother rips him apart, limb by limb, rejoicing, thinking she has killed a lion, and must endure the terrible recognition of what she's done. As if grief cannot exist separately from the one who has lost, who is lost, who wanders disconsolate. Grief snatches the griever surely as any supernatural force, and drags us unwillingly into places we have not been, or did not dare go with other losses before, but must now, now that the burden is too great and smites us hard. Grief changes us, utterly, and can kill. I thought that the intensity of the loss that I was feeling might unleash my own fatal illness; I hoped so, triggering those cancer cells lying dormant in us all, that two years from then I might be dead. I had heard of this happening to other widows who loved and I welcomed the thought. I thought wistfully of *Sati*, the Indian rite in which the widow immolates herself on her husband's funeral pyre, too late. George was cremated directly after his funeral, and the first full intensity of my sorrow did not hit until six months after he died.

Though I could not believe I would reunite with George in an afterworld in which I do not believe, and bridled when anyone suggested such an outlandish thing, my death would bring relief from pain and the storm of inchoate feelings, my relentless sleeplessness, night after night lying trembling awake in bed without any coherent thought, shuddering in terror. If finally, I fell into a dreamless sleep like death, I woke shrieking my sorrow, the puppy trembling at my side. "Don't hurt the dog," I said inside my head, "please, don't hurt the dog," speaking to the agonized one, not me, but all that remained of who I once had been. Nor could I eat. Nor read. Nor watch mindless TV. Nor go anywhere where people might be. There was no distraction. No relief as I tumbled deeper into a well of grief.

There were people who remembered how I used to be, but those people were not me. When I heard from my oldest friend, "You had a life before George. You will have a life after George," I felt betrayed. Even if the first part were true, I was nothing now, and had no life beyond this grief.

I had been strong for so long; what happened? I felt snatched, taken, dragged into an underworld dark and dank. I felt unknown to myself, a sorry stranger, a suppliant. I felt every slight or hurt intensely. I felt wronged, but I could not take comfort from anyone, though comfort was offered by close friends and family. Isolate. I would cry and shriek. At any moment, scenes from our long medical nightmare would appear sharply in my head. Blood, urine, and shit. A needle piercing his stomach. While we both cried, "No!" too late. George moaning in agony on our floor after that final Darzalex shot. Golden liquid in the catheter bag. His arms black and blue from the never-ending search for a vein. His lovely stomach, distended, once I had stroked, where once I had lain my head, there just where stomach met leg, in his groin, grown too tender to be touched. The tube shoved down his nose while I held his hands tight on his chest. The black juices bubbling up. The catheter tube threaded into his urethra and pulled out pushed, again, into his wounded penis, swollen and flaccid. The agonies George suppressed and, at the end, moaned under. I would wake shaking and screaming, feeling what he felt.

I could go numb. I could sometimes mercifully fall into deep sleep as if I had no unconscious self. As if dead. Waking came as a shock. Life an alien state. I did not know how to propitiate Grief, what to offer to appease the devourer, who like the companion ancient deity Eros to whom Grief is most intimately related and without whom there can be no grief, is relentless, immoderate, unthinking, demanding, and dangerous. But there is no such deity, standing unto itself. There is no Grief god to propitiate, there is only the lover who has lost their love.

Early in the afternoon of the day George died, his doctor responded to the text, "he's gone," I'd sent him at 2:08 am. He asked how I was. "How could you be," he added. "I feel I did what I had to do to fulfill the promise of how we lived. The hard part is yet to come," I replied. The morning of the night George died, I knew that much, but nothing more. Grief had not yet emerged from the shadow of death, and grief would take the next six months to fully show itself. Feeding off itself, grief grew stronger. I was, for the immediate moment, and for the few months to follow, until the memorials were over, in a state of shock. I was in a manic phase. Highly, compulsively functioning as I planned first his funeral-cremation ceremony, then the scattering of his ashes, then his public event. The need to memorialize drove me. As long as I could represent his life and his death publicly, I was focused and sure. I was caring for George. The intrusive medical images I could not escape drove me to do more, to feel more superhuman—perhaps as doctors feel, after all, and like them, I was often arrogant.

I was driven to write at all hours of the night and day, and I had a bizarre, egomaniacal sense that I was writing brilliantly, as if I were on speed, page after unread page. The writing at 5 am, puppy-dog walking at 3 am, 6 am, and again at 8, the many long walks at all hours of day and night, unconscious sleeps in the afternoon, churning out words, an endless agitation kept me going. Through October 1, the date of his public memorial at LaMama, there was the necessary work of reading through and editing his last diaries, planning who would speak and the order of the event. I had taken the semester off from teaching. Immersed in his memory, I felt my life had purpose. I still could care for him.

I had been shocked into superhuman mode by the months of increasing high intensity caregiving, and my increasing intimacy with the bodily functions of the man I loved, the glowing urine, the tender penis, which sometimes I let my tongue stroke, or my cheek touch. My intimacy with every aspect of George's death. On his last day of life, I had put my hand between his legs to feel if I needed to clean him; instead of diarrhea, a white viscous liquid stuck to my fingers, about which a nurse and his doctor said different things, but was clearly a sign of his imminent death. I picked up his leg then; it was no longer stiff, but completely limp. I knew he would die within hours. Like someone in a long, losing war against death, I was going berserk, a phrase used to describe soldiers in the thick of battle who suddenly feel invincible, who begin firing wildly, flinging themselves head-first into danger. I was immune to human frailty, as I wiped his bottom those last days, orchestrated visitors, listened to their stories of our past adventures, and laughed with them, sitting next to George on our bed. I was ALIVE. So was he.

With George dead, I called all the shots. I was bold enough to bar people from the private funeral outside in a public cemetery, people I did not like or thought did not like me, people who had ignored us during George's long illness, and now wanted to be present to take part in my intimate mourning. I forbad the first wife and the seventeen relatives she wanted to bring—after she demanded to see George's will and his death certificate the day he died. I told a couple we knew but about whom I had a strange feeling, not to come. And they fired back. "We loved George but we never liked you," in a long, ugly email. This was a joke we had, George and I, "everyone loves you," I would say, "and everyone hates me." It was not entirely untrue. For the past several years, I had handled all the producing aspects of our theater, and I got into all the inevitable quarrels with unions, with artists. Whatever was self-centered, opinionated, and abrasive about my personality, I gave full rein to it now. After all, no one had been through what I had, seen my love out of this world. Like the battle-crazed warrior, I had walked through the valley of the shadow of death and emerged unscathed. Like the soldier with PTSD who flies off the handle at the slightest loud noise, who terrorizes family and friends, so I demanded my will be done.

I'd been in a Zoom grief group for a few weeks. A woman said, "You are doing so much, when do you have time to grieve?" I left the group in a huff. She was right. I was outrunning grief, but like any other marathoner, I would have to stop. I was still living with George as long as I nurtured his memory publicly, on Facebook and with the ceremonies, as long as I was writing furiously in the middle of the night. I was still living his final days. I was still keeping him from harm, enhancing and guarding his legacy. I was fighting off grief. But I had not even glimpsed my adversary yet.

George had a far more balanced temperament than I. "Let it go," he would say. Or "Just keep going," when we did not know how to produce a play, where or with what money. But now, I could let nothing go. I had to maintain control, especially since my actual life was only the chaos of his loss. George, who had been raised in poverty in New York City, nevertheless had the equanimity of the entitled, educated European gentleman he would have been had Hitler not come to power. I was raised in upper middle-class comfort on Chicago's North Shore, but I was my peasant father's daughter, or a shtetl Jew, argumentative, radical, like my mother's Russian side, and when in a heightened state of coping, which both George and I knew well from our work in theater, he would retreat into reflection and I would take action, wrong or right. I would fight, and weep. He would murmur, "Rest perturbed spirit," and hold me close. There was no one to hold me now.

The night George died, I sent death notices out to an email list, including his family in Germany, and I emailed the managing editor of the *New York Times*, whom we knew. He assigned the obituary to a former theater critic, who, nevertheless, had not heard of George. As he researched my husband's life, he became impressed. "Why," he emailed me, hadn't George chosen the commercial career that could have been his, "Why, he might have had a recurring role as a judge on *Law and Order?*" (Like every New York actor, George was on plenty of episodes of *Law and Order*, where he played judges, lawyers, and a Nazi in a wheelchair.) "George wanted to change the world," I wrote back, "and he knew *Law and Order* was same old, same old. It was as simple or foolish as that." Yes, it was. Had he been foolish or wise, had we been? It was too late, now, to change one thing.

I had hoped to bury George in a plain wooden casket in the Bread and Puppet Memorial Grove in Glover, Vermont, where Peter buried his wife Elka the summer before. However, only those who own the land are entitled to burial on private property. Besides, George's body would need to be transported by train, at some cost, and who would follow us from New York to the Northeast Kingdom? So, I found on the internet, quite by random, the undertaker who had handled the green burial of eco-activist and writer, Joel Kovel, whom I knew by reputation. The undertaker recommended a ceremony at nearby and beautiful Greenwood Cemetery (where decades ago, before the grounds were landmarked and restored, before I knew George, I entered through an opening in the broken fence and walked over the tumbled gravestones while pregnant). George would be cremated after the service and I would take his ashes to Vermont. We were not, either of us, in the least observant, but for some reason, I felt that speed was of the essence and that George should be buried, cremated, rather, two days after his death. The funeral was by invitation and, therefore, would be small—in fact, word spread and many, many people showed up.

The undertaker arrived at the house the morning George died, and with a brief prayer, oversaw the removal of George's body from our home. I had not washed George, nor had I removed his catheter. I had simply forgotten to do these things. "You didn't want to hurt him, anymore," his psychotherapist would tell me about the catheter. Perhaps. Why I did not wash his flesh, I did not know. I hadn't thought. Perhaps, if I had had a woman beside me. Someone from hospice, a death doula, to help, to offer warm water and a soft sponge. But there was no one with me but his grieving son.

The funeral under a canopy of trees in Greenwood Cemetery on a blistering hot early August morning was officiated by our close friend, Jan. Though a wonderful poet, she chose a poem by Joy Harjo to read. The doctor arrived on his bicycle in a black suit, sweating in the bitter heat. He said one sentence I barely heard, something about working together with me to keep George alive, and he sat down. I thought he would have gone on for a while, eulogizing George. I was surprised. He had taken the day off work to come. George's granddaughter, Briana, read the poem she had written overnight: "It is so lovely to be an Actor/ in the play we call Earth … It is the greatest part to play/In the final Act of bringing all that you can bring/ What a lovely thing/To finally become everything." Was he now, in fact, a nature god, as he would have most loved to become? Was he everywhere, everything? Who knew? His stepchild, Carrie Sophia, read Rilke's Eighth Elegy, the poem George had read at his brother's funeral, and I read at the grave of our first cocker spaniel. "With its whole gaze/ a creature/ looks out at the open, But our eyes/ are as though turned in/ and they seem to set traps/ all around it/ as if to prevent/ its going free …" Our friend Ynestra read a selection from the last poem he heard, "Ode to the West Wind," and asked the question "how does one make a man like George?" "His mother," I raised my voice to say from my seat in the first row, seated next to George's doctor, whose knee I squeezed. I read for George his favorite pond speech from my play *Extreme Whether* that he had been rehearsing the day his voice cracked. "This is for you, darling," I said as I touched his coffin and stepped to the microphone. It was so hot and the sun was so bright. Our friend, Christen, burst from the crowd and flung herself onto the coffin, unannounced, in Irish Catholic, and performance-art fashion, to shriek, "George, George," and improvise her eulogy. There was Joan Baez, "There but for Fortune Go Your or I," Paul Robeson's "Shenandoah," Pete Seeger's "We Shall Overcome," during which some of us joined hands and sang. We moved his coffin into the waiting station wagon for its slow trip down the hill. I have no memory after that. Did I walk alone? Yes. By myself, I made my way down the hill. How did I let the coffin go by itself into the crematorium without throwing myself on top? But I was determined not to show my emotions in public. I had people coming to the house. I had to act my part. The gracious, accomplished widowed person. It was as if I blanked out. I could not have stood it if I understood what I had done, if I had walked that last road with him. Sent his body into the oven. I veered off before, got inside Patrick's waiting car. His doctor followed him the entire way, to the crematorium.

In early September, I traveled to Vermont, driven by Patrick along with Nesta and Michal, who was producing George's October public memorial at LaMama, to scatter George's ashes in the Bread and Puppet Memorial Grove. With Michal and Cindy Rosenthal, who would emcee, I coordinated readers and speakers and I planned the order of events, their rising and falling, the comic interludes and climactic scene, George's Angel Speech, as if I were creating a play, and, indeed, it played well. The October memorial was held in the big, high-roofed Ellen Stewart Theater. George had been "a darling" of Ellen's. One whom she never refused. He had acted in her theaters many times. I wrote the speech I would deliver, and read it out-loud to myself at least twenty times. Until I could read it through without tears. I refused to cry in public. I did not want to detract from memories of George. I selected parts from his "Brig Log" and a long section from his diaries to be read by actors with whom we had worked, Tommie Moore, Kathleen Chalfant, Rocco Sisto. I chose the video excerpts of George in *I Will Bear Witness, Another Life,* and *Blue Valiant,* three such different roles. Some of his favorite moments and mine. JoAnne Akalaitis read a selection from *Cymbeline*. George had played the King in her production at the Public Theater. A production that was wonderfully inventive and alive, and hated by the critic from the *New York Times*, but which Joe Papp loved and was the reason Joe appointed JoAnne to his place once he died. Many of our collaborators spoke. George's son, Alex, read George's diary entries he selected and his granddaughter Briana again read her poem to George. Over two hundred people gathered that day, his two nieces from different states, students of his and mine I had not seen in years, one of our yoga teachers, old friends we'd lost track of. The memorial was a "success," I was told. It gave a rich, full picture of his life. After any production closes, though this only ran for one afternoon, there comes always the crash.

Alone with my puppy, I broke down, finally. I woke from deep, dreamless sleeps, screaming wildly. I wailed. I could not bear it. I was so grief stricken. Then, I'd fall back into a dreamless sleep like death. I woke terrified to find myself alive. And during the worst of this time, the worst of my sleepless nights and uncontrollable shrieking, my puppy ran away from me three times in Fort Greene Park where we went every morning, sometimes as early as six am, to wander during off-leash hours. I roamed the park like Demeter roaming the earth, crazed by what I lost, my little dog, so dear to me, now, hollering madly, "Percy, come, Percy, come," until the entire park went on alert, and people relayed their sightings and some kind person or another managed to catch my puppy somewhere and walk him back to me. One friend found him crossing DeKalb Avenue, a certain death, but she grabbed him in in the middle of the road. Many mornings in the park, completely distraught, I broke down weeping and shaking in the arms of people I barely knew. I would walk up to strangers and say, "I just lost my husband." Usually, they were kind. Several are friends, now. The "healing circle" that formed around George fell away. The doctor was gone from my life. George's psychotherapist, whom I'd begged to remain counseling me, dropped me, abruptly, after six months, right before Christmas, for reasons of Freudian protocol. I was angry and bereft. I had no one to counsel me. Another of my front teeth broke off at the root in January, the day before I had to return to teach. A month into the new semester, the theater department was abruptly abolished without warning by the college, and though I was on a three-year contract, it would not be honored; I would lose my adjunct teaching job. So my personal loss was suddenly compounded by my lack of teaching work, and the extra income it brought, the structure and camaraderie teaching provided.

If I had been alert and unflinching, even bizarrely cheerful, as George and I edged toward the end of the earth, if I had been overly confident and confrontational in the early months after his death, I was hopeless and terrified now. I taught in a monotone. Before teaching days, my sleepless nights were especially fraught. I wept and screamed in the early mornings. I dragged myself first to the park with my pup, then to the subway and in to school, exhausted. My brother came in February for a few days and found me crying and yelling in sorrow and pain. Unable to form a coherent thought or make a plan. He was kind. He held me carefully while I shrieked. We walked and walked. When he left, after a week, I fell deeper into pain. Grief felt impenetrable, unstoppable, unbearable. George was gone from me utterly. I was alone, depleted and frightened. I thought about suicide. My friend Nesta, also living alone, called me every night. Every night I seemed worse. Unable any longer to write, still unable to read, too tired to think, unable to rest. I joined a new grief group at the behest of my friend, Paula, whose husband had died two months before mine. Now that I had crashed, I showed up on Zoom, haggard, wasted, incoherent; the group members who did not know me at all evidenced concern and fear. I was clearly in a desperate state. The group leader, an Orthodox Jewish nurse, a widow, caring for her mother with dementia, urged antidepressants, which most in the group were on, but I was not ready yet to try. She suggested I go to a dog training class with other people, which I managed to do and which Percy liked. He stopped running away and learned recall. The pup was the only comfort I had. His devotion the only love.

My friend Charlotte, co-founder of Brooklyn for Peace and a retired pediatrician, called me, and, surprised to find me so alone, began to visit me almost daily. I was worse, day by day. Worn and weak, sleepless, I thought of committing myself to a psychiatric institution and begged for her help. I wanted someone to take care of me. On a Sunday, Charlotte's physician husband drove us uptown to the branch of the big hospital where he was still teaching, though he had just retired from practice, and which had a psych ward. We hoped the psychiatric doctor on duty could prescribe something for me. But they are forbidden to prescribe, unless you commit yourself.

"Take off all your jewelry," this from one of the two armed guards looming. I comply, taking off necklace and rings. I am being criminalized. On the cots in the aisle are women naked under loose hospital gowns, swearing, screaming, kvetching. "Drug overdoses," the young psychiatric doctor contemptuously says, "you want to be with them?" If this is what passes for mental health care, I will go without. I reclaim my jewelry from the plastic cup. I am not going to get undressed, sit naked under a thin gown, loosely tied, with armed guards prowling the hall. Then be sent to a psych ward. Since a doctor "gently" abused me as a child, and another when I sought a cervical cap in graduate school stuck his finger unceremoniously, without warning, up my ass, I have had a horror of male doctors and have mainly avoided their touch. Charlotte's husband had gone to his office and he returns, now, wearing his white doctor's coat with his nametag clipped to the pocket. He moves in close to the young psych doctor and he asks, fraternally, for his advice. If I were to be admitted what would the psychiatrist prescribe? "Ativan." Charlotte, Ollie, and I walk back to his office where he writes a prescription by hand as, since his retirement, he no longer has access to the computer system. We drive to the local Brooklyn pharmacy we think most likely to fill a paper script. Charlotte stays with me while we wait. Ollie waits in the car. I swallow my first Ativan. They take me to their house for the afternoon. After being sleepless for weeks, I finally fall asleep on the bed in their spare room. I began to take Ativan every night, though it is addictive.

With sleep, I begin to think about how to deal with my grief. I need help, but of what sort? During my intake Zoom interview with Jewish Family Services, the young Orthodox therapist tells me about her grandmother who lost her great love and says to me about George, "You know you will see him again." I want to scream, what sort of nonsense is she spouting. Talk therapy with the young therapist she assigns me feels useless. She is in training and much too young to understand. "Loving Karen" or "processing your grief" sound like empty platitudes from textbooks. I have no idea how to do such things. Besides, I don't want to do them. I want to die. And, besides that, I don't want to be like the others I've met in the grief groups online: glum and complaining for years after the death of their spouse. I want to go mad. Shriek. Rage. Only my growing puppy calms me, sleeping cuddled next to me, or as he is, right now, under my desk, his head resting gently on my bare foot. When I shake in bed, he lays his body over my chest, presses down, and stays there until I calm. Without this little dog, I'd be dead. The grief group leader keeps advising antidepressants. My new primary care physician, a woman, who is obviously concerned, discusses admittance to a psychiatric unit with me, again. Only my puppy saves me. I can't leave him. She renews my Ativan prescription and prescribes a sleep drug, but it does not work. She listens. I like her, but there is little she can do. She offers antidepressants. They would take a few weeks or months, even, to kick in. I am leery, I fill the prescription, but I don't take them.

My forty-something former neighbors whom I like very much—their third child was born during the pandemic on their bathroom floor, right next to our apartment door, then they moved down the street to a larger apartment—recommend psychedelics, ketamine and psilocybin mushrooms; everyone in their circle, their age, is doing them. Jeralyn is enormously kind and perceptive. She has just had both breasts removed to treat a bad cancer found early with her first mammogram, which she had on a whim just as she stopped breastfeeding. She lived downtown during and after the September 11 attacks, and that is her only risk factor, but it's enough; like everyone, she'd been told the air downtown was safe to breathe. It was not. "You have life inside you, I can see. You are not just your grief," she tells me. They hook me up with a psychotherapist who guides psychedelic experiences. Ivica is young and pretty, smart. I meet her on Zoom. She suggests I try ketamine, first, and then a mushroom trip. I have the antidepressants in my medicine cabinet; I could take them if I wished. But I make the mistake, still in my manic phase, of telling the grief group and the young therapist about my decision to use ketamine. The young therapist shares a note from her supervisor which states such experiences can be "fatal," and the grief group members respond by attacking me for insinuating, as I in fact had, that I don't wish to be hooked "like everyone else" on antidepressants. How arrogant I am. The single man in the grief group, who all the widows dote upon, turns on me so viciously that I leave the Zoom in a huff, and never return to the group. Slowly, I begin to try to wean myself off the life-saving Ativan before I become addicted.

Grief has me firmly in its grip. I had gotten some sleep, thanks to Ativan. Still unable to read a book, unable to concentrate, writing great quantities of incomprehensible prose, still barely getting through teaching my classes. Sleep deprived, screaming in sorrow into my pup's brown and white fur. The beautiful, devoted young dog licking my breasts in the morning, my one sensuous experience with another living being.

Grief demands I give more. Grief demands obeisance. I have to subjugate myself to Grief. I have to go through whatever Grief asks. I chose ketamine because I wish for an experience, perhaps to prove I still live. Grief has taken my life. I am crazed. I want insight. I don't wish to live as I am. I wanted an experience that would shock me back into feeling. I did not want to be numb. I was so alone. So afraid. I thought, perhaps, I could meet up with George in a vision, wherever he was, though I also did not believe he was anymore anywhere. My mind felt diminished. I could not stand the thought George was gone. Vanished. Atomized. Maybe the ketamine would allow him to show himself to me. Perhaps, I could have a vision of George. I turned to ketamine as people in the 19th century held a séance to contact their dead.

I do six ketamine trips with Ivica on Zoom. She plays music while I swirl the bitter pills in my mouth and spit my frothy saliva out into a cup. Each experience is a revelation and, for the first time, I feel the Grief that has frozen me nearly dead begin to loosen its grip. What I had to do was to give myself over to the experience of the sorrow I felt and to all the sorrows that had calcified so long underneath. How many of the tortured feelings I was having were pure grief, how much was the depression I had struggled with all my life, from my earliest awareness of myself as a sad child who didn't deserve to be acknowledged, now exacerbated by the loss of the person who loved me, as a parent might, unconditionally. Each ketamine trip showed me the tangle of my emotions in a visible way then dropped me back into the hot liquid tar of despair, but each trip evidenced I could claw my out for a while.

On my first trip, I see George, dressed in the gray, brown, black and white patterned French shirt I gave him when we first met, that he still wore and which hangs in my closet now. I feel his presence. I see many happy images like flipping through an old photo album of the many photos he took on our trips to Italy and our time at Ursula's magical castle, Civitela Ranieri. I am dressed in the wine and purple colors I wore then. Then, bang, I am hit with the depression. Closing night of the first New York production of *The Beekeeper's Daughter*. I am on stage with the cast, taking a bow, when the words come into my head, "Now I must kill myself." It had actually happened like that. The suicidal depression grabbed me like a claw from under the earth on closing night while I stood on the stage being applauded. I ruined the next production of the play by giving it over to a Croatian director who did not understand it, and by miscasting. Success led to disaster, a pattern. The depression slams into me. I stayed in bed for over a month, then. Did I ruin my life like this? (Years later, George told me he almost left me because I was so depressed, so difficult to be with, and he felt so helpless. If I helped him die, he stayed with me, then, to help me live.)

Ketamine trip number four is a turning. I have wanted to find George in the other world. I have wanted to see if I could get myself there sometime soon. Instead, he comes to me. I watch him bend and contort to fit his pretzel frame into the space just behind my heart. He manages to climb inside. I can consult. I can hear him say, "just let it go," or "just keep going." I can feel his warmth and his love. "I love you badly, madly, but not sadly," he used to croon. This is not the vision I longed for. I had wished to find him in the afterworld, whatever that is. This vision of George inside me ties me here to this earth. It is not being lost in him, but his being inside me. He has not left me entirely. He is not entirely gone. He is no longer completely absent. I will live as a hermit if I must, with a dog at my feet and George inside my heart. On ketamine trip number five we fly. We are two crows, going fast, dipping low over the earth, birds of prophecy—like the owl he turned himself into in my play. And for the first time in weeks, I can sleep without taking Ativan, the anti-anxiety drug I've become hooked on, again. On ketamine trip number six I find us together in Greece, when during a swim after our trip to Dephi, George stepped on a sea urchin. His foot thick with spines. I hold him close while Lydia removes the spines one by one. It happened like that. "Baby George," I sometimes called him. The old man who never grew up and kept all his life the sudden charm of an impish boy. He is inside me, now. This is what I learned from the ketamine.

There remains the psychedelic, mushroom-induced trip. Ivica arrives at my house with an energy healer, dressed in white, carrying a drum and Tibetan bowl that hums. They bring lilacs, lavender, and sage. It is May. I have a play, *Troy Too*, in rehearsal, but have barely been able to attend to its many demands and crises of personnel and funds. The director Avra, from Greece, is staying in my house. She is lovely; we've become friends. It is good have someone staying here, with me, though I asked her to leave for the day. The day after, Lydia will arrive from Greece, at Newark airport. She called while George lay dying. She has been rehearsing on Zoom from Greece with the American cast while she finishes shooting her television show. Now, it is one week before our New York opening. She arrives tomorrow in person to play the modern Hecuba, a homeless woman, in my short verse play about COVID, Climate Change and Black Lives Matter, which Avra has published in her book, *Staging Twenty-First Century Tragedies*. It would be nice if I were able to function.

"The energy here is very pure," the energy healer says; immediately I am relieved, what if she'd said "impure," what could I have done about that, but she did not and I'm anyway distrustful of such blah, blah. The energy here is what it is. How we lived. They bring me the chocolate-flavored mushrooms, of which I ingest many. I had tripped in my youth, LSD and psilocybin. I had had visions. I had seen the trees dancing and the rocks gyrating. I'd come down from these trips feeling a living-breathing member of Gaia, knowing we are alive in a living world and should stop the Vietnam war. This was the social context—the war, the deaths, the assassinations. We tripped, to find the alternative vision. Alive in a living universe. Where all is holy. "Holy, holy," Allen Ginsberg wrote, "holy the cock of the grandfather in Kansas, and we'd sung his words, and mine answering him, "holy the cunt of the grandmother ..." at the Living Theatre Seders. One night, when Julian was alive, Allen suddenly opened the door, just like the Messiah, and stood chanting "Holy" with us.

This day, ten months after George died, I feel devoid of communal surround. Isolate in grief as I've been for so long, so alone. It's not entirely true. I have friends, a small family, a dog; I have a play in rehearsal, in which the speech of the Talking Fish George recorded almost three years ago will be heard. George will act posthumously. He would like that. He and Lydia always wanted to act together; now they will. She will respond to the Talking Fish projected on the wall, as if George, the Fish's voice, were actually there. I like the speech very much, and the production is coming along well. Lydia will stay in my apartment with me as she once stayed with us in the big house. Then, she, George and I spoke endlessly of Greek theater. Then, I was happy, but now I am isolate; desolate is a better word. No one I know understands. Most are terrified. Some have withdrawn.

Ivica brings me more of the chocolate-flavored cubes. There is some ritual drumming by the energy healer, Barbara, a bit of an echo as she rubs the rim of the Tibetan bowl. There is the usual crystal, of course. The admonitions to "let go." I am resisting because I already know, the phrase has already hit me on the inside of my head, "this is an unbearable grief but it must be borne," as if spoken by someone else. *Unbearable*, finally, the word has been said, the problem is clear. I am bearing the unbearable weight of unbearable grief. This is why I seem unable to feel, to react, to experience anything. I'm weighted down by an unbearable grief which nevertheless has to be borne. I'm terrified. I will fall apart if I confront the full weight of this unbearable grief. I will be crushed. (Falling apart is what I've been doing: thinking of suicide, sleep deprived, shrieking ...). Despite the relief of holding George inside, small George inside my chest, where I often rest my hand as I walk, and speak to him, often out loud. I babble as I walk, to George or to the puppy. But mainly I walk alone with my dog on empty sidewalks at odd times.

What does it mean: a trip to the underworld? *Unbearable grief* is where I am going. That much is clear to me from the start. I'm resisting. Who wants to go there? Only love, only love drags us down, Demeter, Orpheus descending, but I'm not a god or a mythic character. I'm a broken woman, a nonentity, invisible. Carrying a grief that is unbearable. I cannot survive such a trip. I am stuck, completely reluctant to begin the necessary descent; there is no way out but through, so I sit immobile on the couch while the healers ply me with quantities of chocolate-flavored mushrooms. My little insightful dog, Percy, is resistant, too. Though he comes from a line of Romantics. Did the original Percy trip? Undoubtedly and with Byron and Mary Shelley, no doubt. This Percy decides to put his body between me and the effects of the shrooms. He lies on my stomach, reinforcing my resistance as I half lie, half sit on the couch, staring straight ahead into the abyss. He is not going to let me go anywhere at all. He gets it. I am looking in my slightly nearsighted way at a blurry collection of photos of George in some of his favorite roles in my plays, crowded together on the top of his mother's inlaid roll top desk, relic of her haute Prussian-Huguenot past. It is handsome but worthless. George once had it appraised; it would cost more to fix its broken parts than it is worth.

For a moment, this desk on its crooked, spindly legs begins to gyrate, a small dance, like the mother to whom it belonged, a spidery dancer, a healer, willowy, the "iron butterfly" her students called her. But the desk fails to leap. It settles down, back into its elegant rickety self; it will not fall apart. This is to be a visionless trip. The underworld is dark, dank, without discernible shapes, empty, vast. I might not survive it. I sit here eating more mushrooms, going nowhere. But I will not survive if I do not descend. I also know. I will remain dead to life, as I have been. A grief unbearable, yet I must bear it.

I do not know, were I to make this dreadful descent, if I could ever come back, but if I do not go where I am bid, I will remain as I am, unbearable even to myself. *A grief unbearable yet it must be borne,* the phrase is all that

I hear, over and over, a voice speaking in my head, from where, the depths of my grief, or from outside of me, an oracular voice from the underground calls. I will go bitter, deformed through the rest of my days, if I do not follow this call. I begin to cry. The energy healer has taken my pup outside for a long walk. She thinks he's been keeping the mushrooms from taking effect, and perhaps so. I cannot move from the couch. I'm frightened, in fact. *A grief that cannot be borne.* Born, perhaps, from me, carried to term, splaying me open in order to live. I know how difficult it is to give birth, how much is demanded in the act, and to give birth to unbearable grief—who in their right mind would wish to do that? Hence, the psychedelic push may be of necessity. I would never do this myself. Gone. Mad, perhaps. People do lose their minds on drugs. But, if I do not take the chance, go where I am bid, I am as if entombed, never to have felt what I could not feel—a grief impossible to bear, that must be borne, and born, externalized. I weep, quietly. I see nothing, nothing for four long hours. The salt tears roll down my cheeks. I cannot stop crying. The underworld exists. I am wandering there, but it is impenetrable. I cannot see in the dark. Through the dankness, I wander, distracted, alone. But I feel my feelings, and unbearable grief is working through me, unbearable, yes. I am terrified. Too frightened to move. I weep silently. No wonder I have gone mad. No wonder I wake shrieking in the early morning, the puppy with me in the bed, howling my rage into the unfair world absent my love, alone but for Percy and the mice who seem to have invaded. George died and all of a sudden, we have mice. I hear them scurrying through the walls. "Don't hit the dog," I murmur as I wail into his fur—and I don't—perhaps, he'll survive the sorrow he absorbs. "Don't hurt the dog," I could not tolerate myself if I did that. The innocent pup who comforts me when I wake screaming.

I do not find George under the earth. I do not take his hand. I do not look back. I find only darkness. I see no illuminating image. No voice echoes through the cavernous space, calling to me. I find no source of wisdom. But the instructions remain clear, you must go down, to the center, where there is nothing but sorrow, unendurable. And endure it.

I weep and I wander in the dark. George is nowhere. He has vanished completely into the universe. He is not down here where I have been sent by his death. Here, where there is no comfort. People say (not me) the dead "are in a better place." I would never say that. I don't believe it and I don't believe them when they say it. I don't believe they believe it themselves. As I descend, I encounter only the weight of my loss, in the darkness. I know Ivica, first, and now, Barbara, have seated themselves on cushions nearby. I know that Percy sometimes lies on my chest. Sometimes licks the tears that run down my face. Sometimes sits away from me, on the far side of the room, head on his paws, watching. I know myself to be alone in what I am enduring, yet I feel myself being seen. My grief cannot be shared, lifted, or comforted, but it can be witnessed. I know I will never find George under the earth. He is gone from me. Utterly. I am not Orpheus, nor is he Eurydice. I am not Demeter, goddess of agriculture; I have no power. There will be no sudden delight. My beloved's hand, briefly in mine. I will not hear his voice before it cracks.

I am wandering through grief for four long hours. I am bearing the unbearable—the weight of my feelings. I had not known I could do this thing, as I had not known I could have lain with him in our bed while he died, or put my hand into his gritty ashes and scattered them to the wind in the Bread and Puppet memorial grove. I did not know, and could not have done. I feel the terror wrenching through me, the horror of loss, fear of utter aloneness, without love. It's not so much not being loved but not being able to love that I fear. I let the sorrow wash over and through me.

The grief had been an external thing, a weight, and now I have let it inside. It had to be borne and born. I had to give myself over as if giving birth to a child, perhaps, giving birth to a new self, myself as container of my grief, which before had battered and sought to slay me. I had not just to walk through but to walk within. The grief had to become part of my blood and bone. It had been weighing me down, battering me from without, now it has had to become who I am and remain, a woman bereaved. I will never not have lost my love.

I had not known I could live and grieve at the same time. Now, I do. The grief is in no way diminished by having experienced it so fully. It is not to be borne, no grief is, yet I am bearing it—as the living must do.

The two women sat with me for hours and did nothing; alongside a dog, they attended. All eyes were on me the entire time. This is what it means to be witnessed. If I died, if my heart stopped as I thought it might from the exertion of grief, I would not be alone. They would come to me and smooth my bent and frozen limbs, curled into myself as I was, immobile. Weeping silently on the couch. They would have seen, and they did see. Wordless, attending. An ageless ritual in which women have sat by the mourner, not offering comfort, but silent accompaniment.

When I ascended, when the underworld was done with me and coughed me up, I found myself ravenously hungry on the living room couch, with the two women and the puppy dog in attendance. The day before I'd made a large pot of bean soup. I offered it. Soon enough, I found myself sitting cross-legged on the couch, eating soup, laughing and talking. It was like that; I found myself where I was not hours before. Here, in this room, now. They had witnessed where I'd gone and needed scant explanation. I felt "myself" suddenly; the self I had been when George was alive. My voice had returned to its fullness. I was breathing deeply. When I next spoke to my daughter, she said, with enormous relief, "Mom, you are back." I had not known she had been so frightened, her mother gone. I had not been able to know anything about the effect I had on anyone else. I had been cut off from life by grief and could inflict only my suffering on those around me. A wonder so many remained so kind, so staunchly loyal. No wonder grief isolates.

It seems odd to say I carry a grief that enriches my life, but I think this is so. How distant I was from people who mourned—in my past life—how much more aware I've become, kinder, perhaps, some days. If I live up to the standards of the new self I found underground, I hope I can say this is so.

I had not thought I could grieve and live, and since I had to make the choice, I chose grief—and begged for death. Or, rather, I had been claimed by my sorrow. And, in fact, I could not live and grieve, both at once, until my trip to the underworld, the very interior of my loss. I must carry what is mine, his loss, without George. He never knew the person I am now—grieving him. Sometimes, walking the dog, I put my hand on my heart where he is and I say, "You fucking bastard, you went and left me alone." I can hear his laughter. Ever since the turning, that fourth ketamine trip when George bent and distorted his beautiful body struggling to become small enough to fit inside my chest, I am able to hold him as close I ever held him while he lived, when photo after photo shows us leaning into each other, looking into each other's eyes.

The weight that could not be borne is a depth I have traveled. George's death, private, at home, outside the medical system, without "benefit" of absent hospice care, was ritualized. We managed, family and friends, to surround him his final week, to retell at his bed the adventures we shared, his eyes alive with remembrance. He opened his arms in embrace. Now, my grief had also been ritualized without doctrine or creed. I had been witnessed, held. I went to the underground and returned—the epic mythical journey.

There was a great economy to the psychedelic trip. One afternoon, frozen on my couch, I traversed the unknown terrain of my grief. It was long, lonely, and terrifying. No doubt, many have walked there before me, held in communities across continents and centuries. No, I did not think I could do it. I feared I would not live through it were I to experience the full weight of my sorrow. I remember my trip to shul with Judith, on Shavuot. How she wailed, fell to the ground, beat her fists. How we women circled her, not interfering, watching. "She will have a good year; she is getting it all out," the anonymous witnesses spoke. Ritual culture. We cannot grieve in isolation, nor, I think, can we adequately grieve in conversation, not in grief groups or private therapy sessions. We need to be free of polite expectation. Wail, scream, cry, sit, immobile, for hours, eyes wide, unable to speak. Extremis needs be allowed. We are not to be calmed. We need to be let go. Grief demands we travel alone into the unknown. We enter a profound isolation when we grieve and must be let be, but we must be seen. Not comforted. Not judged. Not told to get on with it. Not given any of the platitudes. Not even told about what others have suffered. Not dismissed. Each person's way is profoundly solitary. Held in a communal gaze, others' eyes simply upon us, watching over, if we can find or create such a space in our frightened culture.

The next day, I met my Greek friend at the airport. Lydia will play a modern Hecuba, a homeless woman, in my play, *Troy Too*, in which George will also appear, through his voice, in the speech of the talking, plastic-engorged Fish. Lydia was coming to act with George. That had been their mutual wish. I was in the thick of rehearsal, again, and both the director and the leading actor were staying with the little dog, Percy, and me. Isolated all winter, we were glad to have a temporary family. The play became a success, a small production winning high praise. I found myself able to laugh. I bought a fitted, flaming red dress, and an orange and purple jacket. I carried with me my grief, unbearable, borne.

I had crafted this play, *Troy Too*, from found and imagined language at the height of the pandemic in 2020, coinciding with George Floyd's murder and the Black Lives Matter protests up our street. George and I heard the chants, put on our masks and hurried out of the house. Our fists in the air. Our voices rising. We were furious and exhilarated, out of lockdown, on the streets one more time for a cause in which we believed. He was "well" then, on cancer and heart medications, but able to go about, to protest, in Fort Greene Park where we sat with neighbors in silence for eight minutes and forty-six seconds, to the vigil at City Hall in downtown Brooklyn, where George, masked and wearing plastic gloves, took the knee. His fist in the air. In the winter of 2021, he recorded for Christen's then-online series "Experiments and Disorders" at Dixon Place, the tragicomic monologue of the talking Fish, an animal engorged with plastic remnants polluting the ocean, who bemoans his fate. "If I can't breathe, neither can you. That is the tragic irony. I'm just a Fish, get used to it." In *Troy Too*, the audience heard the many nuances of George's wonderfully malleable voice with which he endowed his Fish, a unique character, and I felt the terrible pleasure of hearing that voice once again, distorted though he made it, elongating words in a gravelly tone, "p-p—P—Plassss-tic, say the word."

"I can't breathe" is the recurring phrase in *Troy Too* that unites our common experiences of climate change, police murders, and the COVID pandemic. As Black audience members, as medical professionals, and students thanked me after the performance with tears in their eyes, I realized we are, perhaps, capable again of a shared ritual culture. The collective experience of COVID has led us into the ritual space, and, if so, we might be capable, too, of *Katharsis*, the Greek expression for having gained Clearer Sight through suffering. (Though the world has not gone this way; this is *still* the hope.)

The play was the next best momentary cure I found. It was a ritual mourning experience containing within it seeds of joy, of common feeling. Better, even, than ketamine or a trip to the underworld, was the collective theater experience. I was with my collaborators, again, actors and designers with whom George and I worked for decades.

I was now in remission, so to speak. The success of my play, Avra and Lydia living with Percy and me in the house. The warming weather drove grief into hiding. I cook for a large gathering on the year anniversary of George's death, his Yahrzeit. I have a candle burning. A religious friend with whom I'd lost touch told me he had been saying the Kaddish for George in shul every Shabbat the year through. I invite Jerome to say the Kaddish in our house. George's doctor comes to Yahrzeit gathering. We had agreed to disagree and had renewed our acquaintance, at least for now. I speak about George in front of my guests and I tell them laughing, that George was always losing everything, his hat, scarf, keys, his red-paper, taped wallet. But, I say, George never lost his sense of purpose. I read from a diary entry of his, I found in a small notebook, one of the many he left around the house:

> *Our species should be constantly reminded that we also are equally responsible to others than we. Together and individually, we ultimately contribute what we have to the community of our tribe but ultimately to the world because it turns the wheels of all of life in the wheel of the entire living organism called planet Earth. Each living creature helps to play the role so arrayed by Diversity.*

Jerome says the Kaddish in Aramaic. Alex recites it in English. I tell him, "When the son says the Kaddish for the father, the father's spirit enters the body of the son," a line I had heard from Schlomo Carlebach who officiated at Julian's gravesite. "To be hoped," Alex says with a smile. He had grown more open and gentle, like George, since he had attended George's death.

Three days later, I left for Greece. My brother and his wife Henriette joined us in Athens. We spoke often of George. Lydia and I continued our running conversation about Greek tragedy we'd begun, with George, in 1992, when she stayed in our big house. At night, in Greece, I slept soundly and my dream-life was rich. The last time I'd visited Lydia in Greece I had been with George, of course, and my thirteen-year-old daughter and her best friend, whose mother had recently died of cancer, and who joined us for our summer trip. That was when George stepped on the sea urchin. Lydia is one of Greece's most renowned classical actors, but she was also appearing on Greece's most popular television show and everywhere we went, people, especially young children, approached her, often for her autograph, calling out to her by her television name, "Margarita." During the pandemic, the Greek National Theater's production of *The Persians* was live-streamed around the world from the ancient theater in Epidaurus, a gift to a locked-down world population. Lydia played the Queen, and George and I watched her performance on my computer in Brooklyn; even so it was thrilling. In Greece, touring ancient sites, swimming in the sea, taking a horseback ride, I was prepared to think I was going to be fine. I'd come through the first year of grief, screeching at the wall. But, now, I was relaxed, and happy sometimes. What could go wrong but everything?

We went first to the ancient theater at Epidaurus, where we watched *Oedipus at Colonus*, the final play of the Oedipus cycle in which the old king who is most cursed becomes most blessed as he disappears into the ether. It is a sublime, unforgettable experience to watch any of the Greek tragedies in the ancient stone theater as the light fades, and this play about the death of the old king, a role that would have suited George, had special resonance. The next day, we drove to Eleusis, where, for a millennia-and-a-half, Greek-speaking initiates of all social classes celebrated the Mysteries to Demeter. The vision shared over centuries by all initiates was drug induced by a hallucinogen, ergot of barley, they drank before descending. Like my psilocybin trip, drugs were used, in community, to explore the mystery of death. Not one initiate in the thousands of years the Mysteries were celebrated *ever* revealed the sacred vision all witnessed in the underground cave to which they descended, but all who saw the ultimate mystery unfold before them returned to upper earth assured of their own blessings after death. Aeschylus was accused of revealing the mystery in his trilogy, *The Oresteia*; and he was put on trial, but acquitted. "Sing sorrow, sorrow, but let good win out in the end," is the ancient choruses' recurring refrain. And, perhaps, the experience of the shared, drug-induced vision was indescribable, and that is why no one ever revealed what it was. Or pitch black, like my trip to the underworld. And, perhaps, I was one more initiate over time into what cannot explained, "a grief unbearable that must be borne."

We drove across the Thessalian plain, where the small Athenian army once defeated the invading Persians, to Mt. Pelios, home of the satyr, where Lydia's two-room stone house stands on top of a peak above the Village of St. Georgios, of course. We hiked miles on the mountain tails, talked endlessly about ancient theater and modern life, continuing the discussion we'd begun with George decades earlier. At sunset, we swam in the Adriatic. We went to the museum at Volos where the goddess figurines with their upstretched arms excavated from gravesites date from centuries before the Eleusinian Mysteries, from the seventh century BC and earlier. We ate late dinners of fresh vegetables and fish outside with friends from the village. I was not alone and, as always, in Greece, I felt the resonance of the ancient ritual culture infusing every activity of daily life.

Then I came home.

The second year of grief hit me like a truck. Alone, but reunited with my pup who stayed with a live-in dog sitter and who, a neighbor assured me, missed me while I was gone. It was September, the month in which Julian and my father died, two days and some thirty years apart. I had two sections of environmental justice to teach and though I had taught the class many times, each semester the climate news was worse. Medicane Daniel, the huge storm that blew off the Mediterranean Sea, exacerbated by the hottest year the human world had yet known, struck Mt. Pelion and Thessaly, the rich agricultural land where I had just been. Lydia's small stone house almost slid down the mountain, saved only by roots from the trees that surround it. The storm ruined crops and killed 200,000 animals who floated, bloated, in the dirty water on the same Thessalian plain where once the Athenians repulsed the Persian invasion and saved their fragile democracy. The storm gained force, to devastate Libya, a poor country with bad government whose inhabitants were told to shelter in place while sea walls, dams and houses collapsed. Thousands drowned. I was teaching environmental justice students about this storm, as it happened.

There was no way out but through. Again, I was unable to sleep or to eat, and I started to shake. I would lie in bed for hours, too frightened and weak to get up or shower. I dragged myself into class and taught climate collapse, all too resonant, in a barely audible voice. At home, the pup and I were alone but for my friends Jerry and Jan, with whom Percy and I walked and walked through Brooklyn parks and streets, often when I could not speak. I wept. I shrieked. I was losing weight. I developed the upper respiratory infection that was going around and a hacking cough that got worse over months. I coughed hardest in bed, but I could not get up for days on end. The bed I shared with George, the bed where he died, was the only place that felt safe. I lay trembling at its outer edge, on stale sheets I was too weak to wash. The boiler broke, flooding the living room, and had to be replaced, at considerable cost. Again, the pup cuddled with me, or lay on top of my belly, while I coughed and wailed. "I'd be dead without this dog," I said to myself again and again.

Then came the massacre of October 7, and Israel's endless retaliation began. Each day brought more sorrow and pain to people I did not know but whose grief I could understand. "I cannot go through another war without George," I screamed to myself. Then as the violence intensified, "Perhaps, he's lucky not to have lived to see this." George hated the concept of the chosen people. "Either we all are chosen or no one is," he said. I dragged myself to demonstrations and vigils calling for an immediate ceasefire but I was afraid to be in a crowd, and, shaking, I would have to leave. Sally Ann Parsons, our costume designer for decades, came with me to a public reading from selections of my plays to mark the War Resister's League 100th Anniversary. I was thin and bent, my clothes hung on my frame, my voice stuck in my throat, a public display of a woman in grief, but people were kind.

Sally Ann's therapist agreed to take me on. For the first time, I was able to speak to an accomplished woman my age who had been happily married to a man she admired, and widowed, now, for seven years. "The second year of grief is the worst," she told me, confirming the massive pain I was feeling, "the first year you are the center of attention, by the second year, people expect you to get on with it, but you just now experience the reality of being truly alone." Ruth gave me permission not to "get better" but to feel my feelings. To weep and shriek, lie in bed, to suffer. She was the first person I'd met who did not expect me to heal—until, and unless, I felt everything I needed to feel—a grief that was devastating. Unbearable, but to be borne. In the dog park, I broke down in a Black woman's arms who has a dog named Treasure (we often know the dogs' names, not people's) and she held and comforted me. Damond and his wife, Loyda, close dog-park friends, Jehovah's Witnesses, helped me take George's clothing to Goodwill. But the experience of packing his clothing drove me into hysteria. I called my old friend, Martha, a professor, therapist, and human rights worker, who stayed with me on the phone as I stuffed his clothing into bags, keeping only a few costume pieces from his Victor Klemperer and the first shirt I'd given to him. At the holidays, I visited family; saw my daughter, my grandsons, my brother, John, and his wife and met their friends. And slowly, over months, the therapy began to help; the kindness of strangers, of my small dog, family and friends, began to work. I gave a dinner party on what would have been George's ninety-first birthday, for six people, including George's son and granddaughter. I decided to help Brianna fund her first play, in the memory of her grandfather, who had been so proud of her. I asked other people to donate to Brianna's production in George's memory and they did. I could feel how happy this would have made him, because he was inside me, and that made me happy. Memorializing in these ways was a balm. I attended vigils for a Ceasefire in the freezing cold, outside a congressional office and at the Irish Hunger Memorial. I donated to a Palestinian relief fund. I joined Jewish Voice for Peace. These actions, too, felt like memorializing George. The grief of the world and my grief intertwined.

I took a six-week grief and yoga workshop, on Zoom, with much younger people, several of whom had found their friends dead on the floor from drugs. We were encouraged to grieve, and to show our grief publicly. Grief demands ritual. Without communal witness of one's own story, it may be impossible to process grief. I gave in, finally, to the most prevalent treatments. Psychotherapy and antidepressants. Though the first antidepressants prescribed did not work, after three tries, I was given a prescription that did, and my anxiety lifted, which was an enormous relief. Still, antidepressants and therapy are private, isolating events, though they are mainly all this culture commonly offers—and only to those who can afford them. Communal commemorative rituals need invention, whether hallucinogenic, ceremonies of scattering ashes, celebratory dinner parties, or protests against war, which were my ways of memorializing George. In the middle of one night, I woke and found George's sharp profile in bed next to me. Is it his spirit that comes, or my deep love for him that calls forth such images? Or both, his spirit and my love in concert. Turned out it was only the extra pillow.

Grief is "spiraldic" like a spiral, a gyre, the yoga-grief teacher frequently said. "Turning and turning in the widening gyre, the falcon cannot hear the falconer," Yeats wrote in "The Second Coming," his poem of savage beauty and of despair for the wretched communal-political terrors we face, never more than now. Violence born with "a gaze blank and pitiless as the sun." Grief demands we spiral back inside, again and again, that we go down under, confront the unknown, the unbearable, and grow ourselves into fuller feeling, for the other(s) who suffer(s) unbearable losses and for our own grieving self. If grief does not serve compassion—Compassion, which is Eros without compulsion, Compassion, which is love for the suffering self, and for all selves who suffer—what god does grief serve?

—

Two years after we scattered George's ashes, I am back at the Bread and Puppet farm in Glover, Vermont, with the little dog, grown, who was then a wee pup. "He's a prote*k*shion dog," Peter says, in his German accent, pointing. It has snapped cold in early September, but the day is bright, and Percy and I make our way across the road to the path that leads to the Memorial Grove. From the hill, I can see the dark stand of pine trees in the large meadow below; above its edges, a view of the green mountains. When the procession danced and sang down this road two years ago, I saw none of the land, consumed by the task, my hands into his ashes, their rough pieces of bone. The grove has had a calamity of sorts. Three large pines have hit the earth, falling across some of the older wooden sheds, the small ghost houses of the earlier residents in this place. But George's tree, set slightly apart, in the newer neighborhood of the lost, stands tall and proud. I can feel the density of the spirits here and the younger people, this summer's crop of puppeteers, who knew none of these shades in the flesh, tell me the same—"that grove" they say, in awe. The dense feeling in the air, as if a congregation of vital spirits, is palpable to all. Even with the downed trees, perhaps, also because of them, as all things must finally go to ground, the Spirit life abounds. A silent cacophony of selves. They are here, some part of them, lingering together, and, after all, most of them knew many of them. George knew Judith, Elka Schumann, Grace Paley and others whose houses I cannot find. His memorial is one of the simpler ones and for that reason I like it fine. If George could be anything, he would want to be a tree, and here he is. His wool Irish cap flat against the bark, where I nailed it two years ago, but, now its plaid wool looks like a knob in the tree trunk. Peter has lettered, as I requested, a simple board and nailed it some feet above the hat: George Bartenieff, in black print, January 24, 1933-July 30, 2022. I stare at the dates, almost as if I'd forgotten what they were. The trunk is straight and tall. Its branches high above. Underneath the hat, someone, most likely Peter, has made of curved wood a frame for George's photo, which I'd left in a plain, store-bought one at the base of the tree. He looks now as though he is appearing from the tree, a secret door has opened and out he slips. He stares, sternly, dressed as Uncle, the wry environmentalist he loved to play, "in those days we painted with our tongues," Uncle said about the virgin land, and "we would exit as we'd come, gently, unremarked upon." Peter told me one night on the phone that George seems to move in his frame, as if alive, and the photo, which is a particularly wonderful one taken by Beatriz Schiller of George as Uncle in the 2018 LaMama production of *Extreme Whether*, captures his intensity, his ever-present vitality, and he does, in fact, seem to move in the slanting light of the setting sun. I stand for a while taking in the simplicity of his memorial, the huge pine to which he is now attached and emanates from. If George could become anything, he would wish to be a tree. I hug his tree, and I feel one beat, as if of a very strong heart. An essence within the tree. George's heart beating just once more, against my chest. Why not? As if he had been waiting here these two years for me to come. If George could be anything, he would have wished to become a tree in the forest. He would have wished to have been scattered here, his gray and bony ashes, with his friends and colleagues. I back away from the tree, satisfied.

All week, Peter and two talented puppeteers have been refining short "bed sheet" plays about Gaza. Puppeteers perform in front of bed sheets on which Peter paints angels and devils, and a few choice words. All week, I have been watching the rehearsals develop, watching the puppeteers invent and Peter give short, insightful notes. All week, Peter and I have been muttering, "it is unbearable" to one another, about the genocide growing worse in Gaza. "When it began, I thought I could not live through another war without George," I tell Peter. "Now, I think, he's lucky he did not live to see it." Peter agrees; he is thinking of Elka. The puppeteers have found a poem from Gaza whose words are stark and beautiful, and they have set it to a traditional step song Protestant hymn. (Step song hymns are sung every Tuesday evening after dinner in the Bread and Puppet's theater-barn, with members of the near-by farm community.) "How high can a missile fly/does it graze the moon/can it reach the stars/now orphan child step into my arms/Let me scatter you across the sky/and turn your tears to stars/so that when night falls/ you are not afraid of the dark./ and when bombs chase us here on earth/ I can look up from the rubble/ see your twinkle, see your light/ know that you have outlived the night." Peter. who mainly eschews words in favor of puppets, is also very capable of recognizing language's impact and he is thrilled with this addition, which the hymnal harmonies make even more powerful, sung in the voices of the two young men.

In the 60s and 70s, before I knew either of them, though I knew of their work, George played the title roles in *Woyzeck*, *Diagonal Man* and *Othello*, in Peter's puppet versions. On European tours, "he spoke his part in Polish, Czech, German, French; he didn't know any of those languages," Peter laughs. But George had a keen ear and could endow sounds with meanings. Peter always likes to have one or two accomplished actors among his puppeteers. "What was special about George's acting?" I ask him.

"His immediacy. He was always *there*."

"I will see you, again," the ninety-year-old master puppet artist points his finger at my chest as I am about to leave. "The Memorial Grove is very important." Yes. To memorialize is to pass the stories on, to extend through generations the ties that bind the community of war resisting artists. To memorialize is to put our grief to use in the world. I have come this far in two years. I go in and out, now, from terror to being able to cope. At my best, which is not every day, I am no longer a mass of hysterical fear, clutched tight in my bed, screeching. I have become an elder, enduring, bearing, memorializing grief—for self and world. With the small dog.

Chapter Four:
We Do Not Know
What We Do Not Know

"They killed him," the Chinese herbalist MD Dr. W. emailed me, meaning the allopathic MDs George had attending to him—his oncologist-hematologist, his heart and his infectious disease specialists and the treatments they used. Three antibiotics a day for a year and a half, necessary to ward off another potentially fatal sepsis attack, but toxic. Cancer drugs: Revlimid, thalidomide, Velcade, and Darzalex, none of which George tolerated well or for very long. None of which had the desired effect of driving his cancer numbers down. Only the heart doctor's blood pressure pills kept his atrial flutter flat, seemingly without side effects. "I will be his primary care physician," the hematologist said when I asked him for a referral and so he assumed his double role, both specialist and general practitioner looking after his patient's whole self. "Voodoo medicine," he snapped when I told him about George's nontoxic herbal teas, which cost us $200 to $400 a month, not covered by insurance. The herbalist changed the brew every month to "outsmart" the cancer. Who knows if these teas might have kept George alive without adverse side effects had he stopped toxic Western medical treatments before the final Darzalex shot? There is no research.

George's blood cancer specialist, who was now also his primary care doctor, was mercifully good with our limited funds. The woman who handled his patients' financial information when George began cancer treatment immediately separated George's finances from mine, "I don't want to know a thing about what you have or make," she said. He and I had kept our finances separate in any case. We each contributed our share to running the house. Knowing George was now living on a limited income, his Social Security and Actor's Equity pension, his cancer doctor gave him, without charge, six packets of the very costly thalidomide pills another patient had donated. This drug, originally prescribed to pregnant women supposedly to prevent miscarriages was responsible for serious birth defects in thousands of children. Then, it was discovered to attack certain cancer cells and thalidomide was repurposed as a multiple myeloma drug. Every month George was on it we each had to answer a medical quiz and state we were not seeking to birth a child—at our ages. He could not tolerate thalidomide. He took himself off it after several months in order to act in *Blue Valiant*.

When, in the second year of his treatment, George became a charity patient at the hospital, I threw out the large paper box filled to the brim with exorbitant, unpaid medical bills. I was not to be held liable for George's medical debt I could not have paid without becoming homeless myself. I recognize my luck in a cutthroat, capitalist medical system that has ruined survivors' lives, and am extremely grateful for the concerns of his cancer and primary care doctor and for the fantastic woman who handled his patients' financial records. She allowed me, once widowed, to escape medical bankruptcy.

"I have to speak about a drug I don't like very much," George's doctor said in February 2020, on his way to Banff, Canada. Why would he have to do that? I wondered, but I didn't dare question, then, because the man wasn't feeling well himself and he was ministering to my husband. The doctor stopped by to see George, who was in hospital with diverticulitis, another painful chemotherapy side effect, and, at the same time, he was supervising while a resident administered mild anesthesia and took another bone biopsy. The doctor and I spoke briefly about the coming pandemic. "It's going to be bad," he told me, and I remember I said something I had just learned about the 1919 flu epidemic at the end of World War I—when the whole world was exhausted from an orgy of killing, and the widespread use of poison gas. The doctor would return from his conference in Banff, very ill, with the "worst" hacking cough he'd ever had. He would be out of work for two weeks, an early case of COVID, most likely, from an early spreader event.

George's cancer doctor was my most reliable companion during the pandemic lockdown, when we saw virtually no one except members of the medical profession. I texted him, and he, me, at all hours of the day and night. Whenever George had a medical issue, but also, we texted back and forth about music and art, about Paul Robeson and James Baldwin, about Chartres Cathedral where the doctor went everyday as a young exchange student in France to stand while the evening light poured through its Romanesque windows, and where he returned, alone, after the death of his first wife, whose watercolors he invited me to his office to see and which he sent me photographs of. We spoke about the Midwest, where we both grew up. He in a rural Iowa community; I in suburbs of Chicago. He told me he was the first person in his family to go to college. That his father was a machinist who died of a heart attack when the doctor was in high school, a man who would have liked Donald Trump, his liberal son thought. We both went to state schools, he to the University of Iowa on full scholarship, I to the University of Wisconsin, with a partial scholarship. Both of our fathers had died young. We both ended up at Columbia, I to earn my MFA at the School of the Arts; he for his physician's residency.

George's doctor became the text mail recipient of my childhood horse memories, which bubbled up while I directed *Blue Valiant*. He came to the launch party we gave at Kathy and Henry's large house when we all viewed the film we'd made. The doctor hugged me, spontaneously, "I'm proud of you," he said at the after party. "I'm proud of you, too," I said. We were friends. He took the day off so he might come to George's funeral service, arriving on his bike in ninety-degree heat, wearing a somber black suit. We sat next to each other, like family, my daughter on my other side. Yet, when it came time for him to speak of this man he loved, he could manage only a single sentence. We had worked together, he said, to keep George alive. He could not put his feelings into words, and abruptly sat down, his upset palpable. Accompanying George's coffin on the way to the incinerator, the doctor walked with my friend, Nesta, alongside her wheelchair, "I feel I failed," he said. I was walking alone on the other side of the road. I saw them, but I did not cross the street. I could not accompany George's body to the furnace door to be burnt to ash, but his doctor faithfully did. Alone, so alone. George dead. The doctor gone from my life.

I googled him one day. I was expecting to find the doctor's photo and his five-star rating, but instead a page unanticipated and alarming popped up. It was the Dollars for Docs ProPublica website and on it I read that George's cancer doctor "makes more money than most doctors make" from Big Pharma, well over a million and a third dollars more as of 2018 and counting. I was stunned. Part of President Obama's healthcare plan mandates that doctors report their extra earnings to a government website, and so information once hidden is now public.

Those "conferences" the doctor was always going to, before the lockdown, and then again, immediately after ... that conference in Banf, where his son accompanied him to go skiing, and that drug he "didn't like" but "had to speak about." His fancy hotel in Puerto Rico and the great restaurants he went to in San Juan that he bragged about one day as we stood in the new infusion center hall, waiting for George, his luxury hotels and great meals were perks for the sales conferences where he was hired to speak. Paid for by the pharmaceutical companies that booked his appearance. The "conference" he was at when George was in the ER for seventeen hours before his emergency hernia surgery, and, then, again, the "conference" in Philadelphia he was at while George was being rehydrated in another emergency room the last week of his life those were *not* academic presentations of new research papers, as I had naively supposed. No. He was not a research doctor. These were sales conferences at which he spoke and for which he was paid big bucks by Big Pharma while he extolled the efficacy of the specific cancer drug the company manufactures. Of course, he had prescribed these drugs for his own patients. Of course, he believed what he said. Nevertheless, the doctor I so trusted, had relied upon, and liked so much was moonlighting for Big Pharma. He was similar to a television doctor in an advertisement wearing a white coat, a role George had auditioned for once. George's doctor was on the payroll of pharmaceutical companies, many of them, the Dollars for Docs website informed me. "If you are concerned about this, we advise that you ask the doctor directly." I was stunned. Shocked. I felt betrayed. How had I not known this when it might have mattered to George? To me this way of earning extra money felt inordinately corrupt. The doctor had been cheating on us, as if we were not his first concern; he had other, more lucrative commitments than his hospital practice. He was a shill. Like a snake oil salesman. I was appalled. I was hurt. I felt deceived. I was so raw. George had just died. Now, this. Hadn't we shared an unspoken pledge to devote ourselves selflessly to George?

I took the website's advice; only I did not exactly ask him about the money he was being paid, rather I wrote, "if George had known about your lucrative ties to Big Pharma, he would have gone off treatment earlier." I could hear the conversation in my head. I would have gone to George with this information, fresh from my google search, incensed. I would have blurted out the news. "Your doctor hawks cancer drugs." (Why hadn't I, in fact, done this same search while George was still alive, when the knowledge might have benefited him? I was angry with myself for my lack of due diligence.) We would have expressed our shock, or, more likely, George in his calmly ironic way would have said, as he often did say when I was extremely upset, "but of course, you expected *Better Housekeeping* maybe." George was so much more unflappable than I, more humorous, too, in a pinch. Nevertheless, we would have agreed. I knew this because I knew George. He would have taken himself off treatment before the final Darzalex shot, before his bowels became impacted—perhaps. He might have lived longer, lived better, without the pain and indignities of his last months. We might have been happier had he stopped treatment earlier—as we would have done, I convinced myself, but now it was too late. I asked my two married physician friends what they thought. They are among the most principled people I know. One worked as a pediatrician in public health settings, and now runs Brooklyn for Peace, a forty-year-old peace and justice organization to which I belong. The other, her husband, practiced and taught at a major New York hospital and is involved in a leadership position with the national organization Physicians for Single Payer, advocating for Medicare for all. They had taken me under their care during one of the worst phases of my deepest grief. They were surprised; they did not think doctors did such things. They knew this was not common practice. They did some research and recommended several studies to me. I read them and learned: the majority of doctors refuse to take money from pharmaceutical companies and consider the practice to be unethical. These doctors believe drug companies ought to be forbidden to offer money for drug testimonials. Another study concluded that physicians who do accept extra payments from pharmaceutical companies for appearing at conferences and vouching for the company's drugs tend to make two mistakes: they over-prescribe the specific cancer drugs they are paid to endorse and/or they prescribe the specific drug they are paid to recommend, even if another drug might be proven to have better outcomes. If George's treatment had ended months sooner, while his hernia festered, but weeks before the last disastrous Darzalex shot (a drug his doctor also hawked), what then would have been the result? Bring him in, I'll check him out, and we had gone dutifully to the doctor's office where he dutifully patted George's groin, and cleared him for cancer treatment that week. Had we known what I knew now—George would not have gotten that shot. He would have stopped treatment earlier. What would have happened with George off treatment? Perhaps he would have avoided an impacted bowl. Perhaps he would have had an easier death. Perhaps, a longer life? "They killed him," the Chinese herbalist wrote; his words were still fresh in my mind, despite or because of the fact that they, too, were cruel. Everything felt cruel to me in those months after George died.

My words to the doctor elicited a furious response by return email. One does not dare speak to a doctor as I had dared. I was attacking those "who had tried to help," I agreed with that much. "You have poison in your heart" that "will retard healing," the doctor wrote. He withdrew himself from speaking as planned at George's large public memorial service at LaMama. I said he could still speak, of course. He refused again. I asked him several times. He refused to attend. As I began to spin out-of-control, down the dark well of my grief, his words continued to haunt. Perhaps I did have "poison in my heart." Perhaps I would never heal. Other people, including my oldest friend, rebuked me for how angry I was. Perhaps, George's doctor was right. I had nothing left inside but poisonous rage. So what. I wanted to die. Perhaps I would die from grief—my fury would poison me. Like the wicked witch, I would melt. Perhaps I would be lucky and my poisonous heart would give out. The doctor's diagnosis was correct. Poison in the heart. Terminal disease. I welcomed the thought. I felt such rage.

I lashed out at the doctor whom I had needed so much. I felt he had betrayed my trust. He struck back with fury because he believed he had given so much to us both. He believed, as I had, that we two had been an unusual pair. We each loved George. Perhaps we, too, loved one another a bit. We had worked together to keep George alive. George was dead. We each felt we had failed. We had each lost George, and, therefore, of course, we would lose one another. Good, I thought. Done. But I was deeply hurt. Stunned. After all, I had only accused him of doing what he did. Take extra money from the pharmaceutical industry. I tried to patch things up. I told him we need not agree. He could still speak at the public memorial. He said, "No," definitively. We stopped communicating.

Cancer exists in a silo of personal fear; we are each of us vulnerable, beholden to those who call themselves experts, who live in an arcane world of chemical potions whose full effects no one understands, and which vary from patient to patient. Three weeks before George died, he said to me from his hospital bed, attempting to recover from the hernia surgery he would never recover from, "I do not want anyone to know I have cancer. I feel diminished." We had to tell the Mabou Mines Company that George would not be able to perform at their fiftieth anniversary celebration the excerpt from Goethe's *Faust* he still knew by heart in the original German, and had been rehearsing in his head, from the director JoAnne Akalaitis' acclaimed antinuclear piece, *Dead End Kids*. (JoAnne was also being treated for cancer, everyone knew this, but, somehow, George still felt shamed.) "Can I tell them, we've had a family emergency?" I asked George. "You can tell them that." As an actor, George feared he would not be cast if anyone guessed he had cancer. He told me, again and again, how fast rumors of ill-health fly in the professional world. Who wants to hire someone terminally ill? (Indeed, he was overlooked for several TV roles during the pandemic after a few stunning video auditions, but who knew the reason.) George did not ever want anyone to know how ill he actually was and he acted health brilliantly. Although, of course, people knew. Much of the downtown theater community had seen George in March at LaMama when I spoke at a celebration of the work of performance artist Penny Arcade, and they saw, as I could not, how frail he'd become. He made himself walk the ten blocks from the theater to the reception. He had his first glass of wine in months, and he spoke animatedly to his friends. George fooled no one but me. We were in our own space, ignoring death. While the party went on in the front room of the same restaurant, Pangea, on Second Avenue in the East Village where we had celebrated George's 87th birthday with many friends, and the doctor, too, his wife and his son in attendance, George and I were served a private dinner by the restaurant's owner in the back room.

The American avant-garde, which endorsed our right to self-define who we are and our right to live and love joyously as we self-create, emerged in the 1950s, in direct response to the atomic threat, and to the cancer-causing petrochemical polluting industries that grew up after the war. The avant-garde in which George, Julian Beck, and Barbara Deming played seminal roles is intricately entwined with opposition to the bomb, and to military-industrial ecocide. The great explosion of creativity and of human self-determination that began in the fifties, becoming more inclusive, decade by decade and, which we hold onto now as well as we are able, when human freedoms are increasingly in our country in peril, the radical theater and the arts of self-transformation and nonviolent action, all are driven by an opposing world-view to state violence. The twentieth-century Avant-garde emerged in reaction to the two world wars, the horrors of the concentration camps finally widely perceived and the dropping of the atomic bomb. Against such heretofore-unimaginable terror, the Avant-garde embraced "anything goes" experimentation, random chance, mixing forms, forbidden contents, fluid sexual identity, hallucinogenic drug culture, rock and roll, and free love. The Avant-garde galvanized the artistic world, broke boundaries and intoxicated. It offered a poetic, musical, artistic, sexual frenzy—inclusive, outlandish, open, expansive. The imagination was liberated. Do it now, experiment, create! Defy capitalism and the state. Go to jail for refusing to take part in air-raid drills, go to jail for defying segregation, for insisting upon putting on plays that expose the punitive prison system, go to jail for protesting war after war, for sitting down on a bridge in a white upstate town, facing down white men with guns. And so we lived inventing freedom, for ourselves, our children, for the art worlds and the world. Like the Romantics, like the Transcendentalists, like the Abolitionists, like all the free spirits before us, breaking from toxic violence, envisioning the world anew.

Months after George died, it struck me that our eviction from the large Victorian house we rented and lived in so happily, and cheaply, for twenty-three years, in which we entertained so many friends from around the world with large dinners, Seders, dances around a lit Christmas tree, that our loss of this house might well have triggered the multiple myeloma hidden inside his bone marrow, so hard to detect. He had been a hidden child in Germany; he developed a hidden cancer. Two years after we lost our home, George had his first sepsis attack, a year and a-half later, he was diagnosed with multiple myeloma. First, his parents left him behind on his family's estate. Then, his German family sent him and his brother away to a Steiner school. Then, the two boys were accompanied by a hired nanny on a German luxury liner, where anti-Semitic films were shown after dinner; they crossed the ocean to reunite with parents who hurled shoes and epithets at each other while the boys hid between their beds in the strange place to which they had come. Then, he moved with his mother and brother from the country to the City, which he learned to love but at first he hated, and a life of poverty growing up, with many moves of house. He also moved Theater for the New City from space to space as rents grew too high, until he located and raised the money and found the city building to purchase for the permanent home for the theater he co-founded, where it remains on First Avenue and East Tenth St on the Lower East Side of New York. Then he lost the theater he co-founded, when he could no longer work with Crystal Field, his ex-wife, and she kept control—also suing him for alimony, which he paid monthly for over two decades, so he was broke at his death. George was a hidden child who developed, sometime late in his life, a smoldering, a hidden cancer deep in the marrow of the bone. Did the suppression of all of his losses, then his eviction from what had been "our home" for twenty-three years trigger the onset of his cancer? There is scant research into emotional triggers for runaway cancer cells. What difference would taking past trauma into account make to treating cancer, in any case? But what if we *knew that there must be* a causal connection between trauma and cancer? What then? Would such knowledge help with cancer prevention? Would it help us create less emotionally and chemically toxic environments? Would knowledge of a mind-body-trauma-disease connection lead to more serious efforts at cancer prevention?

Christen Clifford, who acted Admira, the raped woman, in *The Beekeeper's Daughter* and the trophy wife, Tess, in *Another Life*, both opposite George, both in three different productions on two continents, grew up on the shores of Lake Erie. She is a young survivor of cervical, ovarian, and, more recently, breast cancer. She writes when I ask her:

> *Oh yes—I wonder if I got gynecological cancers because I was raped twice as a teenager. Because I had bad sexual experiences. And grew up in Buffalo near Love Canal and not that far from Three Mile Island—Three Mile leaked into Lake Erie in the 70s and I was in that lake every day in the summer. I think of it like Climate Change in my body, the "Anthropocene," the mistakes of greedy humans, accumulated in my womb, where I made and stored my eggs.*
>
> *I feel very lucky that I was able to give birth and breastfeed and nurture and create and grow and love with these body parts before they were sickened, before they developed illness. And yes! George fleeing the Nazis, both of you fleeing the greed of your landlady. I didn't really have many good sexual relationships—I always wanted to and still do—but I didn't always listen to my body.*

Advanced cancer care is good business practice, so why prevent cancer. Just as Exxon, Mobil, Shell, etc. decided it would be bad for their bottom line to leave greenhouse gas-emitting, carcinogenic oil, coal, and gas in the ground. Even though, their own scientists understood as early as 1970, exactly what Rachel Carson knew when she wrote *Silent Spring*, while she suffered from fatal breast cancer, that industrial pollutants are killing the natural world—and poisoning us in the process. "For those in whom cancer is already a hidden or visible presence, efforts to find cures must, of course, continue. For the generations as yet unborn, prevention is the most imperative need," Carson warned in 1965. She was brutally attacked by the petrochemical industry for her groundbreaking book, which nonetheless led Republican President Richard Nixon to found the Environmental Protection Agency in an effort to monitor and reduce the spread of carcinogens.

If one in every three of us will get cancer in a lifetime, that means no one escapes either being stricken or living with and loving one of those stricken, or both, and having, as we all do, many friends and family members struggling with cancer, its treatment options and side-effects. Therefore, the demand for chemical treatments for cancer is endless. One can imagine a future New York City, ravaged by floods and the rising seas, baking under an intolerable sun, the particulates in the air making it difficult to breathe, and with the gleaming cancer infusion centers still standing and functioning, amid the detritus of a climate-changed world.

"You can't cure cancer with chemicals," George's MD Chinese herbalist repeatedly said. I did not disagree, but neither did I know the efficacy of his herbal potions. We were using them on blind trust, more or less, as George blindly, too, submitted to the chemical treatments, because that's all there is. George relied on, and benefitted from, acupuncture, Kundalini yoga, organic diet, and Freudian psychotherapy, too. This was the healing program we put together, which enriched George's life and made him feel better. What if he'd eschewed, at his age, cancer treatment altogether? What if he had gone off treatment earlier?

Why is it so difficult to go off-treatment at the end? Exactly, that is, when the approach of death becomes stunningly clear—and there is no longer a way to forestall it. Because chemical treatment keeps alive the comforting myth that science might triumph? That death will be defeated. That any amount of suffering is worth this struggle to live a bit longer. Can it be so? Susan Sontag, who famously decried any use of illness as metaphor, is a case in point. Flown across the country on a medical jet paid for by her partner, photographer Annie Liebovitz, to receive a bone marrow transplant that her own cancer doctor in New York knew would not work, a blistering treatment administered by a doctor on the West Coast, who did not know her, but who was willing to try it anyway (for pay), Sontag was returned to New York to die in agony. Her cancer doctor held her hand, while her son, David Rieff, paced the edges of the room. Rieff records the scene in his moving memoir, *Swimming in a Sea of Death*. Kept apart from his mother while she clung to the hand of her cancer doctor. "We have to do better for people like Susan," his doctor, bereaved, told the bereaved son.

Sontag's book, *Illness as Metaphor* is justly famous as a cautionary tale, demanding we never see illness as a metaphor for anything at all. Her death offers another sort of warning against the belief in the fiction that more treatment will finally offer up a cure, even at the point the disease is incurable. An extension of life, even when the pain is unbearable. My mother suffered from a similar delusion, and my father, increasingly unable to make any decision for himself, submitted to every possible treatment until his brain was destroyed. George, too, despite what I already knew, stayed on treatment too long. This is a medical system that reads death metaphorically as a "failure" and does not know how to bear witness, offer help, or to allow and facilitate death with grace. Those of us who care for those who have cancer are equally liable to insist upon treatment, at any emotional and physical cost, because we are equally afraid of confronting death. Because, more than anything at all, we all long for more time.

In 2018, the last year for which data was available on the Dollars for Docs website published by ProPublica, George's doctor earned $319,000 from drug companies for speaking about their drugs at sales conferences. He earned the most money, $91,000, for promoting Aliqopa, a drug used to treat leukemia, but he also earned $25,006 in 2018 for promoting Darzalex, the last multiple myeloma drug that George was on and the drug administered by shot to the stomach that caused George so much pain, leaving him mute on our floor. "George is too weak for treatment," I had said, but the doctor ordered treatment, anyway, the one final treatment, as it turned out, for he was never again well enough to tolerate any cancer drugs.

Let's swap the word "protagonist" for "patient." A patient is accepting, uncomplaining, trusting, unquestioning, lacking in agency, subservient to others and willing to endure, also, often willing to try anything, offering body up to the latest experiment even without proof for the benefit of medical science, for the benefit of others not yet ill. Willing to go on any drug trial, if lucky enough to be approved. In other words, a patient is a good sick person. Compliant. Whose sick body can be used for experiment, willingly. A protagonist, in contrast, becomes actively engaged in their personal fate, and sees that fate as partly of their own making. While we all are created by and subjected to many forces beyond our control, and events that happened before we could be fully conscience of what has been done to us, we each have decisions to make nevertheless. The protagonist understands that difficult choices must be theirs. The protagonist understands, like the tragic hero, that often the choice is between two evils. Like Oedipus who says, "And I am on the brink of fateful hearing, yet I must hear," the protagonist chooses to bear full knowledge of their fate. No longer a victim, storm-tossed, but as a hero, whose sacrifice benefits the rest of us. The protagonist would make treatment decisions with a self-determined goal in mind—to live well or to live longer, even, to do so for the benefit of science, and the others who will come after. The protagonist would enter more fully into or disengage with, would be empowered to continue or to stop treatment. Would listen to advice but make up their own mind—knowing that we often cannot know what is best, and that there may be no good option at all. The patient-turned-protagonist would have the final word and would be heard. Their will would override medical experts. The patient-turned-protagonist would have access to knowledge, be treated with respect, with deference, and with admiration by doctors and by caretakers, not as a burden, not as an inert object, not as an unlettered fool, or an experiment. The protagonist would be admired. For the protagonist is in a struggle for their life: struggling to live with cancer, discovering how to live their life after cancer, in remission, with the anxiety and joy of that, or grappling with dying from the disease. The protagonist would be the hero of their story. Not the doctors. If we were to empower cancer patients, allowing them their rightful status as protagonists in what is now a worldwide, industrial-age plague of cancers, the protagonists with cancer would become our teachers, our advocates, and, yes, our heroes. They would show the way—not just in matters of disease and treatment, but of courage. They would demand, from their privileged position as enlightened sufferers, better conditions for us all.

Patients make life easier for doctors. Their rounds can be accomplished quickly, with a pat on the shoulder, if that. Doctors can stare at their computer screens, not look the person they are treating in the eye. Doctors no longer use their hands to diagnose, they rely upon tests; their own intuition, their own sense of touch atrophies. They can abandon the terminally ill. With patients, doctors keep their designation as undisputed experts. They do not have to stop and converse, explain, or question their own position. "Rounds," too, has a dismissive sound. The doctor, often trailed by two or more interns, breezes into the patient's room, displays his knowledge in winks and nods to the attendants, who are novices before the priest, says little to the patient and nothing to the caretaker sitting anxiously in a chair. As the patient sickens, the doctor need not bother to make eye contact. When George was dying, we endured a round like this with his cancer doctor, who was also our friend and confidant, but who now avoided looking at or speaking to me, as I sat stock-still in a chair. Who did not speak directly to George. His female resident, whom I had not met, nor were we introduced, stared into my eyes. I returned her gaze. She was trying to see what I might be feeling, but of course, I barely knew myself what I felt, stunned, terrified, trying to adjust to what was the end of George's life, and no one bothered to ask either George or me how it was for us. Each one of us was afraid. The doctor, too, of our need, of our hurt, of our rage. No one took me aside to talk. No one sat down on the plastic mattress next to George and took his hand and looked into his eyes. We had to ask for palliative care, which did not exist. We had to demand to be released from hospital. I expected his three doctors to come to say goodbye when George was released from the hospital for the final time. No one came. No one tried to speak with George, to inquire what his wishes might be for his death. But, death is neither a disease nor a failure. It is what happens to people. We needed time to adjust. We were all in shock. None of his doctors was like

Peter Schumann, with his boisterous voice, "Put him on," he commanded me when I told him George "was not who he was." And they spoke and laughed one last time. But Peter was in Vermont. We needed a witness close by, family perhaps, but my family was far away. We needed someone who might have seen the pain we were each in, even including the pain of his doctor, and how our fear isolated us, each one from the other. No one in the hospital where we were came to speak with us, no chaplain, rabbi, or priest; no one helped us to speak. I might have hoped for a palliative care doctor or a social worker, but though both existed in the hospital system we were in, and I requested to see both of them, neither acted as an empathic listener or an informed witness. The social worker would only speak with me if George were a Medicaid patient, as her primary function was to secure payments for the hospital from the Medicaid system. The palliative doctor had only the function of writing the release form from hospital so the hospital could no longer be sued, and of turning us over to hospice. Hospice, as it turned out, assumed no function at all; understaffed, they sent no one. I began to think they were a Medicare fraud.

And yet there were moments when the medical nightmare fell away and the human took over, even within the hospital system. Two months before his death, George told his cancer doctor the story of his early life in Nazi Germany, in detail, over two appointments that lasted two hours each. I stood as a silent witness in the back of the room as George, in a wheelchair, spoke and his doctor, seated close to him, looking directly at him, listened intently, with interest and empathy. This was end-of-life care in which medicine had no part to play any longer. This was George's doctor bearing witness to his patient, honoring his patient's needs. George's doctor employing the skill of close listening. I was very moved as I stood in a corner, watching. George felt consequential. His life story meaningful. His doctor, the recipient of George's tale, felt consequential, too. And nevertheless, despite the relationship we three had built, despite or, rather, because of the doctor's admiration of and his love for George, despite what he called George's "brilliance," the transition from George as his patient to George as a dying man, to George dead, was fraught. The doctor also was suffering. "I feel I failed," he told my friend at George's funeral. He did not tell me.

I felt I had failed, too, of course. We were bound, the doctor and I, by our grief, by our loss. It was easier to fight with each other, to cast blame, than to admit how bereft we each felt. There is no protocol for doctor and widow, no way to untangle.

On the year anniversary of George's last cancer treatment, George's doctor and I made contact for the first time since we quarreled. I asked him when he thought George might have "contracted" his myeloma. He replied:

> *Contracted implies contagion, which is not the case. The first time he had protein studies was shortly before I first saw him and at that time he had a three gm M protein which didn't develop overnight. He must have had myeloma six-to-twelve months before the first test was performed. That is less relevant to his outcome than the tolerance for and response to treatment. He did not die of progressive myeloma but neither tolerated treatment very well nor responded as well as hoped. His blood counts dropped on Revlimid and he had problematic side effects on lowest dose thalidomide. Treatment was adjusted to his tolerance and there was less myeloma at the end than when he was diagnosed but more than the average person has after that period of treatment. That was likely due to poor tolerance for treatment but could also reflect inherent disease resistance to treatment. Does that help? If you have another question please ask.*

Interesting that the doctor speaks only of the first two treatments George tried. He leaves out the Velcade treatments and the final Darzalex shot that caused George such pain. Did he do so consciously, or had he blocked the final treatment from his mind? In a following email, the doctor wrote, "in retrospect, if we had known an inguinal hernia would be key to survival, there might have been less cancer treatment." In retrospect, then, we agreed; George should have gone off cancer treatment earlier. The hardest decision to make but one that possibly ought to be made more often in cancer treatment—a decision that, therefore, ought to be made easier to make, if possible.

Every person's life is a poem, and each life must be read individually, as metaphor. To read cancer stories as metaphors for our injured world is emphatically *not* to blame those who have the disease, one in three of us in the United States, one in three who become the protagonists confronting the disease of our age, but, rather, to interrogate a growing cancer industry that is part of our growing climate and military crises. We are animals, and like all animals, we, too, are threatened with extinction by the choices humans make. If we were to interrogate fully both the *traumatic and the chemical-pollutant* causes of cancer, would we become gentler, more able to envision and make the necessary societal changes—protect our environment, eschew violence, form and value strong, nurturant communities in which everyone has enough? If so, would we suffer any less the ills of the lethal cancers that threaten us all?

This book is the story of my bearing witness to cancer and to the attempts by its sufferers to become more fully protagonists in their own cancer treatments, more cognizant of choices—limited though they be—and even if they are unable, finally, to make them. More aware of their need for community. And more creative, even as they weaken. Cancer is such a fearsome adversary, so bent on destruction and murder, that doctors, with their highly specialized skills, often see themselves in a war against "It" in which the person who harbors the disease becomes collateral damage. War metaphors, the "fight against cancer," "battling cancer" are, therefore, not useful. We need another paradigm.

Protagonists at the end of their cancer stories do extraordinary things: they finish books and write poems, keep diaries, tell stories, and confront trauma, with their waning strength. They create unforgettable characters on the stage, like Julian doing Beckett's isolate man and George as seer in *Blue Valiant*. They get arrested for the greater good like Barbara. And like these three, they gather their community around them as they dance toward death. They stay cognizant as much as they can and inform us of the very moment when they lose "sense and language," as George did, a shocking moment of insight he shared—and even, then, in the midst of the desperate loss of all that they are, they remain present. They bestow love with their final smiles, their gaze, their last words, the embrace of their family and friends and they share astonishing grace by letting us stand as close as we dare to the mystery of death as it sweeps them away from us. When we find ourselves still alive and they not, we are humbled, honored, and though lost, privileged to have walked to the edge with them; though left, abandoned, alone and in sorrow, we have been enriched, deepened, and have come closer to life's mysteries. Death never reveals what death is, but death shows us how well we have loved. How well we have been loved, too. Death teaches of love only there is no end.

When George was in hospital in June, I asked Noam Chomsky to tell me about his first wife's death.

> *Carol's cancer was a shock. I urged her to see her doctor because of persistent coughs. They did a chest X-ray and sent her right off for a biopsy. Malignant, then MRIs. All over her brain. I checked carefully with specialists, some who I knew well. All agreed that radical brain radiation was imperative. It was untreatable by any known means, so she was put on an experimental drug that was just in the trial stage. It kept her alive for two years, to everyone's surprise. Two years of steady decline to infancy, also slow collapse of bodily organs. I wanted to keep her at home. Managed, until the end, with occasional stays at the cancer ward at MGH. After a few months, I needed some help. Near the end, twenty-hour-a-day visiting nurses (amazingly wonderful people). It was hard, but I'm glad we did it that way. After the first few months, she didn't really understand what was happening and was often quite happy, like a little child. Liked for me to read her children's books, and since her short-term memory was gone, the same ones over and over. And to look at old family photos, also over and over. Oddly, very warm and intimate days. To the very end. She died peacefully, at home, children nearby.*

A month later, when Noam heard George died at home, he wrote, "So sad. The best way, though. Stay Strong."

Noam, at 94, is suffering from a massive stroke that has left the brilliant linguist unable to speak. He is still alive as I write, in San Paolo, with his second wife, Valeria Wasserman-Chomsky, but our communication over decades has ceased. I was barely out of graduate school and he was a young professor when we met and I interviewed him on the lawn at M.I.T., about his early linguistic theories and his early opposition to the Vietnam War. Language is innate to the human brain. We come wired with syntax, which allows us to engage in complex communications, and to tell our stories. Why, then, so uniquely gifted, are human beings so destructive? *Why Only Us*, and *What Kind of Creatures Are We?* are titles of Noam's last books on linguistics. I made the second title a recurring refrain in the final song of *Other Than We*, in which George played Opa, a Noam-like linguist, and the "Newbies" sang, "What kind of creatures are we, Opa/ What kind of creatures should we be? ... How should we live,/ tell us please./ How should we live?" And as George as Opa lost language and metamorphosed in full view of the audience into his magnificent owl, "whoo, whoo," the bird of wisdom, watching over, the Newbies found their answer for themselves in the air through which he seemed to fly. We will live "with kindness and restraint, with love," they sing. How grateful I am Noam and I shared our stories. As pacifists, we understood that because we oppose violence of all sorts, our task is to be with our beloveds unto death. If we are lucky enough. Death lived together between beloveds, like sex, both bestows and becomes an act of grace. One person dies while the other holds the story inside, the mystery remains alive. Grief, which is love, survives. Death hidden, institutionalized, medicalized, or a violent death due to war, denudes life and diminishes us all. Death engaged, if we are lucky enough to be present, and often our presence *does* depend upon luck, adds to the mystery of our love.

If each one of us is a poem, made up out of events of origin, so to speak, events we had no control over, jangling together, then what we make of the consequential events of our lives, how we transcribe ourselves into the world becomes our unique language of metaphor. We self-create from the original chaos of our circumstances of birth—insofar as we dare to become. George wrote himself into the world as a boy-child of nature, terror, and wonder. Though he lived halfway through his eighty-ninth year, he retained his boy-child-self. This is why, like a curious child, he continued to transform into and out of a sparkling essence he found in each character, even into an owl, even to speak for a fish on stage, post-death. His challenge and gift was to fit himself into the form of characters he imagined so fully that he, himself, seemed to vanish in order to animate them. Astonishing creations he made all his life. His eyes bright with wonder his final days. Until he, too, disappeared. Though, he reappears, now and then. "Sometimes I feel he is so close," I say to Peter Schumann as we return from the Memorial Grove, this time driving in his rickety car, two years after we scattered George's ashes. "I know," he responds speaking about his wife Elka, whose grave is in the same grove, overgrown with flowers. "I will see *you*, again," Peter says to me at the end of our visit. "This grove is *very* important." George's ashes are where they should be, amid the pine trees and memorial structures to so many friends. I can feel him there. The grove is alive with spirits—enough to make one believe these people have not fully left the world. Or, that they remain inside our memories of them.

Exactly one week after George died, at the exact moment in the night, 2:08, I had felt his heart stop, I woke. A red cloud floated a few feet above our mattress where he had lain. A shimmering rectangular, translucent, scarlet shape. It was George, I felt. What remained to me. He had come to share a last radiance, pushing through the barriers of the permeable world; he was there, sparkling as his eyes had.

Acknowledgements

Thanks to our friends and collaborators who knew and loved George and who offered themselves to me in grief. First, to Nina Kamberos, publisher of Laertes Books, Egret Imprint, a press for plays, for so many acts of kindness and support, for being the first reader of this manuscript, and for bringing out an elegant collection of my plays, new and old, *4 by Malpede Plus an Intervention*, ensuring that *Us, Blue Valiant* and other plays remain in print. Thanks to Kathleen Chalfant and Lydia Stryk for reading the early manuscript and for their enthusiasm about this book. Erika Duncan read portions of early drafts and gave me her always-valuable notes, as she has done for virtually everything I have written since we met in 1976. Robert Reiss sent me his grandmother, Anna Poor's memories of Barbara Deming, and he found Erik Bentley's cogent observation about Julian and Barbara. Ilion Troya and Garrick Beck shared valuable memories about the Living Theatre from their privileged positions as Julian's lover and his son. Rose Heredia transcribed George's diaries and urged him to continue to write. Nancy Allen, George's acupuncturist, comforted him and kept him strong. My daughter, Carrie Sophia, understood my grief while dealing with her own and shared with me the joys of Abel and Eben, her sons. My twin brother, John Malpede, his partner, Henriette Brouwers, Ynestra King, Jan Clausen, Martha Bragin, Michal Gamily, and Jerry Gorelnik walked with me, talked with me, even when I could not speak. Beatriz Schiller and Johan Elbers took me away to their country home after George died, and we watched Michael Cacoyannis' Greek tragedies on film every night. Thanks to Patrick Munto who drove George, and drove to Vermont. Charlotte Phillips, Sally Ann Parsons, Mahayana Landowne, Christen Clifford, Oliver Fine, Mary Ting, Cindy Rosenthal, Tony Giovannetti, were there when I needed them most. Folma Hoesch gave me a personal grant so that I could begin this book. Editor Mark Martin offered early advice. Thanks to my neighbors, in Clinton Hill, Brooklyn: Ashish Preshar and Mary Rinaldi, Jeralyn Gerba and Justin Carter, Loyda and Damond Short, Charles McMickens, Mishi Faruqee, Sarah Peck, Jennifer Mninte, Mariah, Henry, Eva and Mateo Deguara-Pagan, Christophe Hascoate and Edgar Garces. Lydia Koniordou with Avra Sidiropoulou flew in from Greece to bring *Troy Too* to blazing life. Basil Twist secured HERE performance space for the production. Ruth Oscharoff has provided the wisest, sustained counsel. Thanks to Jessica Bell, Amie McCracken, Anne S. Epstein, Melissa Slayton of Vine Leave Press for their valuable notes and their commitment to this book. Margarita Yarborough copyedited the earliest version. And of course, to Percy Bysshe Shelley II, liver and white cocker spaniel, my constant companion, the last in a long line of spaniels to comfort George, who does what good dogs do, and for Cleis, Hermes, and Abby, his worthy predecessors. Barry Bryant conducted the long interview with Julian Beck two weeks before his death; the selections reprinted here were first published in *Cancer and Consciousness,* Samaya Press, 1990. "In a Pine Wood" was first published in Dark Matter: *Women Witnessing, #16,* 2023; "Julian Beck" was first published in *The Nonviolent Activist,* November 1985.

Vine Leaves Press

Enjoyed this book?
Go to *vineleavespress.com* to find more.
Subscribe to our newsletter:

www.ingramcontent.com/pod-product-compliance
Ingram Content Group UK Ltd.
Pitfield, Milton Keynes, MK11 3LW, UK
UKHW041459201125
9096UKWH00029B/489